Alastair Wilkins
Editor

Progressive Multiple Sclerosis

Second Edition

Springer

Editor
Alastair Wilkins
Southmead Hospital
University of Bristol
Bristol
United Kingdom

ISBN 978-3-319-65920-6 ISBN 978-3-319-65921-3 (eBook)
https://doi.org/10.1007/978-3-319-65921-3

Library of Congress Control Number: 2017960800

Printed on acid-free paper

This Springer imprint is published by Springer Nature
The registered company is Springer International Publishing AG
The registered company address is: Gewerbestrasse 11, 6330 Cham, Switzerland

Preface

Since the first edition of *Progressive Multiple Sclerosis*, knowledge concerning the disease has advanced significantly. The drive for therapies to address disease progression is active and our understanding of the pathophysiology of the disease grows year on year. This has helped inform development of new treatments, and the hope is that the significant advances in relapsing and remitting disease will be replicated in progressive MS over the coming years. Importantly, the first successful clinical trials in progressive MS are being reported and a novel drug therapy approved and licenced.

The second edition of *Progressive Multiple Sclerosis* is intended to update readers with an overview of the current state of knowledge concerning this common disease. The field is evolving and new concepts have arisen since the publication of the first edition. New chapters on novel therapies and rehabilitation have been added and existing chapters updated. It is hoped that this book will be of use to neurologists, both those in training and those who have practiced for many years. The book composes chapters covering the expanse of knowledge on progressive multiple sclerosis from clinical features and epidemiology through to current and future treatments.

Bristol, UK　　　　Alastair Wilkins

Acknowledgments

The editor would like to acknowledge the hard work and determination of all the authors who contributed to this book.

Contents

Chapter 1
General Introduction: What Is Progressive Multiple Sclerosis?

Alastair Wilkins and Stanley Hawkins

1.1 Introduction

Over the past decade major advances in multiple sclerosis (MS) therapies have occurred, as well as significant increases in our understanding of disease aetiology: over a hundred susceptibility genes have been identified, complex immunological pathways have been mapped out and rapid changes in imaging techniques have vastly added to our understanding of temporal changes occurring in the course of the disease. Numerous large scale drug trials have been conducted and increasingly efficacious treatment options are emerging with effects on relapse frequency, allowing the clinician an array of therapeutic options. Indeed for patients with relapsing and remitting disease, therapies are offering the real prospect of significant disease modification with reduction in disease burden and disability [1]. Yet despite these advances, treatments for those with progressive MS remain limited and, once established, current drug therapies have little influence on the disease course of progressive MS. Patients with progressive disease are often frustrated by the lack of effective disease modifying therapies and often feel 'left behind' when compared to the range of treatments being offered to relapsing patients. This is an understandable frustration and one which is often difficult for patients to comprehend. Having said that, knowledge concerning the disease mechanisms is burgeoning and many research groups are starting to develop strategies to treat disease progression. As time goes on, a clearer understanding of exactly what needs to be treated is

A. Wilkins (✉)
Institute of Clinical Neurosciences, University of Bristol, Southmead Hospital, Bristol, UK
e-mail: Alastair.wilkins@bris.ac.uk

S. Hawkins
Department of Neurology, Royal Victoria Hospital, Belfast, UK

A. Wilkins (ed.), *Progressive Multiple Sclerosis*,
https://doi.org/10.1007/978-3-319-65921-3_1

becoming apparent and improved trial protocols are being developed. At the heart of such strategies is an increasing knowledge of the pathophysiology of disease progression. The second edition of *Progressive Multiple Sclerosis* will review the current state of knowledge concerning disease progression and put it in the context of developing and future therapies for this particular phase of MS. To set the scene, in this chapter some general features of MS will be discussed and definitions and clinical characteristics of progressive MS will be presented.

1.2 Multiple Sclerosis in General

1.2.1 Presentation and Diagnosis of MS

The diagnosis of MS rests heavily on clinical assessment. A history of 'attacks' (relapses or exacerbations) should be sought and consist of episodes typical of acute inflammatory demyelinating events in the CNS with duration of at least 24 h. Such attacks will typically be characterised by visual disturbance (optic nerve); hemisensory change (cerebral white or grey matter); hemiparesis (cerebral white or grey matter); vertiginous symptoms and diplopia (brainstem); or parapa-resis and urinary dysfunction (spinal cord). A detailed neurological history documenting more than one episode of such an attack, coupled with an examination revealing objective clinical evidence for more than one lesion within the central nervous system, is enough to make a diagnosis of MS in the appropriate clinical setting. In general patients presenting in such a manner will, however, have investigations both to confirm clinical suspicions and also to exclude other causes. Magnetic resonance imaging (MRI) is the paraclinical test most commonly employed in MS diagnosis, often combined with spinal fluid analysis and electro-physiological tests.

For the 'typical' patient, the diagnosis may not prove to be too challenging. However, in a number of scenarios the diagnosis may not be immediately clear and may only transpire after a further clinical episode has occurred or additional paraclinical evidence has been obtained. In order to address some of the issues relating to MS diagnosis and also to allow an 'earlier' diagnosis of MS, a number of criteria have been developed. Most notably, in recent times, the McDonald criteria for MS have been developed combining clinical and paraclinical markers of disease dissemination in time and space [2, 3]. Thus, if a patient has two attacks suggestive of an inflammatory central nervous system lesion, but only objective evidence of one lesion on examination, then the diagnosis of MS can be supported by MRI dissemination in space (one or more T2 lesions in at least 2 of 4 CNS areas typically affected by MS (periventricular, juxtacortical, infratentorial or spinal cord). Similarly, when patients have had only one attack but there is objective evidence on examination of two or more lesions, the diagnosis of MS may be supported by MRI evidence of dissemination in time (either new T2 lesion(s) or new gadolinium-enhancing lesion(s) on follow-up MRI; or the simultaneous presence of both an asymptomatic gadolinium enhancing lesion and non-enhancing lesions on the same scan). Regarding a clinically isolated syndrome (CIS; one clinical attack suggestive of CNS inflammation with objective clinical evidence for one lesion on examination), the McDonald criteria require MRI dissemination in both space and time (one or more T2 lesions in at least 2 of 4 CNS areas typically affected by MS (periventricular, juxtacortical, infratentorial or spinal cord) for dissemination in space; and either new T2 lesion(s) or new gadolinium-enhancing lesion(s) on follow-up MRI or the simultaneous presence of both an asymptomatic gadolinium enhancing lesion and non-enhancing lesions on the same scan for dissemination in time).

In summary, the McDonald criteria 'allow' dissemination in space and time to be fulfilled by observing MRI patterns or changes in MRI lesions over time in those patients who would otherwise not meet the clinical criteria for the diagnosis of MS. Whilst earlier diagnosis has been driven by the notion that earlier treatment may lead to a long-term reduction in disability, there is still much to be learnt about the optimal time and type of disease modifying therapies for CIS or 'McDonald criteria MS'.

The diagnosis of primary progressive MS (PPMS) and secondary progressive MS (SPMS) will be discussed later in this chapter.

1.2.2 Aetiological Factors in MS

An exact understanding of the precise cause of MS is still lacking. Despite this, important recent advances in MS aetiology have been made. In many parts of the world MS is a common disorder, the incidence of which is dependent on a number of factors including age, gender, family history and geographical location [4]. These factors, particularly familial risks and the variations in incidence dependent on geographical latitude have provided clues concerning aetiological factors in the disease. Most now accept that underlying the pathogenesis of the disease are combinations of genetic factors leading to disease susceptibility coupled to environmental influences. Of the genetic influences, certain polymorphisms in the human leucocyte antigen (HLA) region of chromosome 6, notably the DRB1*1501 allele, appear to confer the largest portion of the genetic susceptibility [5, 6], but this is only about 12% of the genetic susceptibility. Perhaps not surprisingly a number of other variations in genes regulating the immune system confer disease susceptibility [7]. The relationship between genetic factors and disease course, that is to say what genetic factors regulate aggressiveness of the disease or whether the disease starts as relapsing and remitting or primary progressive, for example, is unknown and only a few genes with putative neuroprotective functions have been implicated in genome wide association screens (GWAS) [7, 8]. Further understanding of the role of individual risk alleles in disease onset and course is likely to be of importance in future years, not least for developing pharmacogenetic strategies and, possibly, improving prognostic information at diagnosis.

Several environmental factors have been suggested as being important in disease initiation, notably Epstein Barr Virus (EBV) and vitamin D levels. The observation that geographical latitude influences disease incidence prompted the search for a link between climate and the disease [9]. Epidemiological studies have suggested that there is an inverse relationship between past sunlight exposure and MS susceptibility [10]. Vitamin D_3 (cholecalciferol) is made in the skin by the action of ultraviolet (B) light on 7-dehydrocholesterol and vitamin D effects are thought likely to explain the majority of the geographical incidence variability in MS. High serum levels of 25-hydroxyvitamin D have been found to have a protective effect against MS [11]. Some studies have shown low serum vitamin D levels may be associated with relapsing and remitting disease with levels particularly low prior to relapse [12, 13]. Conversely, higher levels may be associated with lower relapse frequency [14]. Importantly, the active form of vitamin D (1,25-hydroxyvitamin D) is a potent immunomodulator with a range of immunosuppressive actions [15]. Recently it has been shown that a vitamin D response element is found in the promoter region of HLA-DRB1, which suggests that vitamin D may regulate this key genetic susceptibility locus and thus provides a link between genetic and environmental factors in the disease [16]. Whether vitamin D supplementation to the at-risk population will reduce disease incidence or whether administration of vitamin D to those with MS will modify the disease process is the subject of active research and a number of studies. It is estimated that over 1 billion people worldwide are vitamin D deficient [17]. Further to this, it is not fully established whether the effect of sunlight exposure on MS risk is purely driven through vitamin D elevation or whether sunlight may have other immunological effects.

The widespread nature of vitamin D deficiency and the presence of multiple interacting susceptibility factors have made it difficult to dissect out its precise role in disease onset. Similarly, working out the association of EBV and MS has proved challenging because of the high rates of infection among studied populations. EBV infects approximately 95% of the population of most Western countries, yet rates are higher in MS, with no evidence of previous EBV infection being extremely rare in the disease [18]. Interestingly, the risk of MS appears to be 20-fold greater in those who have had infectious mononucleosis than those who are EBV-negative

[19]. Potential mechanisms by which EBV may induce disease in MS include B-cell clone immortalization, antigenic mimicry and dysregulation of cytotoxic T-cells against EBV-infected B cells [20]. EBV infects B lymphocytes and may immortalize them into memory B cells, capable of prolonged survival in the peripheral circulation [21]. Serological studies have shown that those with higher titres of anti-EBV antibodies have a higher risk of developing MS, compared to those with lower titres [22]. Furthermore, plasma levels of EBV nuclear antigen-1 (EBNA1) increase over time before clinical onset of MS [18, 22]. People who are EBNA1 positive and give a history of clinical infectious mononucleosis are at even greater risk; and an older age of primary EBV-associated Infectious Mononucleosis may confer a higher risk of MS [23]. Studies have suggested that people positive for the HLA-DRB1*1501 and who had high EBNA1 titres are at greatly increased risk of MS, linking genetic and environmental factors in MS susceptibility [24]. Whether EBV has its major effect by inducing peripheral immune changes within circulating lymphocytes, or through direct central nervous system immune dysregulation, is not clear. Currently the evidence for direct EBV infection in the brain or EBV latency within B cells residing in the brain as a cause of tissue injury in MS is unclear. Some groups have reported widespread EBV infection of infiltrating B cells and plasma cells within the brain, although others have not [25, 26]. Determining the role of EBV in MS pathogenesis may lead to strategies to prevent MS, although determining whether some form of vaccination programme will be effective is likely to be highly complex.

Other lifestyle factors appear to influence MS susceptibility, notably smoking and obesity. Smoking increases MS risk and, again, HLA-DRB1 allele status seems to influence susceptibility, with smokers who are HLA-DRB1*15 positive and HLA-A*02 negative at approximately 14 times increased risk of developing MS than non-smokers with neither genetic background [27]. This has a clear and important public health message particularly those at higher risk of MS based on family history and geographical location. Dietary factors in MS have been postulated for many years and numerous 'MS diets' have been touted. No specific diet has been shown in studies to be superior to a standard healthy diet. Alcohol and caffeine intake have also been studied but no firm conclusions or recommendations can be made at this time. The observation that adolescent obesity is associated with increased risk of MS is of importance, given the global obesity epidemic [28]. Onset of obesity in adolescence seems to confer this risk, with no increased risk of MS associated with obesity onset later in life. Again, there is an immunological link: those people with obesity and who are HLA-DRB1*15 positive and HLA-A*02 negative are at increased risk [29]. Obesity decreases the bioavailability of vitamin D and also has immunological consequences that may impact on MS.

1.2.3 Disease Course Patterns in Multiple Sclerosis

Once the disease has started the course may be highly variable between different individuals. The difficulties in providing an accurate prognosis of disease course leads to uncertainty and can contribute significantly to patient anxiety. In addition, discussions concerning the choice of disease modifying therapies can be complex and whether to choose a more potent yet higher risk therapy at disease onset when the prognosis is uncertain makes for difficult decisions. Increasing understanding of disease course and disease phenotypes, gathered mostly from large disease registries, has, however, allowed for better discussions of disease prognosis in recent years.

One of the most intriguing enigmas of MS is why some patients have a rather disease benign course, whereas others may experience an aggressive disease course. Benign MS is a well-recognised entity and is typically defined as a disease subtype in which the patient shows little or no disability or disease progression after many years (Expanded Disability Status Scale (EDSS) < 3 after a minimum of 10 years of disease duration) [30, 31]. The prevalence rates of benign MS quoted in the literature vary widely, possibly reflecting the difficulty of ascertaining data in this population of patients, as well as the use of differing definitions of benign disease [32, 33]. Although benign MS, by definition, is associated with fewer motor (ambulation) problems than other forms of the disease, symptoms in other neurological domains are common and may cause significant morbidity [34]. On the other hand, it is possible that people with MS can live a normal life span without major disability [35].

Prognostic indicators of likely disease activity are often declared early. Particularly in relapsing and remitting disease, a major prognostic indicator is the time between first relapses and the relapse frequency in the first 2 years of disease, such that those with a shorter interval between the first two relapses and those with a higher first-2-year relapse rate show quicker progression through disability milestones [36]. These issues will be discussed further in chapters.

The subject of the following chapters of this book is progressive disease. In brief, disease progression may be either a clinical description of the temporal course of the disease (in general only confidently diagnosed in retrospect); or defined for trial and epidemiological studies as a sustained increase in a specific disability scale over a fixed period of time. Disease progression may be either primary, that is progression from the outset, or secondary, that is progression following a period of relapsing and remitting disease. Standardised definitions of the common clinical courses of MS were proposed by Lublin and Reingold in 1996, based on an international survey of clinicians involved in MS care, and revised in 2013 [37, 38]. A pictorial representation of disease course patterns in MS is given in Fig. 1.1.

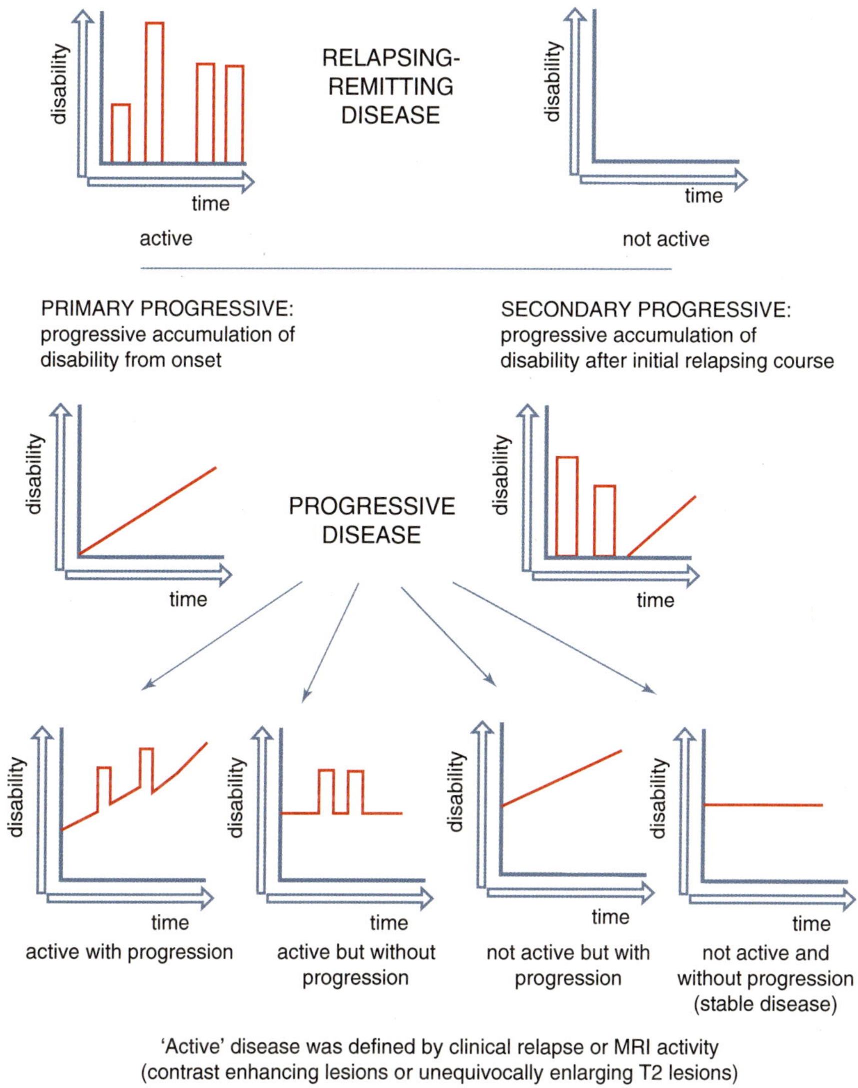

Fig. 1.1 Disease course patterns in MS

1.3 What is Disease Progression?

The clinical course of multiple sclerosis (MS) represents a spectrum. The subdivision of MS, according to the clinical course, has become increasingly important in recent years, since therapeutic clinical trials have shown demonstrable reductions in the frequency of clinical relapses and of inflammatory lesions as demonstrated on magnetic resonance imaging (MRI). Measures of disease progression are more resistant to change and in patients with progressive MS, it has been more difficult to demonstrate positive benefits from therapeutic interventions.

It has long been recognised that although patients may essentially share the diagnostic label of MS, there is considerable variation across a spectrum in terms of clinical phenotype, prognosis, MRI appearances, immunological characteristics and pathology. The nature of the clinical course may also determine the response to disease-modifying therapy and the course itself may be influenced by underlying genetic heterogeneity.

In approximately 85–90% of cases, the onset of MS is marked by relapses and remissions—relapsing–remitting MS (RRMS). With time, an increasing proportion of these patients enter a secondary progressive phase (SPMS), 40% within 10 years and 65% within 25 years. SPMS represents a phase during which there are generally fewer relapses. It is characterised by gradual progression in disability between relapses or without relapses. A minority of patients, 10–15%, do not have relapses at the onset of the disease, but rather, steadily accumulate disability over time [39]. This has come to be described as primary progressive MS (PPMS) [37].

How does the clinician know whether a patient with MS has progressive disease? In a similar way to the initial diagnosis of MS, although paraclinical measures and biomarkers (imaging and otherwise) can help, the diagnosis of progressive disease still remains firmly a clinical one. Neurologists will usually be able to classify the disease subtype of an individual patient based on clinical history and examination, although patients experiencing transition from relapsing and remitting MS to secondary progressive MS may be difficult to fully classify, as will patients experiencing significant numbers of relapses. In reality disease progression is often not confidently diagnosed until some months have passed in these patients and, thus, defining onset of disease progression is often a retrospective exercise [40].

1.4 Clinical Diagnosis of Progressive MS and Differential Diagnosis

The typical patient with relapsing and remitting MS will usually not present too many diagnostic difficulties. Such a 'typical' patient will often be a young woman with a history suggestive of more than one episodes of neurological dysfunction involving separate anatomical domains thus satisfying the concept of 'dissemination in time and space' [3]. Paraclinical investigations, such as MRI scanning and spinal fluid analysis are used to seek alternative explanations or to confirm the clinical suspicion of MS. Diagnosis of progressive disease, however, may be more challenging. In particular, the diagnosis of MS in those with a history suggestive of PPMS, may be demanding. Furthermore, the question patients sometimes ask concerning whether they have entered the progressive phase of the disease after a period of relapsing and remitting disease is, again, often a difficult one to provide a definitive answer to.

In this section, a description of the diagnosis and differential diagnosis of MS that is progressive from outset and a discussion of the clinical diagnosis of secondary progression will be presented.

1.4.1 Primary Progressive MS

1.4.1.1 Definition of PPMS

That patients with MS can follow a progressive as well as a relapsing course has been recognised since the 19th century, but almost a century passed before a clear distinction was made between those in whom the disease is progressive from onset (primary progressive) and those who have progressive deterioration with or without superimposed relapses, following an initially relapsing and remitting course (secondary progressive disease) [41]. It was more recently still that the clinical category of primary progressive MS was clearly defined [2].

Up to the late 1990's the term 'chronic progressive MS' was widely used in the literature. No clear distinction was made between cases that were progressive from the onset and those in whom progression of disability followed clear, distinct clinical bouts, exacerbations or relapses followed by improvement or remission. Over the years, primary progressive patients were undoubtedly included under the heading 'chronic progressive' [42], whilst some have included those having 'periods of general deterioration resembling relapses' [43] and 'no or relatively few attacks' [44] within the category of PPMS. Some cases that have a steady progressive course at the outset have superimposed clinical relapses, and have been called progressive-relapsing and relapsing-progressive. The picture has been further complicated by the addition of another subcategory termed 'transitional MS' [45]. This term has been used in two different settings. The first is to indicate that patients at a certain level of disability will probably become dependent on walking aids before long. The second is what has been referred to as "single attack progressive MS" (SAPMS) [46]. In this latter category patients experience a single relapse and/or remission and then enter a phase of steady progression without superimposed relapses.

A clear framework was brought to the nomenclature in 1996 with the consensus document produced by Lublin and Reingold [2]. They undertook a survey of 125 members of the international MS clinical research community with the twin aims of standardising terminology and facilitating a broader understanding of the recruitment parameters in MS therapeutic trials. Based on the replies received, PPMS was defined as disease progression from onset with occasional plateaus and temporary minor improvements, the essential element being a gradual, nearly continually worsening baseline with minor fluctuations, but no distinct relapses. The consensus of the vast majority of respondents at that time, including those with MRI expertise, was that MRI evidence was not required in distinguishing this clinical category. The terms 'relapsing–progressive' and 'chronic progressive' were considered redundant, the former for not corresponding to a clearly defined population and the latter for being vague. The term 'transitional MS' appears not to have been considered although 'progressive–relapsing' has been recognised as applying to a small group of patients with progressive disease from onset, but who have clear acute relapses, with or without full recovery. Some clarity regarding the prognosis of MS has been described in the literature over the last 10 years, in particular between the two major groups—primary progressive and secondary progressive MS.

The consensus guidelines have not been universally welcomed [47] and some groups have suggested, on the basis of analysis of their own considerable data, that progressive–relapsing patients and PPMS patients were so phenotypically and prognostically similar as to make their separation unnecessary [48, 49].

In 2013 Lublin and colleagues conducted a revision of the 1996 consensus statement [38]. They support the view that PPMS is *"part of the spectrum of MS phenotypes and that any differences are relative rather than absolute"*. They propose that both secondary progressive and PPMS could be "*active or not active*" on the basis of clinically observed relapses or MRI activity and "*with progression or without progression*" on the basis of regular (usually annual) clinical measures of disability. Furthermore, they support the view that the category of progressive relapsing MS be eliminated, since such patients could be classified as "*PP patients with disease activity*".

Now that MS patients are being reviewed more frequently at clinics and that some are having regular MRI scans, there is a suggestion that the proportion of PPMS patients is falling [50]. However since PPMS typically has a later age of onset, the decline could be overestimated [51].

1.4.1.2 Diagnostic Criteria of PPMS

Clarification of the definition of PPMS has clearly been important, but a range of progressive neurological diseases may present in a similar way. This necessitates the application of relevant diagnostic criteria. Over the past 50 years, several diagnostic criteria have been formulated in MS including those of Allison and Millar [52], Schumacher et al. [53] and McDonald and Halliday [54]. From 1983, for 20 years, the Poser criteria [55] were the most widely accepted and applied. The diagnosis of clinically definite MS (CDMS) by these criteria requires the occurrence of at least two attacks. Since PPMS patients, by definition, have a progressive course without relapse or remission, designation of such patients as having CDMS is impossible. Indeed, the absence of attacks also excludes PPMS patients from another of the Poser categories, that of laboratory-supported probable MS.

The limitations of the Poser criteria were highlighted in a study of 111 PPMS patients [56]. Applying the criteria in that population resulted in 37% of patients being considered to have laboratory-supported definite MS, 46% having clinically probable MS and 17% being unclassifiable. This problem was addressed by a consortium led by Thompson with the publication in 2000 of a position paper setting out specific diagnostic criteria for PPMS [57].

Formulated by a panel of investigators involved in a multicentre, serial, clinical and MRI study of PPMS, three categories of PPMS have been proposed. Definite PPMS represents cases where there is adequate clinical and investigative evidence to render the diagnosis definite enough for inclusion in research protocols and clinical trials; probable PPMS reflects cases where there is strong clinical suspicion of the diagnosis, but insufficient evidence to be definite; and possible PPMS, which reflects the existence of only limited evidence to suggest the diagnosis.

The panel recommended a minimum period of clinical progression of at least 12 months and suggest that there should be documented evidence of progression as may be reflected in the Kurtzke Extended Disability Status Scale (EDSS) [58] or on timed walk recordings. It is presumed that other potential mimics of PPMS will have been excluded by thorough investigation. Age limits of 25–65 years have been set for age at onset, in order for the criteria to be applied, the upper limit being higher than that established by the Poser criteria (59 years). In the new criteria, great importance is placed on the identification of abnormal intrathecal synthesis of IgG. Although it might be argued that a patient with a progressive course, compatible MRI and delayed visual evoked responses could scarcely have anything other than PPMS, justification for the cautious approach is derived from studies of oligoclonal band (OCB)-negative presumed MS, where other diagnoses have become apparent on prolonged follow-up [59]. The minimum number of brain lesions required on T2-weighted images is set at nine although if there is at least one lesion seen on spinal MRI, only between four and eight brain lesions are necessary.

In the position paper the authors applied their proposed criteria to a database of 156 PPMS patients, 64% had definite PPMS, 35% had probable PPMS and just 1% had possible disease [57]. Just how typical this population is of PPMS, in general, remains to be seen, given its relatively youthful profile (average age of 40 years) and earlier age at onset (29 years) than is usually typical for this subgroup of patients. As the authors recommend, validation of these criteria is required both in a prospective cohort and with post mortem examination.

The recommendations laid out in the position paper of Thompson and colleagues were incorporated in the 2001 McDonald Criteria [2]. There have been further revisions in 2005 [60] and 2011 [3].

In 2005, the panel recommended revising the McDonald Criteria for diagnosis of primary progressive multiple sclerosis (PPMS) to require, in addition to 1 year of disease progression, 2 of the following 3 findings: positive brain MRI (9 T2 lesions or 4 or more T2 lesions with positive VEP); positive spinal cord MRI (2 focal T2 lesions); or positive CSF (the identification of abnormal intrathecal synthesis of IgG). These criteria reflected the special role of both CSF examination and spinal cord MRI in PPMS, have been found to be practical and are generally well accepted by the neurological community, and have been used as inclusion criteria for PPMS clinical trials. To harmonize MRI criteria within the diagnostic criteria for all forms of MS, while recognizing the special diagnostic needs for PPMS, the 2010 revision panel recommended that the McDonald Criteria requirement of fulfilling 2 of 3 MRI or CSF findings be maintained for PPMS, with replacement of the previous brain imaging criteria with the new MAGNIMS brain imaging criteria for DIS (2 of 3 of the following: ≥1 T2 lesions in at least 1 area characteristic for MS [periventricular, juxtacortical, or infratentorial]; ≥2 T2 lesions in the cord; or positive CSF [isoelectric focusing evidence of oligoclonal bands and/or elevated IgG index]. This consensus-based recommendation is justified by comparing diagnostic criteria for PPMS and by a subsequent reanalysis of these data by Montalban et al. [61]. These two revisions removed the absolute requirement for CSF abnormalities.

1.4.1.3 Clinical Features of PPMS

Patients with PPMS differ significantly in terms of their mode of presentation when compared with initially relapsing–remitting patients. In the Belfast cohort of 111 PPMS patients progressive myelopathy manifesting as motor disturbance occurred in 67.6%, whereas visual loss at onset was uncommon (3.6%) [39]. This contrasts with the initially relapsing–remitting group, where, although the range of symptoms is obviously similar, the relative frequency of motor symptoms at onset is much less and visual symptoms are much more common (16.8% with motor disturbance at onset and 22.3% with visual disturbance at onset). Similar results have been found elsewhere. One study found that 61% of PPMS patients had pyramidal signs and symptoms at onset, whilst only 19% of an RRMS group did so [62]. In another, 79% of primary progressive patients had motor weakness at onset, whereas just 16.5% of relapsing–remitting or secondary progressive cases presented likewise [63]. Other recent studies, have concurred with the observation that motor symptoms at onset occur in the majority of PPMS patients [48, 64].

Clinical presentations other than progressive myelopathy occur in PPMS, although with much lower frequencies. The neurological domains in which disease progression may occur are similar to those occurring in SPMS.

1.4.1.4 Differential Diagnosis of PPMS

As indicated, the commonest presentation of PPMS is with progressive lower limb dysfunction and signs suggestive of a spastic paraparesis. The differential is large and initial investigations in such patients will be aimed at determining whether there is evidence of any structural lesions causing spinal cord compromise or evidence of intrinsic cord lesion(s). Associated symptoms of spinal cord dysfunction, such as urinary dysfunction (urgency, frequency, nocturia, etc.), are common but often do not helpfully discriminate from other differential diagnoses of a spastic paraparesis. Sensory changes are common, but often not as marked as the motor dysfunction and a discrete sensory level is usually absent in MS and may help differentiate from a structural compressive spinal cord lesion. Similarly, the absolute absence of any sensory symptoms may prompt a more extensive search for an alternative diagnosis, such as amyotrophic lateral sclerosis (ALS) or primary lateral sclerosis (PLS) [65]. However, studies have shown that a large proportion of patients presenting with a progressive myelopathy will have an eventual diagnosis of MS [66].

Inflammatory cord lesions may also arise from systemic disorders such as sarcoidosis, systemic lupus erythematosus and Sjogren's syndrome. Importantly neuromyelitis optica (Devic's disease) may present with an inflammatory cord lesion (typically longitudinally extensive over three or more vertebral segments) [67]. Diagnostic criteria have been developed for this condition and differentiating neuromyelitis optica from MS is of importance since prognosis and therapies differ [68].

Of particular note, female carriers of the X-linked adrenoleucodystrophy (X-ALD) gene, may manifest as a progressive spastic paraparesis often in third or fourth decade and family history of leucodystrophy should warrant further investigations with very long chain fatty acid analysis or genetic testing in this setting [69, 70].

The differential diagnosis of a progressive spastic paraparesis of adult onset is given in Table 1.1.

Table 1.1 Differential diagnosis of a progressive spastic paraparesis in an adult

• Extrinsic structural lesions causing spinal cord compromise
– Degenerative cervical spine disease/cervical spondylosis
– Extrinsic tumour such as meningioma
– (Epidural abscess)
• Intrinsic structural lesions causing spinal cord compromise
– Syringomyelia
– Intrinsic tumour of spinal cord, such as ependymoma
• Inherited conditions
– Iereditary spastic paraplegia (HSP; multiple genetic sub-types with either autosomal dominant, autosomal recessive or X-linked)
– Leucodystrophies including adrenoleucodystrophy (mostly adrenomyeloneuropathy phenotype or female carriers of X-ALD) and Krabbe's disease
– Spinocerebellar ataxias
– Friedreich Ataxia
– Cerebrotendinous xanthomatosis
• Metabolic causes
– Vitamin B12 deficiency
– Rarely inborn errors of metabolism: phenylketonuria, homocysteine remethylation defects, tyrosine hydroxylase deficiency, arginase deficiency, polyglucosan body disease
• Other inflammatory conditions
– Neuromyelitis optica
– Sarcoidosis
– Systemic lupus erythematosus
– Other CNS vasculitides
• Infectious diseases
– Tropical spastic paraparesis (human T-cell lymphotrophic virus type 1)
– Human immunodeficiency virus (HIV)
– Syphilis
– Cerebellar
– Schistosomiasis
• Neurodegenerative conditions
– Motor neuron diseases: primary lateral sclerosis and amyotrophic lateral sclerosis
• Vascular disease
– Spinal dural arteriovenous fistula
– Diffuse cerebral small vessel disease
– CADASIL
• Toxic causes
– Lathyrism
– Konzo

Clinical presentations other than spastic paraparesis occur in PPMS, although with much lower frequencies. The neurological domains in which disease progression may occur are similar to those occurring in SPMS. Progressive visual loss should raise suspicion of Leber's hereditary optic neuropathy (LHON) and lead to mitochondrial DNA testing [71]. Progressive ataxia occurs as a presenting feature in some patients, although may often be associated with features of a spastic paraparesis. The differential diagnosis is broad and a search for other causes of cerebellar dysfunction (including metabolic disturbances (such as alcohol excess), vascular disease, a structural lesion within the posterior fossa, paraneoplastic disease or one of the inherited ataxias) must be undertaken. The differential diagnosis of progressive ataxia in adults is given in Table 1.2:

Table 1.2 Differential diagnosis of progressive ataxia in adults

• Metabolic disturbances
– Alcohol excess (including Wernicke-Korsakoff syndrome)
– Drug induced e.g. phenytoin, carbamazepine, barbiturates
– Hypothyroidism
– Vitamin deficiency e.g. vitamin E, vitamin B12
– Inflammatory disease
– Multiple sclerosis
– Central nervous system or systemic vasculitides
– Sarcoidosis
• Vascular disease
– Including subcortical vascular disease
• Neoplastic and paraneoplastic
– Cerebellar tumour (e.g. Von Hippel Lindau disease), meningioma or metastasis
– Paraneoplastic cerebellar degeneration
• Infections
– Creutzfeld Jakob Disease
– Human immunodeficiency virus (HIV)
– Whipple's disease
• Inherited metabolic disorders
– Wilson's disease
– Leucodystrophies
– Lysosomal storage disorders
– Mitochondrial disorders e.g. MELAS, MERFF, NARP
• Neurodegenerative conditions
– Multiple system atrophy
– Normal pressure hydrocephalus
• Other inherited ataxias
– Friedreich Ataxia
– Other autosomal recessive ataxias, such as ataxia telangiectasia and ataxia with oculomotor apraxia (I and II)
– Autosomal dominant ataxias: including spinocerebellar ataxia (SCA) types 1–7, 10–15, 17, 28; dentatorubralpallidoluysian atrophy (DRPLA); POLG mutations; episodic ataxia (types 1 and 2)
– X linked ataxia: Fragile X tremor-ataxia syndrome
• Autoimmune conditions
– Ataxia with anti-glutamate decarboxylase (GAD) antibodies
– Sjogren's syndrome
– Coeliac disease
• Structural anomolies
– Cranio-vertebral junction anomalies (Arnold Chiari malformations)

In a similar vein, cognitive dysfunction occurs in PPMS, although, again, usually accompanied by other neurological manifestations. Disturbances in verbal memory, attention, verbal fluency and spatial reasoning have been documented in populations of patients with PPMS [72, 73]. Differences between cognitive function in PPMS and SPMS patients have been noted, although the significance of these observations remains unclear [74–76].

1.4.2 Clinical Diagnosis of Secondary Progressive Disease

There are, as yet, no clear clinical, biomarker or imaging criteria that can define the transition point between RRMS and SPMS. Several committees and advisory groups have come up with diagnostic criteria and considerations for the diagnosis of SPMS. The Lubin and Reingold definitions mentioned above defined SPMS as 'progressive accumulation of disability after initial relapsing course, with or without occasional relapses and minor remissions' [37]. In 2013, these definitions were revisited and refined descriptors were proposed which included consideration of disease activity [38]. Thus, SPMS was defined as 'progressive accumulation of disability after initial relapsing course and either: active with progression; active but without progression; not active but with progression; or not active and without progression (stable disease)'. 'Active' disease was defined by clinical relapse or MRI activity (contrast enhancing lesions or unequivocally enlarging T2 lesions). They suggested the term 'progressive relapsing MS' should not be used and this phenotype could be incorporated within the categories listed above.

Database studies, such as MSBase, have been used to evaluate the feasibility and utility of standardising the definition of SPMS [77]. This prospective observational study looked at a pool of SPMS diagnostic categories based on combinations of seven criteria and found the best performing definition to be: 'disability progression by 1 EDSS step in patients with EDSS ≤ 5.5 or 0.5 EDSS steps in patients with EDSS ≥ 6 in the absence of relapse, and a minimum EDSS score of 4 and pyramidal functional systems (FS) score of 2 and confirmed progression over 3 months, including confirmation within the leading FS.'

Natural history studies regarding risk of progression have been hugely informative and rely upon the use of defining disability using specific scales. Secondary progression follows the RRMS in the majority of cases and it is likely that over 80% of (untreated) RRMS patients will eventually enter a secondary progressive phase, with risk of progression increasing incrementally dependent on the length of time since diagnosis [78–80]. The majority of epidemiological studies were conducted predominantly in patients who are treatment naïve or in patients who have received early less efficacious disease modifying therapies. Now that disease modifying therapies have been available for some time, understanding the evolution of disability in this 'treatment era' is of significance in determining the efficacy of therapies on progressive disease [81].

Away from large scale epidemiological studies, when faced with deterioration in an individual patient, it is useful to make a clinical diagnosis of disease stage in order to prognosticate, plan for long term care and, importantly, decide on the suitability of disease modifying therapy. Most physicians seeing patients with an initial diagnosis of RRMS would define secondary progression as period of sustained deterioration in neurological function without remission [37]. Once a given level of disability has been sustained for 6 months, the likelihood of reversibility (in treatment-naive patients) is likely to be negligible [82]. Deterioration may occur as a result of relapse activity and delineating relapse from progression at the point of onset of neurological worsening may be difficult. The speed of change in neurological function may give a clue to the onset of progression: if deterioration in neurological status is rapid this suggests a relapse; whereas slow deterioration would generally be regarded as disease progression [83]. Another important observation on disease progression in MS is that for a given patient, progression of the disease appears to occur at a steady rate [84]. Furthermore, in patient populations once progression has 'set in', further rates of progressive decline appear to happen in a uniform (and slowly progressive) way, and in a way that appears independent of previous clinical disease course [85–87]. Thus, the pattern of deterioration is highly indicative of progression and may delineate from relapse. However, the course of the disease may only become clear over time and may only become apparent after a period of retrospective analysis.

Progressive clinical deterioration can occur in a number of neurological domains, of which the most important will be discussed in more detail below. Usually a fairly-stereotyped clinical pattern emerges of an 'upper motor neuron syndrome' causing impaired ambulation and spasticity, with variable degrees of superimposed ataxia and cognitive impairment. In addition, bladder and bowel dysfunction, fatigue, mood disturbance and paroxysmal symptoms such as trigeminal neuralgia often occur. These will also be discussed further in Chap. 7 with a description of symptomatic therapies.

1.4.2.1 Progressive Motor Dysfunction in SPMS

The clinical diagnosis of disease progression rests heavily on observing changes in motor function and the commonly used disability scales reflect this [58]. Undoubtedly the reason for this is that motor deficits are more straightforward to document and are picked up during a standard neurological examination. The use of natural history studies employing the Expanded Disability Status Scale (EDSS) has provided information on mean levels of motor dysfunction progression within MS populations (see below).

A common manifestation in disease progression is reduced ambulation. Natural history studies often define ambulation difficulties in terms of: limited walking but without aid (correlating to EDSS 4); walking with unilateral aid (stick/cane; correlating to EDSS 6); and wheelchair bound (correlating to EDSS 7). Time to reach these milestones have been studied in some detail in population databases [88]. Of note, progression through disability milestones occurs at a slow rate. For instance in the Lyon Multiple Sclerosis Cohort, time median times from EDDS4 to reach EDSS 6 and EDSS 7 were 5 and 12 years, respectively, and from EDSS 6, median time to reach EDSS 7 was 4 years [79, 89]. Furthermore, reaching a disability milestone appears to some extent to be dependent on age at onset of the disease, such that those with earlier onset of disease tend to reach fixed levels at an earlier age [90]. Further discussions of the natural history studies utilising EDSS measurements will be presented in later chapters.

1.4.2.2 Progressive Cognitive Dysfunction in SPMS

Cognitive dysfunction is common in progressive MS and is an important predictor of quality of life in the disease [91]. The prevalence rates of memory difficulties in MS appears to be of the region of 40–65% [92]. Cognitive dysfunction has been particularly noted in progressive MS and occurs at higher frequency than in RRMS [74, 93]. Domains of cognition relating to learning and recall of new information, as well as working memory appear to be particularly affected [94]. Other changes in cognition such as executive function, semantic memory, visuospatial skills and language function also occur [95, 96]. Importantly, cognitive defects negatively impact significantly on rehabilitation potential in MS [97]. Cognitive problems also contribute to reduced employment and social interaction which may have significant impact on quality of life [98].

A thorough history is required to determine whether depression is a contributing factor, since depression commonly causes defects in memory and attention [99]. Depression is the most frequent psychiatric manifestation of MS with a prevalence of 40–60% and therapeutic intervention may lead to considerable improvements [100, 101]. In addition, fatigue impacts upon cognitive ability in MS, although the precise relationship of fatigue to specific cognitive domains is unclear [102].

Detailed assessment of cognitive profiles in patients with MS may be best performed by neuropsychologists. Of the cognitive batteries available, the Minimal Assessment of Cognitive Function in MS (MACFIMS) battery may be of particular use [103]. MACFIMS is composed of seven neuropsychological tests, assessing five cognitive domains commonly impaired in MS (processing speed/working memory, learning and memory, executive function, visual-spatial processing, and word retrieval), supplemented by a measure of estimated pre-morbid cognitive ability [94, 104].

1.4.2.3 Progressive Ataxia in SPMS

Ataxia is thought to occur in about 80% of patients with established MS, with symptoms particularly prevalent in those with progressive disease [105, 106]. Postural and intention tremors are common features of advanced disease and are thought to arise predominantly as a consequence of cerebellar or thalamic disease [107–109]. Cerebellar dysarthria is also relatively common in those with advanced secondary progressive disease. The cerebellum is involved in cognitive processing and there is some evidence that involvement of the cerebellum may be linked to defects in cognitive processes in MS [110]. Cerebellar pathology has been linked to deficits in verbal fluency, working memory and attention, as well as executive dysfunction [111]. Interestingly, cognitive profiles of people with MS who have cerebellar lesions differs to those without cerebellar involvement [112].

Changes in cerebellar architecture are seen in autopsy brain specimens of patients with a history of chronic SPMS, with widespread demyelination and changes in Purkinje cell phenotype [113, 114]. In addition MRI studies have confirmed extensive cerebellar involvement in progressive MS [115, 116]. Persistent cerebellar dysfunction has been linked with magnetic resonance spectroscopy markers of axonal loss [117]. Interestingly, some researchers have suggested that cerebellar dysfunction in MS may be linked to an acquired channnelopathy, since changes in sodium channel subtypes have been observed [118]. This observation has been the basis of the suggestion that modulation of cerebellar ion channels may ameliorate ataxic symptoms in MS [119].

1.5 Disability Scales Used to Monitor Progressive MS

The Expanded Disability Status Scale (EDSS) remains the most commonly used method of quantifying disability in MS (Table 1.3) [58]. It was developed from the earlier Disability Status Scale (DSS) by dividing into two each step from DSS 1 to 9 and thus effectively creating a 20 point scale [120]. It encompasses a complementary set of scales for eight functional systems (FS; pyramidal, cerebellar, brain stem, sensory, bowel and bladder, visual, cerebral and "others"; Table 1.4). When performing the EDSS the clinician grades according to history and neurological examination in the appropriate grades of the FS. An overall score is assigned by combining the different FS grades with the ability to walk. As such, up to 3.5, the scale is largely dependent on impairment in functional systems, whereas disability in the higher grades is mainly determined by ambulation. EDSS steps 1.0–4.5 refer to people with MS who are ambulatory. EDSS steps 5.0–9.5 are defined by the impairment to ambulation.

Although used for the majority of epidemiological studies and treatment trials, it is not without its limitations. The scale relies on some degree of subjectivity, particularly in relation to ambulation and bladder or bowel function, and the ability to define whether the patient is able to walk specific distances often relies upon estimations, since accurately assessing a patient's ability to walk 500 m in a clinic may not be possible [121]. Inter-rater reliability is highly important, that is whether two independent examiners ascribe the same score to a patient, and some studies have suggested this to be rather low [122–124]. One of these studies estimated that 95% of the independent observers would score within 1.5 EDSS units of the "correct" value. Since treatment trials often use primary outcome measures of an EDSS change of half or one point (sustained for 3 months), inter-rater reliability and precision in allocating scores becomes hugely important and may be a major component in the 'failure' of certain trials.

Table 1.3 Expanded disability status scale (adapted from reference)

0	Normal neurological exam (all FS grade 0)
1.0	No disability, minimal signs in one FS (one FS grade 1)
1.5	No disability, minimal signs in more than one FS (more than one FS grade 1)
2.0	Minimal disability in one FS (one FS grade 2, others 0 or 1)
2.5	Minimal disability in two FS (two FS grade 2, others 0 or 1)
3.0	Moderate disability in one FS (one FS grade 3, others 0 or 1) though fully ambulatory; or mild disability in three or four FS (three/four FS grade 2, others 0 or 1) though fully ambulatory
3.5	Fully ambulatory but with moderate disability in one FS (one FS grade 3) and mild disability in one or two FS (one/two FS grade 2) and others 0 or 1; or fully ambulatory with two FS grade 3 (others 0 or 1);or fully ambulatory with five FS grade 2 (others 0 or 1)
4.0	Ambulatory without aid or rest for ≥500 m; up and about some 12 h a day despite relatively severe disability consisting of one FS grade 4 (others 0 or 1) or combinations of lesser grades exceeding limits of previous steps
4.5	Ambulatory without aid or rest for ≥300 m; up and about much of the day, characterised by relatively severe disability usually consisting of one FS grade 4 and combination of lesser grades exceeding limits of previous steps
5.0	Ambulatory without aid or rest for ≥200 m (usual FS equivalents include at least one FS grade 5, or combinations of lesser grades usually exceeding specifications for step 4.5)
5.5	Ambulatory without aid or rest ≥100 m
6.0	Unilateral assistance (cane or crutch) required to walk at least 100 m with or without resting
6.5	Constant bilateral assistance (canes or crutches) required to walk at least 20 m Without resting
7.0	Unable to walk 5 m even with aid, essentially restricted to wheelchair; wheels Self and transfers alone; up and about in wheelchair some 12 h a day
7.5	Unable to take more than a few steps; restricted to wheelchair; may need some help in transferring and in wheeling self
8.0	Essentially restricted to bed or chair or perambulated in wheelchair, but out of bed most of day; retains many self-care functions; generally has effective use of arms
8.5	Essentially restricted to bed much of the day; has some effective use of arm(s); retains some self-care functions
9.0	Helpless bed patient; can communicate and eat
9.5	Totally helpless bed patient; unable to communicate effectively or eat/swallow
10.0	Death due to MS

The scale also mixes measurement in different domains of disability and that which is measured at one end of the scale is different to the other end of the scale. In addition, some domains of disability are poorly represented, such as cognition. Progression in the EDSS is also not linear, and progression from 1 to 5 occurs much more quickly than from 5 to 7, which, again, may have implications for trial design [125]. Despite this, the EDSS has clinical use, since a particular score is able to convey a description of disability in a similar way that the Medical Research Council (MRC) grade of muscle strength does in a standardised and universally accepted manner.

A variety of other assessment scales are in use. Of these, the Multiple Sclerosis Functional Composite (MSFC) was used in the International MS Secondary Progressive Avonex Controlled Trial (IMPACT) as a primary outcome measure for disease progression [126]. The MSFC was developed in order to address some of the limitations of the EDSS and to move away from the emphasis this scale puts on ambulation as a marker of disability. The MSFC consists of three items: a timed walk of 25-foot (T25FW; measuring ambulation); a 9-hole peg test (measuring upper limb function); and a paced auditory serial addition test at 3 s intervals (used as an indicator of cognitive function) [127, 128]. Component scores are transformed into *z*-scores by standardising to a reference population and the individual scores are

Table 1.4 Functional systems used in assessing EDSS (adapted from reference)

Pyramidal systems	**Visual functions**
0 normal 1 abnormal signs without disability 2 minimal disability: patient complains of fatigability or reduced performance in strenuous motor tasks and/or MRC grade 4 in one or two muscle groups 3 mild to moderate paraparesis or hemiparesis: usually MRC grade 4 in more than two muscle groups or MRC grade 3 in one or two muscle groups; movements against gravity are possible; severe monoparesis: MRC grade 2 or less in one muscle group 4 marked paraparesis or hemiparesis: usually MRC grade 2 in two limbs; moderate tetraparesis: MRC grade 3 in three or more limbs; monoplegia: MRC grade 0 or 1 in one limb 5 paraplegia: MRC grade 0 or 1 in all muscle groups of the lower limbs; hemiplegia; marked tetraparesis: MRC grade 2 or less in three or more limbs 6 tetraplegia: MRC grade 0 or 1 in all muscle groups of the upper and lower limbs	0 normal 1 disc pallor and/or mild scotoma and/or visual acuity (corrected) of worse eye less than 20/20 (1.0) but better than 20/30 (0.67) 2 worse eye with large scotoma and/or maximal visual acuity (corrected) of 20/30 to 20/59 (0.67–0.34) 3 worse eye with large scotoma or moderate decrease in fields and/or maximal visual acuity (corrected) of 20/60 to 20/99 (0.33–0.2) 4 worse eye with marked decrease of fields and/or maximal visual acuity (corrected) of 20/100 to 20/200 (0.2–0.1); grade 3 plus maximal acuity of better eye of 20/60 (0.3) or less 5 worse eye with maximal visual acuity (corrected) less than 20/200 (0.1); grade 4 plus maximal acuity of better eye of 20/60 (0.3) or less 6 grade 5 plus maximal visual acuity of better eye of 20/60 (0.3) or less
Cerebellar systems	**Brainstem functions**
0 normal 1 abnormal signs without disability 2 mild ataxia 3 moderate truncal or limb ataxia 4 severe truncal ataxia and severe ataxia in three or four limbs 5 unable to perform coordinated movements due to ataxia X pyramidal weakness (MRC grade 3 or worse in limb strength) interferes with cerebellar testing	0 normal 1 signs only 2 moderate nystagmus or other mild disability 3 severe nystagmus; marked extraocular weakness or moderate disability of other cranial nerves 4 marked dysarthria or other marked disability 5 inability to swallow or speak

Table 1.4 (continued)

Sensory function	Bowel and bladder function
0 normal 1 vibration or figure-writing decrease only, in one or two limbs 2 mild decrease in touch or pain or position sense and/or moderate decrease in vibration in one or two limbs; mild vibration or figure-writing decrease alone in three or four limbs 3 moderate decrease in touch or pain or position sense and/or essentially lost vibration in one or two limbs; or mild decrease in touch or pain and/or moderate decrease in all proprioceptive tests in three or four limbs 4 marked decrease in touch or pain or loss of proprioception, alone or combined, in one or two limbs; or moderate decrease in touch or pain and/or severe proprioceptive decrease in more than two limbs 5 loss (essentially) of sensation in one or two limbs; or moderate decrease in touch or pain and/or loss of proprioception for most of the body below the head 6 sensation essentially lost below the head	0 normal 1 mild urinary hesitancy, urgency and / or retention 2 moderate urinary hesitancy and / or urgency and/or rare urinary incontinence 3 frequent urinary incontinence 4 in need of almost constant catheterisation 5 loss of bladder function 6 loss of bowel and bladder function
Cerebral (or mental) functions 0 normal 1 mood alteration (depression and/or euphoria) alone (does not affect EDSS step) 2 mild decrease in mentation 3 moderate decrease in mentation 4 marked decrease in mentation (Chronic brain syndrome moderate) 5 dementia or chronic brain syndrome—severe or incompetent	

averaged to create the composite score. Scores for individual items may be used or the composite. The MSFC has the advantage that it is easy to administer and can usually be performed more quickly than the EDSS. The MSFC was designed specifically for use as an outcome measure for clinical trials and validation against EDSS, quality of life measures (QoL) and MRI markers have demonstrated its validity, reliability and sensitivity to change [129–133]. THE MSFC has also been used as a secondary outcome measure for a number of disease modifying drug trials [134–139].

The importance of evaluating treatments using measurements that are important to patients has led to development of patient-based outcome measures, notably, for multiple sclerosis, the MSIS-29 [140]. The 29 items in the questionnaire-based scale measure 20 physical items (e.g. 'In the past 2 weeks how much have you been bothered by difficulties using your hands in everyday tasks?') and nine psychological items (e.g. 'In the past 2 weeks how much have you been bothered by worries relating to your MS?'). Patients respond with a subjective assessment of how their illness affects them on a scale of 1 (not at all) to 5 (extremely).

The Multiple Sclerosis Severity Score (MSSS) was developed to attempt to integrate disability and disease duration in order to give an indication of disease severity [141]. In this system, a patient with a high EDSS after a short disease duration would be classified with a higher MSSS score (and by implication a more 'severe' disease), compared to a patient with the same EDSS but a much longer disease duration. It is useful as a 'single assessment' indicator of disease severity and may have a number of research applications, such as genetic studies analysing the link between susceptibility genes and disease phenotypes [142], as well as epidemiological studies in the disease [143].

1.6 Current Treatments for Multiple Sclerosis

The treatment options available for patients with MS have changed considerably in the past two decades and large numbers of trials of novel therapies are underway. The majority of studies and trials have been performed in RRMS and most trials have used reduction on annualised relapse rates (ARR) as the primary outcome measure. Using ARR reduction as an easily definable outcome measure is perhaps one reason that the trials in RRMS have borne fruit. As will be discussed in future chapters, using clinical measures to determine reduction in disease burden in progressive MS is challenging. Early RRMS trials lead to the licensing of the widely used 'injectable' disease modifying therapies (DMTs) of β-interferon (βIFN) and glatiramer acetate (GA) with their well-known effect of reducing ARR by approximately one-third [144–147]. Despite their modest effects on ARR reduction, these drugs were generally tolerated (albeit with their unpleasant route of administration) and have been extensively used in RRMS. More recently monoclonal antibody therapies such as natalizumab and alemtuzumab have been shown to dramatically reduce relapse rates in RRMS and have demonstrated superiority of the former in relapse reduction [137, 148]. However, the incidence of complications of these drugs, notably the risk of progressive multifocal leukoencephalopathy (PML) with natalizumab; and the high incidence of autoimmune disorders with alemtuzumab, makes careful consideration of risk/benefit profiles an important consideration when discussing the use of these agents in individual patients. Even more recently, ocrelizumab has been shown to be effective in RRMS and, interesting, has shown effects in primary progressive MS (which will be discussed in later chapters) [149, 150]. Three novel oral agents with better efficacies than βIFN or GA have provided a further class of DMTs for use in RRMS. These drugs are fingolimod, a sphingosine 1-phosphate modulator whose primary action in MS is to reduce lymphocyte entry into the brain; dimethyl fumarate, which activates nrf2 anti-oxidant responses; and teriflunomide, which impairs clonal expansion of activated lymphocytes [151–153]. Despite each drug having specific side effects and associated risks, the ARR reduction is generally better than the early injectables and have the added benefit of being oral therapies.

Regarding progressive MS, however, options for disease modification are much more limited. The hope that drugs used to reduce relapse frequency might be effective in established progressive disease has, largely, proven to be unfounded. The likely reasons for this and a review of DMT drug trials relating to progressive MS are presented in subsequent chapters. Despite these trial failures, the evidence gleaned from them has, in association with epidemiological, pathological and MRI evidence, been hugely informative in determining pathophysiological mechanisms in progressive disease and has set the scene for a new generation of therapies specifically targeting disease processes occurring in progressive MS. These issues, along with general descriptions of progressive MS will be discussed in detail throughout this book.

References

1. Lizak N, et al. Highly active immunomodulatory therapy ameliorates accumulation of disability in moderately advanced and advanced multiple sclerosis. J Neurol Neurosurg Psychiatry. 2017;88(3):196–203.
2. McDonald WI, et al. Recommended diagnostic criteria for multiple sclerosis: guidelines from the International Panel on the diagnosis of multiple sclerosis. Ann Neurol. 2001;50(1):121–7.
3. Polman CH, et al. Diagnostic criteria for multiple sclerosis: 2010 revisions to the McDonald criteria. Ann Neurol. 2011;69(2):292–302.
4. Ramagopalan SV, et al. Multiple sclerosis: risk factors, prodromes, and potential causal pathways. Lancet Neurol. 2010;9(7):727–39.
5. Bronson PG, et al. CIITA variation in the presence of HLA-DRB1*1501 increases risk for multiple sclerosis. Hum Mol Genet. 2010;19(11):2331–40.
6. Lincoln MR, et al. A predominant role for the HLA class II region in the association of the MHC region with multiple sclerosis. Nat Genet. 2005;37(10):1108–12.
7. Sawcer S, et al. Genetic risk and a primary role for cell-mediated immune mechanisms in multiple sclerosis. Nature. 2011;476(7359):214–9.
8. McAuley JL, et al. Comprehensive follow-up of the first genome-wide association study of multiple sclerosis identifies KIF21B and TMEM39A as susceptibility loci. Hum Mol Genet. 2010;19(5):953–62.
9. Kurtzke JF. Geographic distribution of multiple sclerosis: an update with special reference to Europe and the Mediterranean region. Acta Neurol Scand. 1980;62(2):65–80.
10. van der Mei IA, et al. Past exposure to sun, skin phenotype, and risk of multiple sclerosis: case-control study. BMJ. 2003;327(7410):316.
11. Munger KL, et al. Serum 25-hydroxyvitamin D levels and risk of multiple sclerosis. JAMA. 2006;296(23):2832–8.
12. Mowry EM, et al. Vitamin D status is associated with relapse rate in pediatric-onset multiple sclerosis. Ann Neurol. 2010;67(5):618–24.
13. van der Mei IA, et al. Vitamin D levels in people with multiple sclerosis and community controls in Tasmania, Australia. J Neurol. 2007;254(5):581–90.
14. Simpson S Jr, et al. Higher 25-hydroxyvitamin D is associated with lower relapse risk in multiple sclerosis. Ann Neurol. 2010;68(2):193–203.
15. Lemire JM, et al. Immunosuppressive actions of 1,25-dihydroxyvitamin D3: preferential inhibition of Th1 functions. J Nutr. 1995;125(6 Suppl):1704S–8S.
16. Ramagopalan SV, et al. Expression of the multiple sclerosis-associated MHC class II Allele HLA-DRB1*1501 is regulated by vitamin D. PLoS Genet. 2009;5(2):e1000369.

17. Holick MF. High prevalence of vitamin D inadequacy and implications for health. Mayo Clin Proc. 2006;81(3):353–73.
18. Sundstrom P, et al. An altered immune response to Epstein-Barr virus in multiple sclerosis: a prospective study. Neurology. 2004;62(12):2277–82.
19. Ascherio A, Munger KL. Environmental risk factors for multiple sclerosis. Part I: The role of infection. Ann Neurol. 2007;61(4):288–99.
20. Salvetti M, Giovannoni G, Aloisi F. Epstein-Barr virus and multiple sclerosis. Curr Opin Neurol. 2009;22(3):201–6.
21. Niller HH, Wolf H, Minarovits J. Regulation and dysregulation of Epstein-Barr virus latency: implications for the development of autoimmune diseases. Autoimmunity. 2008;41(4):298–328.
22. Levin LI, et al. Temporal relationship between elevation of epstein-barr virus antibody titers and initial onset of neurological symptoms in multiple sclerosis. JAMA. 2005;293(20):2496–500.
23. Ascherio A, Munger KL, Lunemann JD. The initiation and prevention of multiple sclerosis. Nat Rev Neurol. 2012;8(11):602–12.
24. Sundqvist E, et al. Epstein-Barr virus and multiple sclerosis: interaction with HLA. Genes Immun. 2012;13(1):14–20.
25. Serafini B, et al. Dysregulated Epstein-Barr virus infection in the multiple sclerosis brain. J Exp Med. 2007;204(12):2899–912.
26. Willis SN, et al. Epstein-Barr virus infection is not a characteristic feature of multiple sclerosis brain. Brain. 2009;132(Pt 12):3318–28.
27. Hedstrom AK, et al. Smoking and two human leukocyte antigen genes interact to increase the risk for multiple sclerosis. Brain. 2011;134(Pt 3):653–64.
28. Munger KL, Chitnis T, Ascherio A. Body size and risk of MS in two cohorts of US women. Neurology. 2009;73(19):1543–50.
29. Gianfrancesco MA, et al. Obesity during childhood and adolescence increases susceptibility to multiple sclerosis after accounting for established genetic and environmental risk factors. Obes Res Clin Pract. 2014;8(5):e435–47.
30. Thompson AJ, et al. A clinical and laboratory study of benign multiple sclerosis. Q J Med. 1986;58(225):69–80.
31. Hawkins SA, McDonnell GV. Benign multiple sclerosis? Clinical course, long term follow up, and assessment of prognostic factors. J Neurol Neurosurg Psychiatry. 1999;67(2): 148–52.
32. Poser S, Wikstrom J, Bauer HJ. Clinical data and the identification of special forms of multiple sclerosis in 1271 cases studied with a standardized documentation system. J Neurol Sci. 1979;40(2–3):159–68.
33. Costelloe L, et al. Long-term clinical relevance of criteria for designating multiple sclerosis as benign after 10 years of disease. J Neurol Neurosurg Psychiatry. 2008;79(11):1245–8.
34. Correale J, Peirano I, Romano L. Benign multiple sclerosis: a new definition of this entity is needed. Mult Scler. 2011;18(2):210–8.
35. Skoog B, et al. A representative cohort of patients with non-progressive multiple sclerosis at the age of normal life expectancy. Brain. 2012;135(Pt 3):900–11.
36. Scalfari A, et al. The natural history of multiple sclerosis: a geographically based study 10: relapses and long-term disability. Brain. 2010;133(Pt 7):1914–29.
37. Lublin FD, Reingold SC. Defining the clinical course of multiple sclerosis: results of an international survey. National Multiple Sclerosis Society (USA) Advisory Committee on Clinical Trials of New Agents in Multiple Sclerosis. Neurology. 1996;46(4):907–11.
38. Lublin FD, et al. Defining the clinical course of multiple sclerosis: the 2013 revisions. Neurology. 2014;83(3):278–86.
39. McDonnell GV, Hawkins SA. Clinical study of primary progressive multiple sclerosis in Northern Ireland, UK. J Neurol Neurosurg Psychiatry. 1998;64(4):451–4.
40. Katz Sand I, et al. Diagnostic uncertainty during the transition to secondary progressive multiple sclerosis. Mult Scler. 2014;20(12):1654–7.
41. Mc AD, Compston N. Some aspects of the natural history of disseminated sclerosis. Q J Med. 1952;21(82):135–67.

42. Goodkin DE, et al. Low-dose oral methotrexate in chronic progressive multiple sclerosis: analyses of serial MRIs. Neurology. 1996;47(5):1153–7.
43. Hillert J, et al. An immunogenetic heterogeneity in multiple sclerosis. J Neurol Neurosurg Psychiatry. 1992;55(10):887–90.
44. Weinshenker BG. Natural history of multiple sclerosis. Ann Neurol. 1994;36(Suppl):S6–11.
45. Filippi M, et al. Transitional progressive multiple sclerosis: MRI and MTI findings. Acta Neurol Scand. 1995;92(2):178–82.
46. Kremenchutzky M, et al. The natural history of multiple sclerosis: a geographically based study 9: observations on the progressive phase of the disease. Brain. 2006;129(Pt 3):584–94.
47. Weinshenker BG. Progressive forms of MS: classification streamlined or consensus overturned? Lancet. 2000;355(9199):162–3.
48. Kremenchutzky M, et al. The natural history of multiple sclerosis: a geographically based study. 7. Progressive-relapsing and relapsing-progressive multiple sclerosis: a re-evaluation. Brain. 1999;122(Pt 10):1941–50.
49. Andersson PB, et al. Multiple sclerosis that is progressive from the time of onset: clinical characteristics and progression of disability. Arch Neurol. 1999;56(9):1138–42.
50. Westerlind H, et al. A significant decrease in diagnosis of primary progressive multiple sclerosis: a cohort study. Mult Scler. 2016;22(8):1071–9.
51. Cutter GR, Salter A, Marrie RA. Declines in the diagnosis of primary progressive MS: a critical change in phenotype or critical measurement error? Mult Scler. 2016;22(8):983–5.
52. Allison RS, Millar JH. Prevalence of disseminated sclerosis in Northern Ireland. Ulster Med J. 1954;23(Suppl. 2):1–27.
53. Schumacker GA, et al. Problems of experimental trials of therapy in multiple sclerosis: report by the panel on the evaluation of experimental trials of therapy in multiple sclerosis. Ann N Y Acad Sci. 1965;122:552–68.
54. McDonald WI, Halliday AM. Diagnosis and classification of multiple sclerosis. Br Med Bull. 1977;33(1):4–9.
55. Poser CM, et al. New diagnostic criteria for multiple sclerosis: guidelines for research protocols. Ann Neurol. 1983;13(3):227–31.
56. McDonnell GV, Hawkins SA. Application of the Poser criteria in primary progressive multiple sclerosis. Ann Neurol. 1997;42(6):982–3.
57. Thompson AJ, et al. Diagnostic criteria for primary progressive multiple sclerosis: a position paper. Ann Neurol. 2000;47(6):831–5.
58. Kurtzke JF. Rating neurologic impairment in multiple sclerosis: an expanded disability status scale (EDSS). Neurology. 1983;33(11):1444–52.
59. Zeman AZ, et al. A study of oligoclonal band negative multiple sclerosis. J Neurol Neurosurg Psychiatry. 1996;60(1):27–30.
60. Polman CH, et al. Diagnostic criteria for multiple sclerosis: 2005 revisions to the "McDonald Criteria". Ann Neurol. 2005;58(6):840–6.
61. Montalban X, et al. Primary progressive multiple sclerosis diagnostic criteria: a reappraisal. Mult Scler. 2009;15(12):1459–65.
62. Bonduelle M, Albaranes R. Statistical study of 145 cases of multiple sclerosis. Sem Hop. 1962;38:3762–73.
63. Cottrell DA, et al. The natural history of multiple sclerosis: a geographically based study. 5. The clinical features and natural history of primary progressive multiple sclerosis. Brain. 1999;122(Pt 4):625–39.
64. Noseworthy J, et al. Multiple sclerosis after age 50. Neurology. 1983;33(12):1537–44.
65. Jeffery DR. Chronic progressive myelopathy: diagnostic analysis of cases with and without sensory involvement. J Neurol Sci. 1996;142(1–2):153–6.
66. Cazzullo CL, et al. Clinical picture of multiple sclerosis with late onset. Acta Neurol Scand. 1978;58(3):190–6.
67. Wingerchuk DM, et al. The spectrum of neuromyelitis optica. Lancet Neurol. 2007;6(9):805–15.
68. Wingerchuk DM, et al. Revised diagnostic criteria for neuromyelitis optica. Neurology. 2006;66(10):1485–9.

69. O'Brien TJ, Gates PG, Byrne E. Symptomatic female heterozygotes for adrenoleukodystrophy: a report of two unrelated cases and review of the literature. J Clin Neurosci. 1996;3(2):166–70.
70. Wilkins A, et al. Very long chain fatty acid levels in patients diagnosed with multiple sclerosis. Mult Scler. 2009;15(12):1525–7.
71. Yu-Wai-Man P, et al. Inherited mitochondrial optic neuropathies. J Med Genet. 2009;46(3):145–58.
72. Camp SJ, et al. Cognitive function in primary progressive and transitional progressive multiple sclerosis: a controlled study with MRI correlates. Brain. 1999;122(Pt 7):1341–8.
73. Camp SJ, et al. A longitudinal study of cognition in primary progressive multiple sclerosis. Brain. 2005;128(Pt 12):2891–8.
74. Denney DR, Sworowski LA, Lynch SG. Cognitive impairment in three subtypes of multiple sclerosis. Arch Clin Neuropsychol. 2005;20(8):967–81.
75. Denney DR, et al. Cognitive impairment in relapsing and primary progressive multiple sclerosis: mostly a matter of speed. J Int Neuropsychol Soc. 2004;10(7):948–56.
76. Wachowius U, et al. Cognitive impairment in primary and secondary progressive multiple sclerosis. J Clin Exp Neuropsychol. 2005;27(1):65–77.
77. Lorscheider J, et al. Defining secondary progressive multiple sclerosis. Brain. 2016;139(Pt 9):2395–405.
78. Weinshenker BG, et al. The natural history of multiple sclerosis: a geographically based study. 2. Predictive value of the early clinical course. Brain. 1989;112(Pt 6):1419–28.
79. Confavreux C, et al. Relapses and progression of disability in multiple sclerosis. N Engl J Med. 2000;343(20):1430–8.
80. Weinshenker BG, et al. The natural history of multiple sclerosis: a geographically based study. I. Clinical course and disability. Brain. 1989;112(Pt 1):133–46.
81. University of California, San Francisco MS-EPIC Team, et al. Long-term evolution of multiple sclerosis disability in the treatment era. Ann Neurol. 2016;80(4):499–510.
82. Confavreux C, et al. Clinical progression and decision making process in multiple sclerosis. Mult Scler. 1999;5(4):212–5.
83. Kurtzke JF. Clinical definition for multiple sclerosis treatment trials. Ann Neurol. 1994; 36(Suppl):S73–9.
84. Fog T, Linnemann F. The course of multiple sclerosis in 73 cases with computer-designed curves. Acta Neurol Scand Suppl. 1970;47:3–175.
85. Leray E, et al. Evidence for a two-stage disability progression in multiple sclerosis. Brain. 2010;133(Pt 7):1900–13.
86. Confavreux C, Vukusic S, Adeleine P. Early clinical predictors and progression of irreversible disability in multiple sclerosis: an amnesic process. Brain. 2003;126(Pt 4):770–82.
87. Debouverie M, et al. Natural history of multiple sclerosis in a population-based cohort. Eur J Neurol. 2008;15(9):916–21.
88. Vukusic S, Confavreux C. Natural history of multiple sclerosis: risk factors and prognostic indicators. Curr Opin Neurol. 2007;20(3):269–74.
89. Confavreux C, Vukusic S. Natural history of multiple sclerosis: a unifying concept. Brain. 2006;129(Pt 3):606–16.
90. Confavreux C, Vukusic S. Age at disability milestones in multiple sclerosis. Brain. 2006; 129(Pt 3):595–605.
91. Langdon DW. Cognition in multiple sclerosis. Curr Opin Neurol. 2011;24(3):244–9.
92. Calabrese M, et al. Cortical pathology and cognitive impairment in multiple sclerosis. Expert Rev Neurother. 2011;11(3):425–32.
93. Bergendal G, Fredrikson S, Almkvist O. Selective decline in information processing in subgroups of multiple sclerosis: an 8-year longitudinal study. Eur Neurol. 2007;57(4): 193–202.
94. Strober L, et al. Sensitivity of conventional memory tests in multiple sclerosis: comparing the Rao Brief Repeatable Neuropsychological Battery and the Minimal Assessment of Cognitive Function in MS. Mult Scler. 2009;15(9):1077–84.

95. Laatu S, et al. Sematic memory deficit in multiple sclerosis; impaired understanding of conceptual meanings. J Neurol Sci. 1999;162(2):152–61.
96. Drew M, et al. Executive dysfunction and cognitive impairment in a large community-based sample with Multiple Sclerosis from New Zealand: a descriptive study. Arch Clin Neuropsychol. 2008;23(1):1–19.
97. Langdon DW, Thompson AJ. Multiple sclerosis: a preliminary study of selected variables affecting rehabilitation outcome. Mult Scler. 1999;5(2):94–100.
98. Rao SM, et al. Cognitive dysfunction in multiple sclerosis. II. Impact on employment and social functioning. Neurology. 1991;41(5):692–6.
99. Feinstein A. Mood disorders in multiple sclerosis and the effects on cognition. J Neurol Sci. 2006;245(1–2):63–6.
100. Chwastiak L, et al. Depressive symptoms and severity of illness in multiple sclerosis: epidemiologic study of a large community sample. Am J Psychiatry. 2002;159(11):1862–8.
101. Harel Y, Barak Y, Achiron A. Dysregulation of affect in multiple sclerosis: new phenomenological approach. Psychiatry Clin Neurosci. 2007;61(1):94–8.
102. Parmenter BA, Denney DR, Lynch SG. The cognitive performance of patients with multiple sclerosis during periods of high and low fatigue. Mult Scler. 2003;9(2):111–8.
103. Benedict RH, et al. Minimal neuropsychological assessment of MS patients: a consensus approach. Clin Neuropsychol. 2002;16(3):381–97.
104. Benedict RH, et al. Validity of the minimal assessment of cognitive function in multiple sclerosis (MACFIMS). J Int Neuropsychol Soc. 2006;12(4):549–58.
105. Kurtzke JF, et al. Studies on the natural history of multiple sclerosis. V. Long-term survival in young men. Arch Neurol. 1970;22(3):215–25.
106. Swingler RJ, Compston DA. The morbidity of multiple sclerosis. Q J Med. 1992;83(300): -325–37.
107. Alusi SH, et al. A study of tremor in multiple sclerosis. Brain. 2001;124(Pt 4):720–30.
108. Pittock SJ, et al. Prevalence of tremor in multiple sclerosis and associated disability in the Olmsted County population. Mov Disord. 2004;19(12):1482–5.
109. Koch M, et al. Tremor in multiple sclerosis. J Neurol. 2007;254(2):133–45.
110. Weier K, et al. Contribution of the cerebellum to cognitive performance in children and adolescents with multiple sclerosis. Mult Scler. 2016;22(5):599–607.
111. Tedesco AM, et al. The cerebellar cognitive profile. Brain. 2011;134(Pt 12):3672–86.
112. Weier K, et al. Cerebellar abnormalities contribute to disability including cognitive impairment in multiple sclerosis. PLoS One. 2014;9(1):e86916.
113. Kutzelnigg A, et al. Widespread demyelination in the cerebellar cortex in multiple sclerosis. Brain Pathol. 2007;17(1):38–44.
114. Craner MJ, et al. Annexin II/p11 is up-regulated in Purkinje cells in EAE and MS. Neuroreport. 2003;14(4):555–8.
115. Calabrese M, et al. Magnetic resonance evidence of cerebellar cortical pathology in multiple sclerosis. J Neurol Neurosurg Psychiatry. 2010;81(4):401–4.
116. Anderson VM, et al. MRI measures show significant cerebellar gray matter volume loss in multiple sclerosis and are associated with cerebellar dysfunction. Mult Scler. 2009;15(7): 811–7.
117. Davie CA, et al. Persistent functional deficit in multiple sclerosis and autosomal dominant cerebellar ataxia is associated with axon loss. Brain. 1995;118(Pt 6):1583–92.
118. Waxman SG. Cerebellar dysfunction in multiple sclerosis: evidence for an acquired channelopathy. Prog Brain Res. 2005;148:353–65.
119. Waxman SG. Acquired channelopathies in nerve injury and MS. Neurology. 2001;56(12): 1621–7.
120. Kurtzke JF. Natural history and clinical outcome measures for multiple sclerosis studies. Why at the present time does EDSS scale remain a preferred outcome measure to evaluate disease evolution? Neurol Sci. 2000;21(6):339–41.
121. Willoughby EW, Paty DW. Scales for rating impairment in multiple sclerosis: a critique. Neurology. 1988;38(11):1793–8.

122. Amato MP, et al. Interrater reliability in assessing functional systems and disability on the Kurtzke scale in multiple sclerosis. Arch Neurol. 1988;45(7):746–8.
123. Francis DA, et al. An assessment of disability rating scales used in multiple sclerosis. Arch Neurol. 1991;48(3):299–301.
124. Goodkin DE, et al. Inter- and intrarater scoring agreement using grades 1.0 to 3.5 of the Kurtzke Expanded Disability Status Scale (EDSS). Multiple Sclerosis Collaborative Research Group. Neurology. 1992;42(4):859–63.
125. Hobart JC, et al. Rating scales as outcome measures for clinical trials in neurology: problems, solutions, and recommendations. Lancet Neurol. 2007;6(12):1094–105.
126. Cohen JA, et al. Benefit of interferon beta-1a on MSFC progression in secondary progressive MS. Neurology. 2002;59(5):679–87.
127. Fischer JS, et al. The Multiple Sclerosis Functional Composite Measure (MSFC): an integrated approach to MS clinical outcome assessment. National MS Society Clinical Outcomes Assessment Task Force. Mult Scler. 1999;5(4):244–50.
128. Cutter GR, et al. Development of a multiple sclerosis functional composite as a clinical trial outcome measure. Brain. 1999;122(Pt 5):871–82.
129. Cohen JA, et al. Use of the multiple sclerosis functional composite as an outcome measure in a phase 3 clinical trial. Arch Neurol. 2001;58(6):961–7.
130. Miller DM, et al. Clinical significance of the multiple sclerosis functional composite: relationship to patient-reported quality of life. Arch Neurol. 2000;57(9):1319–24.
131. Kalkers NF, et al. MS functional composite: relation to disease phenotype and disability strata. Neurology. 2000;54(6):1233–9.
132. Goldman MD, Motl RW, Rudick RA. Possible clinical outcome measures for clinical trials in patients with multiple sclerosis. Ther Adv Neurol Disord. 2010;3(4):229–39.
133. Kragt JJ, et al. Responsiveness and predictive value of EDSS and MSFC in primary progressive MS. Neurology. 2008;70(13 Pt 2):1084–91.
134. Kappos L, et al. Effect of early versus delayed interferon beta-1b treatment on disability after a first clinical event suggestive of multiple sclerosis: a 3-year follow-up analysis of the BENEFIT study. Lancet. 2007;370(9585):389–97.
135. Montalban X. Overview of European pilot study of interferon beta-Ib in primary progressive multiple sclerosis. Mult Scler. 2004;10(Suppl 1):S62. discussion 62-4
136. Wolinsky JS, et al. Glatiramer acetate in primary progressive multiple sclerosis: results of a multinational, multicenter, double-blind, placebo-controlled trial. Ann Neurol. 2007;61(1):14–24.
137. Polman CH, et al. A randomized, placebo-controlled trial of natalizumab for relapsing multiple sclerosis. N Engl J Med. 2006;354(9):899–910.
138. Kappos L, et al. A placebo-controlled trial of oral fingolimod in relapsing multiple sclerosis. N Engl J Med. 2010;362(5):387–401.
139. Goodman AD, et al. Fampridine-SR in multiple sclerosis: a randomized, double-blind, placebo-controlled, dose-ranging study. Mult Scler. 2007;13(3):357–68.
140. Hobart J, et al. The Multiple Sclerosis Impact Scale (MSIS-29): a new patient-based outcome measure. Brain. 2001;124(Pt 5):962–73.
141. Roxburgh RH, et al. Multiple Sclerosis Severity Score: using disability and disease duration to rate disease severity. Neurology. 2005;64(7):1144–51.
142. Briggs FB, et al. Genome-wide association study of severity in multiple sclerosis. Genes Immun. 2011;12(8):615–25.
143. Kister I, et al. Rapid disease course in African Americans with multiple sclerosis. Neurology. 2010;75(3):217–23.
144. The IFNB Multiple Sclerosis Study Group. Interferon beta-1b is effective in relapsing-remitting multiple sclerosis. I. Clinical results of a multicenter, randomized, double-blind, placebo-controlled trial. Neurology. 1993;43(4):655–61.
145. PRISMS (Prevention of Relapses and Disability by Interferon beta-1a Subcutaneously in Multiple Sclerosis) Study Group. Randomised double-blind placebo-controlled study of interferon beta-1a in relapsing/remitting multiple sclerosis. Lancet. 1998;352(9139):1498–504.

146. Johnson KP, et al. Copolymer 1 reduces relapse rate and improves disability in relapsing-remitting multiple sclerosis: results of a phase III multicenter, double-blind placebo-controlled trial. The Copolymer 1 Multiple Sclerosis Study Group. Neurology. 1995;45(7):1268–76.
147. Jacobs LD, et al. Intramuscular interferon beta-1a for disease progression in relapsing multiple sclerosis. The Multiple Sclerosis Collaborative Research Group (MSCRG). Ann Neurol. 1996;39(3):285–94.
148. Coles AJ, et al. Alemtuzumab vs. interferon beta-1a in early multiple sclerosis. N Engl J Med. 2008;359(17):1786–801.
149. Montalban X, et al. Ocrelizumab versus placebo in primary progressive multiple sclerosis. N Engl J Med. 2017;376(3):209–20.
150. Hauser SL, et al. Ocrelizumab versus interferon beta-1a in relapsing multiple sclerosis. N Engl J Med. 2017;376(3):221–34.
151. Cohen JA, et al. Oral fingolimod or intramuscular interferon for relapsing multiple sclerosis. N Engl J Med. 2010;362(5):402–15.
152. Gold R, et al. Placebo-controlled phase 3 study of oral BG-12 for relapsing multiple sclerosis. N Engl J Med. 2012;367(12):1098–107.
153. O'Connor P, et al. Randomized trial of oral teriflunomide for relapsing multiple sclerosis. N Engl J Med. 2011;365(14):1293–303.

2.2 Primary Progressive Multiple Sclerosis

2.2.1 Disease Frequency

Primary progressive MS commonly comprises between 7.9% [4] and 21.7% [5] of total MS cohorts. However, there has been considerable variability in reports of PPMS frequency [4–19]. The highest recorded was from a detailed Dutch study in the 1980s reporting a PPMS frequency of 37% [6]. The reasons for this unusually high figure are unclear, but highlight the difficulties inherent in epidemiological studies of PPMS as a result of changes to the definition of PPMS over time, and differences between prospectively collected data compared to retrospective or cross-sectional data. It is also important to consider the temporal relationship of epidemiological studies to the publication of consensus definitions of clinical course in MS in 1996 [20], which defined primary progressive and progressive relapsing courses for the first time. Caution should therefore be exercised in making comparisons with epidemiological studies published prior to this date, as classification of disease phenotype is likely to be more heterogenous and difficult to translate to modern consensus definition. However, a more recent survey of the same Dutch population in 2007 found that the proportion of patients with PPMS was still 31.3% [14].

Study source should also be considered; as hospital based series are more likely to be biased towards more severe cases [21], which is likely to result in a higher proportion of patients with PPMS. The London Ontario dataset, which was one of the first large MS cohorts used to describe natural history, is a large clinic-based cohort with two subgroups: one group of patients seen from onset of disease, and one from Middlesex County where it was estimated that over 90% of the MS population was recorded in the dataset [10, 22]. Despite similar methodologies, the percentage of patients diagnosed with PPMS in the "seen from onset" group was half that identified in the total cohort [22], suggesting that retrospective diagnosis of PPMS may overestimate prevalence. This is thought to be the result of amnestic bias, since if patients are not seen at onset of disease, earlier episodes of transient neurological dysfunction may be forgotten or remain unreported. More contemporary studies in Caucasian dominant populations generally report a prevalence of 10–15% [8, 9, 12, 13, 16, 17, 19], which is considered a more appropriate estimate of the true frequency of PPMS. However, evidence from selected epidemiological studies suggests that PPMS is less common in other ethnic groups, even after taking into account the lower overall MS prevalence in these populations. Recent studies have estimated the frequency of PPMS in Asia at between 3% [19] and 5.7% [15, 18]. As yet the reason for this difference in early disease course remains unexplained, but remains an interesting contrast to the persistently high frequency in the Dutch population [14], and raises the possibility of local variation (either genetic or environmental) modifying disease phenotype in specific populations.

2.2.2 Clinical Features

Age at onset of MS is highly variable, and PPMS is no different. PPMS patients tend to be older at onset than those with relapsing onset MS (ROMS) [23], and the mean age at onset of first symptoms is in the late 30s [10, 12, 14, 24] or early 40s [4, 11, 13, 16, 17, 25], in contrast to ROMS where mean age of onset is around a decade earlier [12, 22]. As a result PPMS is rare in paediatric-onset MS, with reported percentage between 0% [26] and 2.6% [7, 14, 27]. We have reported on our own series from south east Wales, and found only one of 111 (0.9%) paediatric onset patients had PPMS [28]. The largest paediatric onset case series to date is from Lyon, France [29]. This study comprised 394 patients, and was able to interrogate clinical phenotype of paediatric onset MS in more detail by age at onset, comparing patients with onset <12 years with those with onset between 12 and 16 years, and found that all nine observed cases with PPMS were in the group aged 12–16 years at onset [29]. Conversely, there is a strikingly higher proportion of patients with late-onset MS who have a progressive onset, reported as between 37% [30] and 54.5% [31] in population-based studies. The only study reporting a younger age at onset was a retrospective hospital-based case series from Iran [15]. This study found a mean age at onset of 31, which is closer to the mean age at onset in ROMS patients in Caucasian case series. Although only a single small study, so that caution should be used in interpreting these results, it once again suggests a role for modification (genetic or environmental) of disease phenotype in certain populations.

There is a general consensus that the gender ratio in PPMS is more balanced than in ROMS [4, 8, 10, 12, 13, 16, 17, 24, 25], with a slight preponderance of females affected so that gender ratio is between 1.1:1 [16, 17] and 1.8:1 [8]. This is in contrast to ROMS where gender ratio is between 2:1 and 3:1 [5, 8, 11, 12, 22], although one study observed that gender ratios in PPMS increase again with older age so that over the age of 50 it becomes close to 2:1 [10].

Motor weakness is the most commonly reported onset symptom in PPMS, with between 38.9% [10] and 69.3% [16] of patients experiencing such symptoms and is significantly more frequent than in patients with ROMS [9, 11, 12, 14]. Additionally, studies reporting combined motor and sensory symptoms as long tract dysfunction have observed 84% of PPMS patients presenting with this constellation of symptoms [12, 17]. Cerebellar symptoms have also been observed more frequently than in ROMS [11, 17], but optic neuritis [11, 12, 14, 17] and brainstem symptoms [12, 14, 17] are less common. It has also been reported that in ROMS patients symptoms of MS are age-dependent, with optic neuritis most common before the age of 30 and lower limb motor weakness increasingly prevalent with age [32]. This raises the possibility that the differences that are seen in presentation of PPMS are a consequence of the older age at onset rather than a fundamental difference in the underlying pathological process. This is further supported by studies which have examined sensory symptoms independently of motor weakness, and found that frequency of sensory symptoms is similar in PPMS and ROMS [11, 14].

2.2.3 Progression of Disability

The initial consensus definitions of MS disease course distinguished between a primary progressive course and a progressive relapsing course, where a patient in whom disability progression was present from onset nonetheless had distinct superimposed relapses [20]. However, updated definitions from 2014 have removed the progressive relapsing course as a classification [2]. This decision was based on epidemiological studies showing that although a large minority (between 12.6% [4] and 38.6% [12]) of PPMS patients also have discrete relapses superimposed on progression, there is no difference in sex ratios [4, 12, 13, 17], presenting symptoms [4, 12], or long-term outcome [4, 12, 13, 17, 33], suggesting that there is no reason to consider PPMS and PRMS as separate entities [2]. The current consensus definitions describe a progressive course from onset (PPMS), which may be active or inactive (i.e. with or without relapses), and with or without progression (i.e. stable or increasing level of disability) [2].

The Expanded Disability Status Scale (EDSS) [33] is a measure of disability in MS. Disability is scored between 0 (no disability) and 10 (death from MS), where scores below 4 are based on detailed neurological examination of functional systems, and scores above 4.0 are based predominantly on mobility and ability to self-care. Although there are well-documented limitations of the EDSS score, it remains the most widely used method to assess disability in MS. The most commonly used disability endpoint in longitudinal studies of PPMS is median time from onset of disease to EDSS 6.0, and in patients with PPMS this is reported to be between 6 [8] and 15 [25] years. Most studies suggest a median time to EDSS 6.0 of approximately 10 years [4, 10, 13, 17] (Table 2.1). However, it is important to note that there is a great deal of variation, with 25% of PPMS patients reaching EDSS 6.0 within 5.0–7.3 years, but 25% having not yet reached this milestone even after 15–25 years of follow-up [11, 13]. The British Columbia cohort from Canada is the single-centre study with the longest time to EDSS 6.0 of 14 years [11, 16]. Although this may suggest local factors (either genetic or environmental) which promote a more indolent disease course in this population, methodological issues offer an alternative explanation: This study excluded patients who had reached the specified disability outcome before their first visit to the clinic, which is likely to have led to over-representation of patients with less aggressive disease. Another study has reported a comparable time to EDSS 6.0 [25], but it is unusual in that it is a very large multi-centre study utilising data from the MSBase Registry, which contains data on 18,885 MS patients from 25 countries. The MSBase Registry is a web-based registry established in 2006. Participating clinicians submit data from their clinics or private practice on a voluntary basis [25]. This is an interesting new development in MS research, utilising techniques of big data and data science to address epidemiological questions. However the registry is not population-based and so is liable to biases in patient selection. Additionally, there are significant amounts of missing data (in the study referred to above, data was missing from 3059 patients, i.e. 16.2%), suggesting caution should be used in interpretation.

Table 2.1 Comparison of time and age to EDSS or DSS endpoints in studies of PPMS using survival analysis

			Time (age) to endpoint (years)				
Study	Country	N	3.0	4.0	6.0	7.0	8.0
Runmarker and Andersen (1993) [8]	Sweden	36	–	–	6	–	–
Andersson et al. (1999) [4]	USA	83	–	–	8	–	–
Cottrell et al. (1999) [10]	Canada	216	4	5	8	15	18
Simone et al. (2002) [26]	Italy	114	–	9.33 (48.2)	–	–	–
Confavreux et al. (2006) [12]	France	282	–	0	7.1 (53)	13.4 (63.1)	–
Debouverie et al. (2007) [13]	France	359	–	3	9.9	17.0	–
Koch et al. (2009) [16]	Canada	552	–	–	14.0 (58.6)	–	–
Leray et al. (2010) [5]	France	445	2 (41.9)	–	10 (52.1)	–	–
Harding et al. (2014) [17]	UK	234	–	8.1 (54.7)	9.6 (57.3)	–	20.7 (69.3)
Ribbons et al. (2015) [25]	Multinational	1366	–	–	15	–	–

Traditionally PPMS has been considered to confer poor prognosis compared to ROMS patients, and it is certainly true that median time to disability milestones is significantly shorter than in ROMS: ROMS patients take around 10 years longer to reach EDSS 3.0, 4.0 and 6.0 than those with PPMS [5, 12, 17, 26], and around 20 years longer to reach EDSS 7.0 or 8.0 [12, 17]. PPMS patients also have a 78% chance of progressing more rapidly to EDSS 6.0 than ROMS patients [11]. However, when age at reaching the same milestones is considered, PPMS patients are a similar age to ROMS patients [5, 17, 34]. This suggests that overall lifetime prognosis is no worse than for ROMS patients and when the later age at onset for PPMS is taken into account, may even be considered to be better as PPMS patients spend more time disease- and disability-free. This is illustrated in Fig. 2.1, showing survival curves for the south east Wales MS cohort for time to and age at EDSS 4.0, 6.0 and 8.0, updated as of January 2017.

Although there are now a number of studies that have examined prognosis by using fixed EDSS disability milestones as an endpoint, there are fewer that have used mortality. PPMS has been found to confer a relatively increased risk of death [35–43], and survival times from onset of disease are shorter than in ROMS [35, 36, 40–42]. One study from Ontario, Canada, compared age at death in 216 PPMS patients, of whom 101 had died: 71 of MS related causes and 30 of other causes (mainly cardiac) [10]. Age at death was 58.8 in those dying of MS-related causes, and 66.8 in those who died from other causes, suggesting that patients with more severe MS may be more likely to die earlier. However, in studies that have compared age at death in patient subgroups, PPMS patients are reported to survive to a similar age as ROMS patients [17, 38, 40], consistent with age dependent disability milestones and once again suggesting that PPMS may not confer an overall survival disadvantage.

2.2.4 *Prognostic Factors*

Few studies have examined prognostic factors affecting progression within PPMS patients. Given the substantial variation in time to fixed disability milestones [11, 13], it would be useful to be able to stratify prognosis more accurately. There is largely a consensus with respect to sex, where no association with time to disability milestones has been observed [4, 5, 10, 13, 16, 17, 25]. Indeed, the MSBase Registry was able to examine annual rate of change in EDSS, and found that whilst males with ROMS had a faster rate of change in EDSS score than females with ROMS, there was no difference in rate of change for PPMS patients by sex [25].

Less consistently, age at onset has been observed to be associated with outcome in some studies [16, 17, 44], but not others [4, 5, 10, 13]. In those studies identifying an association, older age at onset was associated with shorter time to EDSS 4.0 [17], 6.0 [16, 17], and 8.0 [17], with similarities to the pattern observed in ROMS patients [34] once again supporting the concept that PPMS may not be a distinct pathological entity.

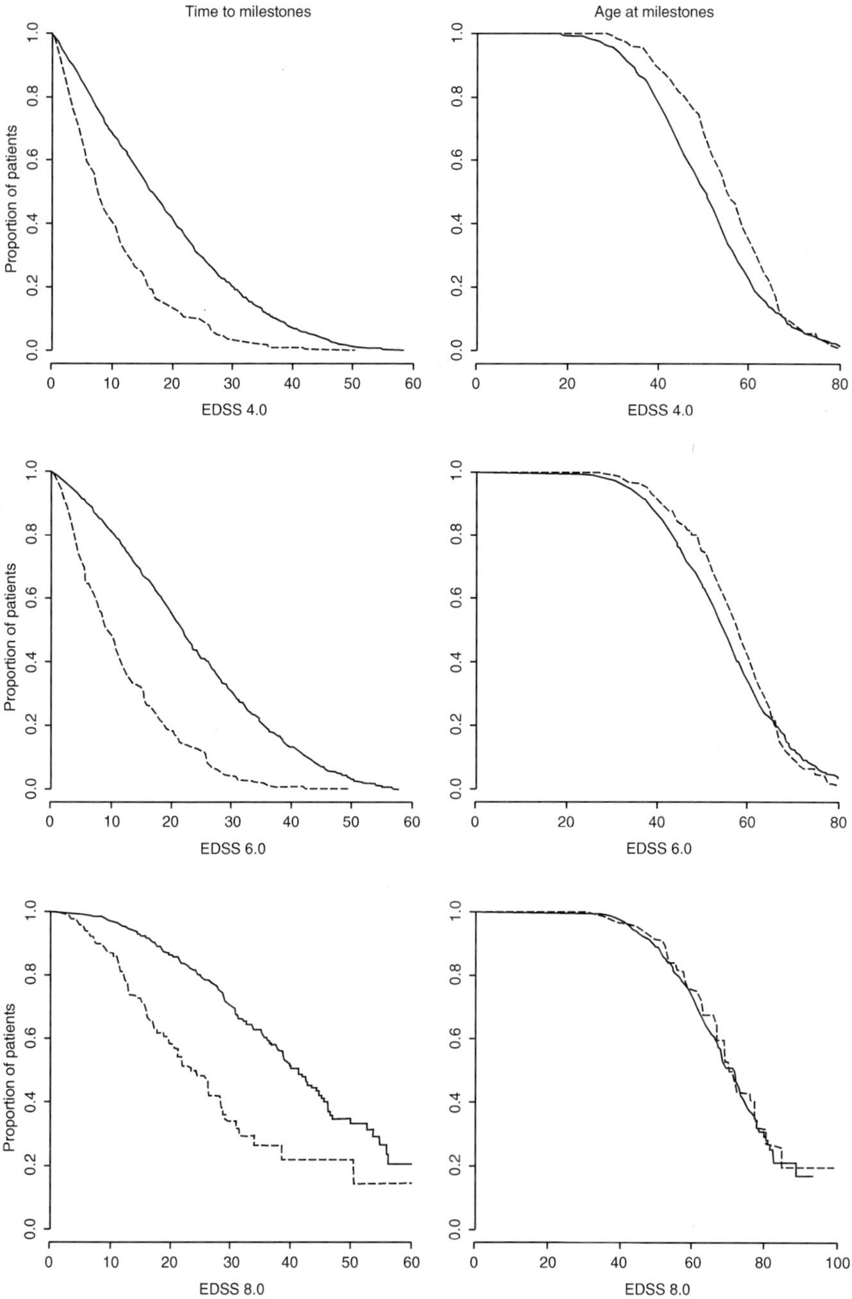

Fig. 2.1 Time to and age at EDSS milestones in the south east Wales MS cohort, by disease course (relapsing onset: unbroken line, primary progressive: *dotted line*)

Time to early disability milestones can be used as a marker of how aggressive the early stages of disease are, and this has been found to be associated with time to later disability milestones in several studies [10, 11, 13]. Time to EDSS 6.0 has been found to predict time to EDSS 7.0 [13] and EDSS 8.0 [11], as has time to EDSS 3.0 [10]. Given that mean EDSS at presentation of PPMS is commonly over 5.0 [4, 17], time to EDSS 6.0 may be a more useful marker in clinical practice. Leray et al. examined the relationship between time to EDSS 3.0, and time from EDSS 3.0 to 6.0 in ROMS and PPMS patients in northwestern France, and found that time from EDSS 3.0 to EDSS 6.0 is similar for all patients, irrespective of how long it took to reach EDSS 3.0 [5]. They concluded that this suggested disability progression is related to some process other than neuroinflammation, and probably related to neurodegeneration.

Finally, several studies have examined whether there is a predictive value of symptoms at onset of disease, and results are conflicting. The study from Ontario, Canada reported that polyfocal symptoms at onset of MS predicted a shorter time to death: patients with three or more neurological symptoms at onset had a median time from onset to death of 13.5 years, while those with one system involved at onset survived for 33.2 years [10]. A smaller study from California found that polyfocal symptoms at years 3, 4, or 5 predicted time to EDSS 6.0 and 6.5 [4]. However, in our study in south east Wales, there was no association of polyfocal symptoms at onset with any EDSS milestone following adjustment for relevant co-variates [17]. There has also not been any consistently reproduced association of specific symptoms at onset of disease. In the British Columbia cohort, sensory symptoms at onset were associated with longer time to and older age at EDSS 6.0 [16], and in an Italian study pyramidal or sphincter symptoms at onset were associated with time to EDSS 4.0 [26]. It is possible that the heavy reliance of EDSS on mobility is an indirect cause of these associations, as those without motor weakness will tend to have a lower EDSS score. In addition, the fact that these observations are reported in single cohorts but do not appear to be universally applicable suggests that they are likely to have less clinical utility in practice.

2.3 Secondary Progressive Multiple Sclerosis

2.3.1 Disease Frequency

Compared to PPMS, fewer studies have specifically investigated secondary progressive MS (SPMS), and fewer still have examined progression of disability and prognosis. This may be in part because the diagnosis of SPMS remains a retrospective clinical assessment, and there remain no reliable imaging or serum markers of conversion to secondary progression [2]. Nonetheless, some conclusions about its epidemiology and natural history may be drawn from the current literature. Table 2.2 summarises previous studies of SPMS.

Table 2.2 Comparison of previous studies of SPMS

Study	Country	n ROMS	n SPMS (%)	Follow up (years)	Time to SPMS (yrs)	Age at SPMS
Bergamaschi et al. (2001) [45]	Italy	186	34 (18)	7	7.7	
Simone et al. (2002) [26]	Italy	596	143 (24)	6.3	6.9	
Eriksson et al. (2003) [46]	Sweden	220 CIS	160 (73)	25	19	
Confavreux et al. (2006) [12]	France	1562	496 (32)	17.6		39.5
Kremenchutzky et al. (2006) [47]	Canada	824	622 (76)	27	7.7–10.3	39.4–40.9
Koch et al. (2008) [48]	Netherlands	571	268 (47)	16	23.3	
Debouverie et al. (2008) [21]	France	2518	933 (37)	14	20	
Koch et al. (2009) [16]	Canada	5207	1821 (35)	20.5	21.4	53.7
Leray et al. (2010) [5]	France	1609	618 (38)	13.1	16	40.4
Harding et al. (2014) [17]	U.K.	1897	879 (46)	15.9		42.4
Tedeholm et al. (2015) [49]	Sweden	212	176 (83)	50	12	
Manouchehrinia et al. (2016) [50]	Sweden	10,835	3671 (34)	17	23	57.4

Conversion from relapsing-remitting MS (RRMS) to SPMS is estimated to occur at 2–3% per year [51], and so in general the longer the period of follow-up in any given study, the greater the proportion of patients who have converted. Weinshenker et al. reported that after 5 years 12.1% of patients had converted, and this proportion increased to 41.3% after 10 years, 57.6% after 15 years, 65.6% up to 25 years, and 88.9% after more than 25 years [22]. Fifty year follow up of a Swedish incidence cohort has recently been published, and similarly found that 83% of patients with ROMS had converted to SPMS [49]. In addition, 52% of the ROMS patients were still alive, of whom 14% remained non-progressive, 22% were progressive but still ambulatory, and 16% were progressive and unable to mobilise [49]. Some commentators have speculated that if all ROMS patients were followed up for long enough they would convert to SPMS [51], but this degree of follow up has never been achieved.

Recent attempts by specialist groups have been made to refine the definition of secondary progression in order to improve the understanding of this disease subtype and to improve study comparison [2], although this remains in an early stage of development. Initial observations suggested that conversion to SPMS should not equate to reaching a specific EDSS score since in a cohort from France 41.8% of patients were deemed to have entered secondary progression before reaching EDSS 3.0, implying that progression may begin at different disability levels [5]. The MSBase registry has examined this in more detail, suggesting that the best definition of SPMS should be an increase in EDSS (defined as an increase of 1.5 points if the EDSS score prior to conversion was 0, of 1.0 points if EDSS prior to conversion was 1.0–5.5, and of 0.5 points if prior EDSS was ≥5.5), confirmed after three months, and with an overall EDSS at confirmation of ≥4.0, and a pyramidal system score of ≥2.0 [52]. However, the clinical utility of this has not yet been formally tested.

2.3.2 Clinical Features

Clinical features at onset of disease are generally similar to those of patients with ROMS who have not yet converted. In particular no difference has been observed for age at onset [12, 33, 47, 51, 53] or symptoms at first presentation [12, 53]. Several studies have observed a higher proportion of males in SPMS patients compared to RRMS patients who have not converted [12, 47, 53]. Finally, in a French cohort, 40% of SPMS patients continued to have relapses even after conversion to secondary progression [12, 51].

2.3.3 Conversion to Secondary Progression

Some imprecision is necessarily incorporated into estimates of time to secondary progression, as there is often no specific event that delineates conversion to progression, and furthermore it is a retrospective assessment of disability over preceding months or years [2]. Nonetheless, most studies have observed a median time from onset of MS to conversion to secondary progression of approximately 20 years [5, 16, 21, 46, 48, 50, 53], although some studies have observed a shorter interval [26, 47], whereas age at conversion to secondary progression has been reported to be between 39 [12, 47, 51] and 53 years old [16]. In the Ontario, Canada cohort, SPMS patients were further divided into those who had a single event before subsequently developing secondary progressive MS (SAP), and those who had multiple relapses before converting to secondary progression (SP). Age at conversion to SPMS was similar for both groups (39.4 years for SP and 40.9 years for SAP) [47], suggesting that number of relapses in the early stages of disease may not necessarily predict long-term outcome.

Several studies have examined factors that predict conversion to secondary progression [16, 21, 46–51, 53, 54], and a relative degree of consensus regarding important prognostic factors has been achieved. Most have observed that males convert more rapidly to SPMS than females [16, 21, 50, 51, 53], and are younger at conversion to SPMS [16, 53]. Age at onset has also been associated with risk of conversion to SPMS, with those who are younger at onset of MS taking longer to convert to SPMS [16, 21, 23, 45, 46, 48, 53], although they are also younger at conversion to SPMS [16, 53]. Furthermore, there is evidence of an interaction of sex and age at onset [49]. Complete recovery from the onset event is associated with a longer time to SPMS [21, 45, 46, 49], while polyfocal symptoms at onset have been associated with a shorter time to SPMS [21, 45, 47, 49].

In order to refine prediction of conversion to SPMS, which still remains imprecise, alternative modelling approaches have been developed [45, 49, 54]. One approach has been to combine features of early disease to produce a severity score, with favourable factors comprising complete remission from the first event, sensory symptoms at onset, and monofocal symptoms at onset. This score was strongly associated with hazard of converting to SPMS, though the effect was attenuated in men compared to women [49]. The findings of this approach are similar to those obtained in a study using a Bayesian model, which is a probabilistic approach aiming to incorporate the considerable degree of uncertainty that is inherent in predicting secondary progression in MS. This found that age, polyfocal symptoms at onset, sphincter or motor symptoms at onset, and degree of recovery from onset event were all important early predictors of conversion to SPMS [45]. Finally, a quite different model that has recently been developed uses the composite of current age, a descriptor of the most recent relapse (presence of sensory symptoms and the degree of recovery), and an interaction between the descriptor of the most recent relapse and the time since that relapse [54]. This is interesting because it takes a continuous approach to calculation of risk, implying that the probability of converting to SPMS is not set at onset of disease but is modified as time goes on and other events intervene.

2.3.4 Progression of Disability

Median time from SPMS conversion to EDSS 6.0 is between 4.0 [51] and 8.2 years [53], and median time from onset of MS to EDSS 6.0 is around 12.5 years [12, 47]. Tremlett et al. observed that in almost half of SPMS patients in British Columbia,

EDSS 6.0 had been reached either before conversion to SPMS, at the time of conversion to SPMS, or before the first clinic visit so that data on their disease course prior to this was not available. This is consistent with observation from other series that SPMS may begin at relatively low EDSS scores [5, 47]. Median time from SPMS conversion to EDSS 8.0 has been reported between 13.6 [47] and 17.1 years [17]. Median age at EDSS 7.0 has been reported as 53.3 years [12], and at EDSS 8.0 65.9 years [17].

2.3.5 *Prognostic Factors*

In general, outcome following conversion to SPMS has not been studied in great detail, and further work to understand progression would be of value. However, association of some clinical factors with outcomes in SPMS has been identified. Age has been observed to be associated with time to disability milestones [49, 53], and furthermore appears to interact with sex, with females progressing more rapidly than men from SPMS to EDSS 8.0, so that both sexes reach EDSS 8.0 at a similar age [53]. Several studies have also identified an association between time to convert to SPMS, and time from SPMS conversion to EDSS milestones [46, 51, 53], and slower progression of disability if EDSS score is low at conversion to SPMS [46, 53]. In the Lyon cohort, patients with superimposed relapses have been observed to take a longer time to reach EDSS 7.0 [51], although a more detailed study in British Columbia noted that the impact of relapses on disability diminished with time [55]. Finally, the severity score identified in the Gothenberg cohort is associated with time to EDSS 6.0, 7.0 and 10.0, as well as conversion to SPMS [49].

2.4 Comparison of Primary and Secondary Multiple Sclerosis

Direct comparison of SPMS and PPMS can be problematic, as ROMS cohorts slowly convert to SPMS over time, so that demographics of this group will change depending on the duration of follow-up of the study. This is in contrast to PPMS, which is more clearly defined from onset of disease. Tremlett et al. have analysed this in the MS cohort of British Columbia, Canada, and shown that sex ratios, age at onset, and onset symptoms vary in SPMS groups by the duration of follow up [56]. This therefore needs to be kept in mind when considering studies that have directly compared the two groups.

2.4.1 *Demographics and Clinical Features of Early Disease*

Most [14, 47, 56] but not all [12] studies have observed a higher proportion of males with PPMS compared to SPMS. Detailed interrogation of the British Columbia cohort reveals an increasing proportion of males with SPMS over time. However it should be noted that even if all ROMS patients eventually converted to SPMS, the proportion of male PPMS patients would still remain higher [56]. Age at onset of MS is consistently lower for SPMS patients than PPMS [14, 47], but is similar to PPMS if age at onset of progression is considered instead [12, 14, 47]. There are some caveats to this: patients with ≥3 relapses in the first 2 years of disease have been found to convert to secondary progression at a younger age than either those with fewer relapses, or those with PPMS [57], and in the British Columbia cohort age at conversion to SPMS was older than age at onset of PPMS [56]. At first presentation, PPMS patients are more likely to have motor symptoms and less likely to have optic neuritis than SPMS [14, 56], but at onset of progression both groups predominantly experience motor symptoms [12, 47].

2.4.2 Progression of Disability

Overall, findings on progression of disability in SPMS and PPMS are mixed. Some studies have reported similar age at disability milestones for both groups [47, 56], while others have found that PPMS patients are older at reaching milestones compared to SPMS [12, 17]. In the Ontario cohort, the number of symptoms involved at onset of disease was found to predict survival time in both SPMS and PPMS [10, 47]. In general it does not appear that PPMS confers a poor prognosis as compared to SPMS; at worst prognosis is similar and may even be better. This is supported by a recent study from France, showing that MS patients take a similar time to go from DSS 3.0 to DSS 6.0, regardless of initial disease course or time taken to reach DSS 3.0 [5]. Taken together, this suggests that once progression is established, it continues at a similar rate in all patients, unrelated to the events that led up to the onset of progression.

2.5 Additional Considerations

Studies of familial MS have observed that there is concordance for disease course within affected families [58–60], with the effect being most strongly observed for siblings with PPMS [60]. Conversely, studies of PPMS have identified that a substantial minority of PPMS patients have a positive family history of MS: 10.6% in Ontario [10], 20.4% in British Columbia [61] and 24.4% in Groningen [62]. These figures are higher than would be expected given population-based recurrence rates, even after age-adjustment (as older age at onset of PPMS inflates risk for relatives by allowing more time for them to develop disease). Those patients with familial PPMS are younger at onset of disease [61, 62], though there is no difference in sex ratios or symptoms at onset [61]. No differences have been observed for risk of or time to secondary progression [62, 63], and more generally in ROMS no difference in long-term outcomes has been identified in patients with familial MS compared to those with sporadic disease [63]. Taken together these results suggest the possibility of a genetic contribution to disease course, although recent large-scale genome wide association studies have not identified genetic markers associated with PPMS [64].

The advent of ocrelizumab has heralded a new era in progressive MS, as it is the first treatment shown to be effective at reducing progression of disease. The ORATORIO study found that fewer patients had confirmed disability progression at 24 weeks, and improvements were also shown in T2 lesion volume load and total brain volume [65]. Given this step forward, it is of value to review the contribution of epidemiological studies to trial planning in progressive MS. This has been examined in PPMS in the cohort from Ontario, Canada, and our own cohort from south Wales, but not in SPMS in any cohort. Sustained accumulation of disability (SAD) is a commonly used endpoint in clinical trials in MS, and has been defined as an increase of 1.5 EDSS points if starting EDSS is 0, 1.0 EDSS points if starting EDSS is 1.0–5.5, and 0.5 EDSS points if starting EDSS is ≥6.0 [66]. However, time spent at different EDSS points differs: it takes a median of 1.3 [67] to 1.6 [17] years to progress from EDSS 4.0 to 5.0, 4.0 [67] to 5.1 [17] years to progress from EDSS 6.0 to 7.0, and 11.5 years to go from EDSS 8.0 to EDSS 9.0 [10]. This variation in time spent at each EDSS level means that chance of SAD will vary depending on the exact score. Although the difference in definition of SAD depending on starting EDSS level attempts to account for this, there remains substantial variation within each group. Data from the epidemiological studies in Canada and Wales have therefore been used to calculate sample size requirements for putative clinical trials. These data suggest that recruitment will ideally be targeted at those with lower starting EDSS scores [17] and that several hundred patients would need to be recruited [17, 67] (necessitating multicentre collaboration). In addition trials of less than one year would be too short in duration to detect any difference in progression, as most untreated patients could be expected to remain stable with respect to EDSS scores for more than one year [67]. As a result early trials were underpowered to detect any effect on disability [68]. However, the ORATORIO trial effectively addressed these issues and included 732 patients from multiple centres in north America and Europe, followed up for 2.3 years. It is to be hoped that this represents the first step in developing new treatments which can address the problem of neurodegeneration and progression in MS, which until recently has been problematic.

References

1. Charcot J. Lectures on the diseases of the nervous system (chapter). In: Disseminated sclerosis: its symptomatology. London: New Sydenham Society; 1877. p. 209–17.
2. Lublin FD, Reingold SC, Cohen JA, et al. Defining the clinical course of multiple sclerosis: the 2013 revisions. Neurology. 2014;83(3):278–86.
3. Compston A, Coles A. Multiple sclerosis. Lancet. 2008;372(9648):1502–17.
4. Andersson PB, Waubant E, Gee L, Goodkin DE. Multiple sclerosis that is progressive from the time of onset: clinical characteristics and progression of disability. Arch Neurol. 1999;56(9):1138–42.
5. Leray E, Yaouanq J, Le Page E, et al. Evidence for a two-stage disability progression in multiple sclerosis. Brain. 2010;133(7):1900–13.
6. Minderhoud JM, van der Hoeven JH, Prange AJ. Course and prognosis of chronic progressive multiple sclerosis. Results of an epidemiological study. Acta Neurol Scand. 1988;78(1):10–5.

7. Phadke JG. Clinical aspects of multiple sclerosis in north-east Scotland with particular reference to its course and prognosis. Brain. 1990;113(6):1597–628.
8. Runmarker B, Andersen O. Prognostic factors in a multiple sclerosis incidence cohort with twenty-five years of follow-up. Brain. 1993;116(1):117–34.
9. McDonnell G, Hawkins S. An epidemiologic study of multiple sclerosis in Northern Ireland. Neurology. 1998;50(2):423–8.
10. Cottrell DA, Kremenchutzky M, Rice GP, et al. The natural history of multiple sclerosis: a geographically based study. 5. The clinical features and natural history of primary progressive multiple sclerosis. Brain. 1999;122(4):625–39.
11. Tremlett H, Paty D, Devonshire V. The natural history of primary progressive MS in British Columbia, Canada. Neurology. 2005;65(12):1919–23.
12. Confavreux C, Vukusic S. Natural history of multiple sclerosis: a unifying concept. Brain. 2006;129(3):606–16.
13. Debouverie M, Louis S, Pittion-Vouyovitch S, Roederer T, Vespignani H. Multiple sclerosis with a progressive course from onset in Lorraine-Eastern France. J Neurol. 2007;254(10):1370–5.
14. Koch M, Mostert J, Heersema D, De Keyser J. Progression in multiple sclerosis: further evidence of an age dependent process. J Neurol Sci. 2007;255(1–2):35–41.
15. Maghzi AH, Etemadifar M, Saadatnia M. Clinical and demographical characteristics of primary progressive multiple sclerosis in Isfahan, Iran. Eur J Neurol. 2007;14(4):403–7.
16. Koch M, Kingwell E, Rieckmann P, Tremlett H. The natural history of primary progressive multiple sclerosis. Neurology. 2009;73(23):1996–2002.
17. Harding KE, Wardle M, Moore P, et al. Modelling the natural history of primary progressive multiple sclerosis. J Neurol Neurosurg Psychiatry. 2014;86(1):13–9.
18. Jena S, Alexander M, Aaron S, et al. Natural history of multiple sclerosis from the Indian perspective: experience from a tertiary care hospital. Neurol India. 2015;63:866–73.
19. Piccolo L, Kumar G, Nakashima I, et al. Multiple sclerosis in Japan appears to be a milder disease compared to the UK. J Neurol. 2015;262(4):831–6.
20. Lublin FD, Reingold SC. Defining the clinical course of multiple sclerosis: results of an international survey. National Multiple Sclerosis Society (USA) advisory committee on clinical trials of new agents in multiple sclerosis. Neurology. 1996;46(4):907–11.
21. Debouverie M, Laforest L, Van Ganse E, Guillemin F. Earlier disability of the patients followed in multiple sclerosis centers compared to outpatients. Mult Scler. 2008;15(2):251–7.
22. Weinshenker BG, Bass B, Rice GP, et al. The natural history of multiple sclerosis: a geographically based study. 1. Clinical course and disability. Brain. 1989;112(1):133–46.
23. Stankoff B, Mrejen S, Tourbah A, et al. Age at onset determines the occurrence of the progressive phase of multiple sclerosis. Neurology. 2007;68(10):779–81.
24. McDonnell G, Hawkins S. Clinical study of primary progressive multiple sclerosis in Northern Ireland. J Neurol Neurosurg Psychiatry. 1998;64(4):451–4.
25. Ribbons KA, McElduff P, Boz C, et al. Male sex is independently associated with faster disability accumulation in relapse-onset MS but not in primary progressive MS. PLoS One. 2015;10(6):e0122,686. published online. http://journals.plos.org/plosone/article?id=10.1371/journal.pone.0122686
26. Simone IL, Carrara D, Tortorella C, et al. Course and prognosis in early-onset MS: comparison with adult-onset forms. Neurology. 2002;59(12):1922–8.
27. Boiko A, Vorobeychik G, Paty D, Devonshire V, Sadovnick D, University of British Columbia MS Clinic Neurologists. Early onset multiple sclerosis: a longitudinal study. Neurology. 2002;59(7):1006–10.
28. Harding KE, Liang K, Cossburn MD, et al. Long-term outcome of paediatric-onset multiple sclerosis: a population-based study. J Neurol Neurosurg Psychiatry. 2013;84(2):141–7.
29. Renoux C, Vukusic S, Mikaeloff Y, et al. Natural history of multiple sclerosis with childhood onset. N Engl J Med. 2007;356(25):2603–13.
30. Delalande S, Seze JD, Ferriby D, Stojkovic T, Vermersch P. Late onset multiple sclerosis. Rev Neurol (Paris). 2002;158(11):1082–7.

31. Tremlett H, Devonshire V. Is late-onset multiple sclerosis associated with a worse outcome? Neurology. 2006;67(6):954–9.
32. Cossburn M, Ingram G, Hirst C, Ben-Shlomo Y, Pickersgill T, Robertson N. Age at onset as a determinant of presenting phenotype and initial relapse recovery in multiple sclerosis. Mult Scler J. 2012;18(1):45–54.
33. Kremenchutzky M, Cottrell D, Rice G, et al. The natural history of multiple sclerosis: a geographically based study 7. Progressive-relapsing and relapsing-progressive multiple sclerosis: a re-evaluation. Brain. 1999;122(10):1941–50.
34. Confavreux C, Vukusic S. Age at disability milestones in multiple sclerosis. Brain. 2006;129(3):595–605.
35. Phadke JG. Survival pattern and cause of death in patients with multiple sclerosis: results from an epidemiological survey in north east Scotland. J Neurol Neurosurg Psychiatry. 1987; 50(5):523–31.
36. Leray E, Morrissey S, Yaouanq J, et al. Long-term survival of patients with multiple sclerosis in west France. Mult Scler J. 2007;13(7):865–74.
37. Grytten Torkildsen N, Lie S, Aarseth J, Nyland H, Myhr K. Survival and cause of death in multiple sclerosis: results from a 50-year follow-up in western Norway. Mult Scler J. 2008; 14(9):1191–8.
38. Smestad C, Sandvik L, Celius E. Excess mortality and cause of death in a cohort of Norwegian multiple sclerosis patients. Mult Scler. 2009;15(11):1263–70.
39. Hader WJ. Disability and survival of multiple sclerosis in Saskatoon, Saskatchewan. Can J Neurol Sci. 2010;37(1):28–35.
40. Kingwell E, van der Kop M, Zhao Y, et al. Relative mortality and survival in multiple sclerosis: findings from British Columbia, Canada. J Neurol Neurosurg Psychiatry. 2012;83(1):61–6.
41. Leray E, Vukusic S, Debouverie M, et al., 2015, Excess mortality in patients with multiple sclerosis starts at 20 years from clinical onset: data from a large-scale French observational study. PLoS One, 10(7): e0132,033. Published online. 10.1371/journal.pone.0132033
42. Jick SS, Li L, Falcone GJ, Vassilev ZP, Wallander MA. Epidemiology of multiple sclerosis: results from a large observational study in the UK. J Neurol. 2015;262(9):2033–41.
43. Sandi D, Zsiros V, Fvesi J, et al. Mortality in Hungarian patients with multiple sclerosis between 1993 and 2013. J Neurol Sci. 2016;367:329–32.
44. Koch MW, Greenfield J, Javizian O, Deighton S, Wall W, Metz LM. The natural history of early versus late disability accumulation in primary progressive MS. J Neurol Neurosurg Psychiatry. 2014;86(6):615–21.
45. Bergamaschi R, Berzuini C, Romani A, Cosi V. Predicting secondary progression in relapsing-remitting multiple sclerosis: a Bayesian analysis. J Neurol Sci. 2001;189(1–2):13–21.
46. Eriksson M, Andersen O, Runmarker B. Long-term follow up of patients with clinically isolated syndromes, relapsing-remitting and secondary progressive multiple sclerosis. Mult Scler J. 2003;9(3):260–74.
47. Kremenchutzky M, Rice GPA, Baskerville J, Wingerchuk DM, Ebers GC. The natural history of multiple sclerosis: a geographically based study 9: observations on the progressive phase of the disease. Brain. 2006;129(3):584–94.
48. Koch M, De Keyser J, Tremlett H. Timing of birth and disease progression in multiple sclerosis. Mult Scler. 2008;14(6):793–8.
49. Tedeholm H, Skoog B, Lisovskaja V, Runmarker B, Nerman O, Andersen O. The outcome spectrum of multiple sclerosis: disability, mortality, and a cluster of predictors from onset. J Neurol. 2015;262(5):1148–63.
50. Manouchehrinia A, Beiki O, Hillert J. Clinical course of multiple sclerosis: a nationwide cohort study. Mult Scler J. 2016:1352458516681197. doi:10.1177/1352458516681197. [Epub ahead of print]
51. Vukusic S, Confavreux C. Prognostic factors for progression of disability in the secondary progressive phase of multiple sclerosis. J Neurol Sci. 2003;206(2):135–7.
52. Lorscheider J, Buzzard K, Jokubaitis V, et al. Defining secondary progressive multiple sclerosis. Brain. 2016;139(9):2395–405.

53. Tremlett H, Zhao Y, Devonshire V. Natural history of secondary-progressive multiple sclerosis. Mult Scler J. 2008;14(3):314–24.
54. Skoog B, Tedeholm H, Runmarker B, Odn A, Andersen O. Continuous prediction of secondary progression in the individual course of multiple sclerosis. Mult Scler Rel Disord. 2014;3(5): 584–92.
55. Tremlett H, Yousefi M, Devonshire V, Rieckmann P, Zhao Y. Impact of multiple sclerosis relapses on progression diminishes with time. Neurology. 2009;73(20):1616–23.
56. Tremlett H, Zhao Y, Devonshire V. Natural history comparisons of primary and secondary progressive multiple sclerosis reveals differences and similarities. J Neurol. 2009;256(3):374–81.
57. Scalfari A, Lederer C, Daumer M, Nicholas R, Ebers G, Muraro P. The relationship of age with the clinical phenotype in multiple sclerosis. Mult Scler J. 2016;22(13):1750–8.
58. Robertson NP, Clayton D, Fraser M, Deans J, Compston DA. Clinical concordance in sibling pairs with multiple sclerosis. Neurology. 1996;47(2):347–52.
59. Oturai AB, Ryder LP, Fredrikson S, et al. Concordance for disease course and age of onset in Scandinavian multiple sclerosis coaffected sib pairs. Mult Scler. 2004;10(1):5–8.
60. Hensiek AE, Seaman SR, Barcellos LF, et al. Familial effects on the clinical course of multiple sclerosis. Neurology. 2007;68(5):376–83.
61. Koch M, Zhao Y, Yee I, et al. Disease onset in familial and sporadic primary progressive multiple sclerosis. Mult Scler J. 2010;16(6):694–700.
62. Koch M, Uyttenboogaart M, Heerings M, Heersema D, Mostert J, De Keyser J. Progression in familial and nonfamilial MS. Mult Scler J. 2008;14(3):300–6.
63. Ebers GC, Koopman WJ, Hader W, et al. The natural history of multiple sclerosis: a geographically based study. 8. Familial multiple sclerosis. Brain. 2000;123(3):641–9.
64. IMSGC. Genetic risk and a primary role for cell-mediated immune mechanisms in multiple sclerosis. Nature. 2011;476(7359):214–9.
65. Montalban X, Hauser SL, Kappos L, et al. Ocrelizumab versus placebo in primary progressive multiple sclerosis. N Engl J Med. 2017;376(3):209–20.
66. CAMMS223 Trial Investigators, Coles AJ, Compston DAS, et al. Alemtuzumab vs. interferon beta-1a in early multiple sclerosis. N Engl J Med. 2008;359(17):1786–801.
67. Cottrell DA, Kremenchutzky M, Rice GP, Hader W, Baskerville J, Ebers GC. The natural history of multiple sclerosis: a geographically based study. 6. Applications to planning and interpretation of clinical therapeutic trials in primary progressive multiple sclerosis. Brain. 1999;122(4):641–7.
68. Zajicek J, Ball S, Wright D, et al. Effect of dronabinol on progression in progressive multiple sclerosis (CUPID): a randomised, placebo-controlled trial. Lancet Neurol. 2013;12:857–65.

Chapter 3
The Neuropathology of Progressive Multiple Sclerosis

Nikos Evangelou, Simon M.L. Paine, and Emma C. Tallantyre

3.1 Introduction

Multiple sclerosis is fundamentally an inflammatory demyelinating illness affecting the brain and spinal cord. The typical clinical feature of relapsing and remitting episodes of neurological disability reflects this pathological hallmark. However, some of the earliest neuropathological descriptions of MS made reference to atrophy of the brain and spinal cord as well as microscopic axonal injury [1, 2] (see Kornek and Lassmann, 1999 for a comprehensive account on the historical reporting of axonal pathology in MS [3]). Likewise, it has long been recognised that most patients with relapsing-remitting MS will ultimately experience progressive accumulation of disability (secondary progression), while in others the accrual of disability is progressive from onset (primary progression). Advances in immunomodulatory therapy have revolutionised the care of patients with relapsing-remitting MS. Meanwhile, until recently, progressive forms of the illness remain stubbornly resistant to emerging therapies in a manner more in keeping with a neurodegenerative disease, although over the last few years a number of agents have shown positive results in SPMS and PPMS trials. In recent years, a new light has been thrown on the neuropathology of MS, with focus often shifting towards neuro-axonal and grey matter pathology as possible correlates of progressive, irreversible disability. In this

N. Evangelou
Division of Neurosciences, School of Medicine, University of Nottingham, Nottingham, UK

S.M.L. Paine
Department of Pathology, Nottingham University Hospital, Nottingham, UK

E.C. Tallantyre (✉)
Department of Clinical Neurology, University Hospital of Wales, Cardiff, UK
e-mail: emmatallantyre@hotmail.com

A. Wilkins (ed.), *Progressive Multiple Sclerosis*,
https://doi.org/10.1007/978-3-319-65921-3_3

chapter, we hope to describe the hallmark white matter inflammatory demyelination of MS, to report on the relatively recent studies of neuro-axonal and grey matter pathology as seen in the progressive forms, and to reflect on the possible pathological correlates of progressive disability.

3.2 Limitations of Neuropathological Studies

Neuropathology studies play a key role in uncovering the pathogenesis of MS. Contemporary *in vivo* imaging techniques have the capacity to provide a quantitative analysis of the entire CNS. However, understanding the histopathology underlying each imaging marker is crucial in order to appropriately interpret the data. Furthermore, even the most sensitive imaging tools cannot rival the detailed resolution afforded by histopathological methods. Unfortunately, neuropathological study is associated with several limitations.

Early studies of the neuropathology of MS relied on histochemical methods, in particular Nissl stains, to demonstrate neuronal and glial cells, silver stains to demonstrate neuronal processes and luxol fast blue or Weils to demonstrate myelin [4]. The more recent introduction of immunohistochemical methods (IHC) offered a more specific approach and allowed information to be gleaned regarding the functional status of a cell e.g. those primed for apoptosis or those with interrupted axonal transport. These capabilities are particularly useful for the study of neurodegeneration. However, as histopathological techniques have advanced, the availability of human tissue for study has remained scarce. It is therefore unreasonable to expect sample sizes anywhere near those of large imaging studies. Similarly, matching of subjects between representative groups is often approximate at best.

The vast majority of neuropathology studies are performed using CNS tissue derived from MS patients at autopsy. Such tissue is often derived from patients with long disease duration and severe disability and so represents the end stage of the disease. Furthermore, clinical information has usually been collected retrospectively, if available at all, without any standardised method of clinical assessment. Brain biopsy, performed during diagnostic neurological investigation, creates an opportunity to study neuropathology in living patients who often have shorter disease durations and less severe disability and on whom concurrent clinical assessments can be performed. On the other hand, invasive brain biopsy is only usually undertaken in cases of atypical or aggressive disease not fitting clearly with MS. While it has been shown that many biopsy patients go on to develop clinically definite MS [5], some have a monophasic illness and even those who develop MS are unlikely to be representative of the MS population as a whole.

Both pathological and imaging studies in MS until recently failed to fully explore the relevance of functional anatomical connectivity of inter connecting structures. The last few years the imaging literature has seen an explosion of connectivity studies that luckily has affected already the histopathology research. This new approach offers the potential to guide further studies of disease mechanisms in MS [6].

Perhaps the greatest limitation histopathology is its ability to uncover a mere snap shot of events as they stood at the time of death or biopsy. Certain findings, for example the degree and nature of inflammation, must therefore be interpreted with caution in the context of an illness which is so long in duration, which may have been modified by therapy, and which evolves so dramatically in its phenotype.

Nevertheless, histopathology unveils features of the disease that even the most contemporary of imaging techniques could not hope to match. It is, therefore, with these caveats in mind that we explore the available data and evaluate how neuropathological study can inform on progressive MS.

3.3 White Matter Lesions

The classical features of white matter lesions in MS are loss of myelin accompanied by varying degrees of immune cell infiltration, oligodendrocyte and axonal loss, remyelination and gliosis. Blood vessels within the lesions may show perivascular fibrosis or blood-brain barrier deficits but may also appear normal. Characterisation of white matter lesions in MS has led to an appreciation that they can be differentiated according to their degree of immune cellular infiltration. It is generally accepted that early in their evolution, lesions are active, reflected by diffuse lymphocyte infiltration, oedema and the presence of macrophages/microglia throughout the lesion. Lesions showing mixed active and inactive components, thought to be older in age, display a hypocellular centre, with macrophages/microglia limited to the lesion border. Inactive lesions are those almost completely lacking in macrophages/microglia [7], often with astrocytic scarring.

White matter lesions in the brains and spinal cords of patients with progressive MS are predominantly inactive in their appearance [8]. These lesions tend to have well demarcated edges separating them from surrounding white matter, a small number of perivascular or parenchymal T-cells and plasma cells and few or no oligodendrocytes [9, 10]. However, a significant number of lesions in individuals with progressive MS do show evidence of ongoing inflammatory activity. Frischer et al. performed an extensive analysis of 2476 white matter plaques using 1220 tissue blocks from 120 MS autopsy cases. They found that the features of white matter MS lesions vary with time. Active plaques predominate in early MS, but are also common in SPMS patients with relapses. However, among SPMS patients without attacks, active plaques are rarely found; inactive plaques predominate. Mixed active/inactive lesions, featuring microglial activation and on going axonal injury, are almost exclusively seen among individuals with progressive MS, irrespective of the presence of recent relapses. The authors conclude that a transition from active white matter demyelination to slow expansion of pre-existing plaques in progressive MS is likely to contribute to disease progression [8].

One group has found patients with progressive MS to have a higher density of plasma cells within white matter lesions (as well as in the meninges and normal appearing white matter) than patients with acute or relapsing disease [11]. Astrocytes tend to be fibrous in appearance in long standing lesions, although occasional large astrocytes are seen. Fibrous gliosis is evident within many lesions in progressive MS [9, 12].

The white matter surrounding lesions in progressive MS tends to contain ramified microglia and foamy macrophages (without myelin degradation products) and a greater number of oligodendrocytes than within the lesion itself. In addition, however, the periplaque white matter also frequently contains clusters of microglia that are positioned along myelinated fibres and are associated with striking C3d deposition. These microglial nodules appear as knots of several microglia/macrophages. They usually adopt a star-shaped configuration and surround individual myelinated or partially demyelinated nerve fibres. The microglial nodules tend not to be seen within the white matter lesions themselves [9].

Moderate to intense IgG deposition can be seen throughout the demyelinated lesions of patients with both early and progressive MS, extending several centimetres into the surrounding white matter. IgG deposition is mostly associated with demyelinated axons, plasma cells and seen within the plasma of blood vessels but is less often associated with microglia, macrophages and astrocytes. However, this pattern of IgG deposition is a non-specific finding common to several neurological diseases where there is disruption of myelin. In a similar way, degenerating myelin in MS and other neurological diseases shows non-specific deposition of C3d and C9neo. The microglial nodules seen in periplaque white matter, on the other hand, appear specific to MS (though not specific to progressive MS) [9, 13].

Dispute exists over whether the immunological features of active demyelination differ between different patients and in particular between different disease courses. One group, who studied plaques showing evidence of active demyelination within an extensive collection of autopsy and biopsy specimens, reported four separate patterns of inflammation. The pattern of inflammation was reported to be constant within all the active lesions of one individual but to vary between individuals. While no straight forward relationship existed between lesion type and clinical course, one of the four lesion types was confined to three patients with PPMS. This lesion pattern was characterised by T-cell and macrophage infiltration, an absence of IgG and complement deposition and an absence of oligodendrocytes within the lesions and periplaque white matter. The authors hypothesised that the lesion type observed may relate to phenotypic differences between MS patients [14]. On the other hand, other groups have not found similar heterogeneity in early MS lesions and therefore speculate that any variation in histological appearance may simply reflect variations in lesion age [15, 16].

Certain white matter areas have been noted to exist in MS brains where axons have myelin sheaths that are thin in comparison to normal white matter but not completely absent. These pale areas are referred to as "shadow plaques". At least some such areas are likely to represent areas of remyelination [16]. A few studies suggest that remyelination can be extensive during early MS but is less common at longer disease durations [9, 10, 13]. That said, one study analysing white matter lesions in 36 patients with progressive MS found 42% of lesions to have some signs of remyelination. The degree of remyelination appeared fairly consistent across several lesions within the brain of one individual suggesting that the capacity for remyelination is determined individually [17].

The low potential for remyelination in patients with progressive MS is likely to be explained by a failure of oligodendrocytes to repopulate a demyelinated lesion. As mentioned above, chronic demyelinated lesions tend to be almost devoid of mature oligodendrocytes. Repopulation of the demyelinated area is dependent on migration and differentiation of oligodendrocytes precursor cells to the region. Although oligodendrocyte precursor cells are present in higher numbers than oligodendrocytes in the white matter demyelinating lesions of progressive MS, their numbers decrease with increasing age of the patient, increasing disease duration and decreasing macrophage populations. Moreover, the oligodendrocyte precursor cells tend to appear quiescent [18, 19]. Interestingly, the number of oligodendrocyte precursor cell within white matter lesions appears to be even lower in the spinal cord than in the brain [18]. Immature oligodendrocytes are frequently seen within white matter demyelinating lesions in early MS [10]. On the other hand, patients with longstanding progressive MS show low numbers of immature oligodendrocytes. The majority of those oligodendrocytes that are present in lesions of progressive MS possess markers indicating maturity but have a small nucleus containing clumped nucleochromatin, little cytoplasm and lack myelin forming processes. These oligodendrocytes are likely to be the few that survived the demyelinating process but no longer function as normal. The remainder of the visible oligodendrocytes have an immature appearance and are likely to be derived from oligodendrocyte precursor cells. However, few are engaged in myelination [19].

Leakage of the blood-brain barrier is another classical component of MS white matter demyelinating lesions, which explains the appearance of contrast enhancement on MR imaging. However, while blood-brain barrier leakage is a recognised feature of early demyelinating lesions, several histological studies have suggested that low-grade blood-brain barrier disruption persists in white matter lesions late into the disease [20–23]. Given that fibrinogen leakage can induce activation of microglia [24], chronic low-grade blood-brain barrier leakage could play a role in perpetuating low-grade inflammatory activity in progressive MS. However, the relationship between blood-brain barrier leakage and inflammation in chronic MS appears more complicated as another study revealed apparent blood-brain barrier leakage in vessels which did not have perivascular cuffs of immune cells as well as blood vessels with perivascular cuffs which did not have evidence of blood-brain barrier breakdown [25].

Axonal loss is well recognised to occur within white matter demyelinating lesions in MS and may differ according to disease course. Markers of acute axonal injury suggest that this is most prevalent during the early stages of relapsing-remitting MS. Acute axonal injury does appear to occur within long standing white matter lesions in progressive MS but with a lower incidence [26–29]. Although overall levels of inflammation are low in white matter lesions of patients with progressive MS, acute axonal injury still appears to correlate with the degree of inflammation even in this patient group [11]. Analysing axonal number is best achieved in the spinal cord where axonal anisotropy allows for easier quantification. Studies of axonal density in spinal cord lesions confirm that patients with progressive MS show striking axonal loss compared with surrounding white matter [30–32].

3.3.1 Diffuse White Matter Pathology

The white matter beyond discrete demyelinating lesions is also abnormal in multiple sclerosis. What is often referred to as the normal appearing white matter in MRI studies, can be demonstrated to possess features of disease when examined under the microscope. Diffuse changes within the normal appearing white matter seem most extensive in progressive subtypes of multiple sclerosis. In particular, patients with progressive MS appear to have diffuse low grade inflammation in the white matter comprising perivascular cuffs of monocytes, T-cell infiltration and microglial activation (Fig. 3.1) [33]. One group has also found higher numbers of plasma cells in the non-lesional white matter in the brains of patients with progressive MS than in those of patients with acute or relapsing disease [11]. Perhaps related is the diffuse low grade disruption to the blood-brain barrier [21, 22]. Furthermore there is evidence of low grade axonal damage which exceeds that seen in patients with relapsing-remitting MS [33]. Further diffuse pathology in the white matter of patients with progressive MS include relatively low density of myelin and excessive fibrillary gliosis [34].

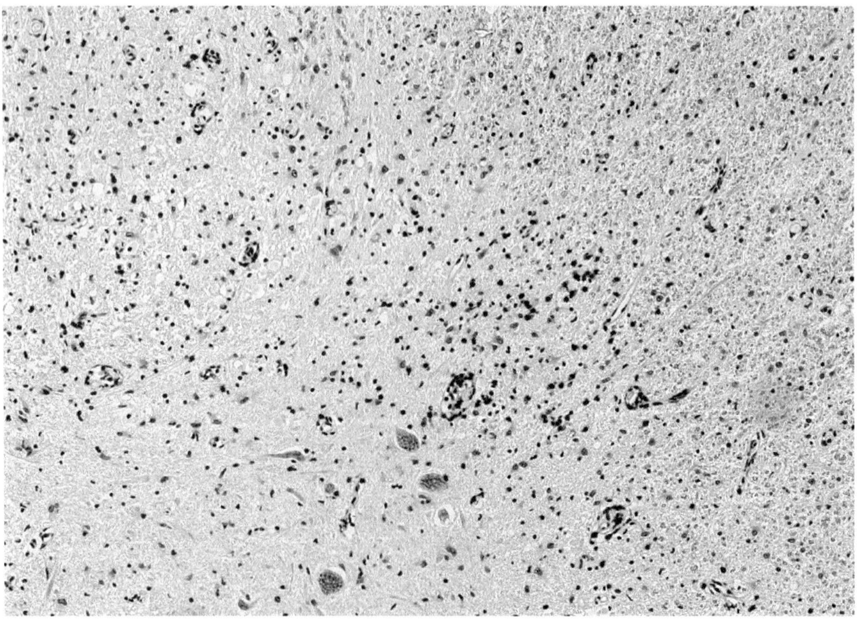

Fig. 3.1 T-cell marker shows the presence of lymphocytic cuffing around venules at the lesion border and in the normal appearing white matter

3.4 Grey Matter Lesions

The presence of grey matter demyelination in MS has been reported since as early as the end of the nineteenth century [35–38]. Brownell and Hughes' autopsy study, conducted on 22 cases of MS, acknowledged the presence of grey matter demyelination although the authors found most lesions involved both white matter and cortex at the leucocortical junction while only 5% of lesions seen in the cerebral hemispheres were truly intra-cortical [39]. Later, Lumsden also reported further on the existence of cortical demyelination with some individual subjects showing extensive regions of demyelinated cortex [40]. These studies are likely to have considerably underestimated the extent of grey matter demyelination, as more recent histopathological studies show that IHC methods targeting myelin basic or proteolipid proteins (MBP and PLP) are far more sensitive than the histochemical methods they employed [41, 42].

Grey matter demyelination affects the cerebral and cerebellar cortices, deep grey matter structures of the brain and also the grey matter of the spinal cord. Several studies have revealed that the extent of cortical demyelination varies greatly between individuals [33, 42, 43]. Patients with relapsing-remitting disease appear to have a limited amount of cortical demyelination, around 2–3% of their cortical area [33, 43]. In contrast, patients with progressive MS demonstrate more extensive demyelination, involving around 12–25% of their cerebral cortical area [33, 42, 43]. Extensive demyelination of the cerebellar cortex has also been found to be a hallmark of patients with progressive versus relapsing-remitting MS [44]. In some patients with progressive MS, there is evidence of very extensive cortical demyelination of a subpial type (referred to as generalised subpial demyelination). In such patients up to 50–60% of the entire cortical area may be demyelinated [42, 43].

Cortical demyelination appears to show regional variation, being most extensive in the cingulate gyrus followed by the temporal cortex, frontal cortex and parietal cortex [42, 43, 45]. This pattern of regional variation may relate to restricted CSF flow as regions deep within the cortical folds are particularly affected [46]. Indeed the hippocampus has been shown to be affected by demyelination in patients with MS [47]. In the deep grey matter, lesions are most frequently detected in the hypothalamus and caudate and in view of their connectivity they may play a role in cognition and behaviour of MS patients [48]. However, compared with cerebral structures, the extent of demyelination has been found to be highest in the cerebellum and grey matter of the spinal cord where typically 40–50% of the grey matter is demyelinated in patients with long standing MS (Fig. 3.2) [44, 45]. All levels of the spinal cord appear equally affected by grey matter demyelination [49].

Overall the extent of grey matter demyelination, expressed as a proportion of area, appears greater than the extent of white matter demyelination although there is a chance this may be affected to some extent by sampling bias. Interestingly, the extent of grey matter demyelination appears unrelated to the degree of white matter demyelination in individuals and those subjects with a heavy burden of cortical demyelination may show little white matter demyelination [33, 42, 49–51].

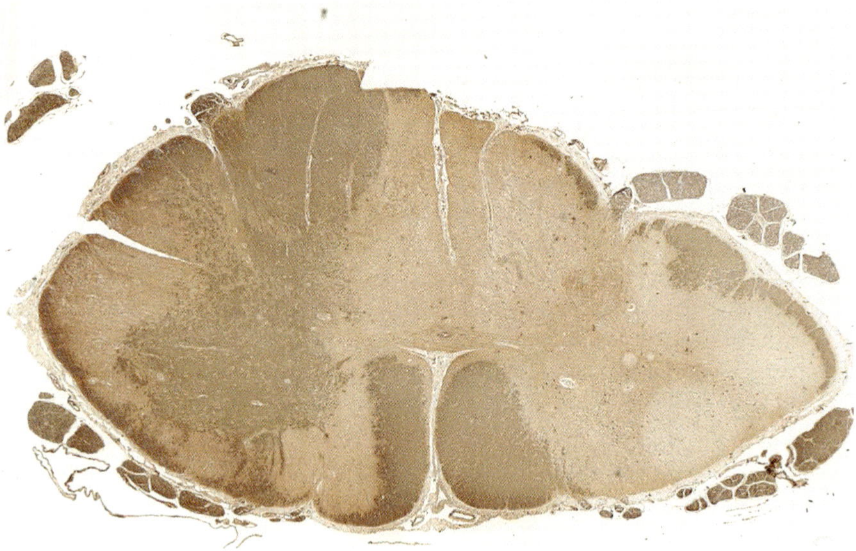

Fig. 3.2 Cervical spinal cord section from a patient with progressive MS showing multiple white and grey matter lesions with varying degree of demyelination

The morphology of lesions within the cerebral cortex seems to be fairly stereotyped. A scheme of classification proposed by Peterson et al. categorises grey matter lesions as falling into three main groups: type 1 lesions involve both grey and white matter, their centre often appearing to fall within sub-cortical white matter; type 2 lesions are located within grey matter but do not extend to the surface of the brain nor to the leucocortical junction; type 3 are subpial lesions that often involve long stretches of cortex of several neighbouring gyri [52].

In those studies using IHC, similarities have emerged in the relative contribution of the different lesion types to the overall burden of cortical demyelination. Less than a third of demyelination affecting the cortex appears to simultaneously involve white matter (type 1 lesions) while the remainder is entirely intra-cortical [12, 42, 43, 45, 50, 52–54]. Of the purely intra-cortical demyelination, type 3 demyelination accounts for the vast majority of lesions (around 50–70% by number or 75% by area) [42, 45, 50, 52–54]. In contrast, in the cerebellum and spinal cord more lesions involve both grey matter and white matter concurrently [45]. Nevertheless, the majority of cerebellar cortical lesions also adopt a subpial morphology with demyelination extending to a variable depth within the granular layer [44].

The finding of different morphological lesion types has led some to hypothesise that different cortical lesions possess different mechanisms of pathogenesis [52]. It has been postulated that factors arising from the CSF or meninges invoke subpial demyelination [33, 52]. In keeping with this hypothesis is the more recent finding that B-cell follicles, possibly representative of tertiary lymphoid tissue, can be identified within the meninges of some MS subjects, particularly adjacent to subpial plaques [55, 56]. These aggregates comprise B-cells, T-cells, plasma cells, macrophages and a network of follicular dendritic cells. Their morphological appearance, the presence of proliferating B-cells and the expression of lymphoid homing chemokines, all strongly support the idea that these structures represent ectopic lymphoid follicles. Similar structures are seen in the thyroid, synovial tissue and salivary glands of patients with Hashimoto's Thyroiditis, Rheumatoid Arthritis and Sjogrens disease respectively. It is proposed that lymphoid neogenesis in chronic autoimmune diseases leads to perpetuation of a compartmentalised immune response [57]. Interestingly, lymphoid follicles appear to occur in the brains of around 40–50% of patients with SPMS but have not been identified in the meninges surrounding the same patients' spinal cords or the cerebellum [55, 58, 59]. Patients with lymphoid follicles seem more likely to have an aggressive disease course (younger ages of onset, irreversible disability and death) and also demonstrate more extensive cortical pathology. In particular, proximity between meningeal lymphoid follicles and subpial cortical lesions has been reported. This translates to a five-fold higher extent of cortical demyelination in patients with versus without lymphoid follicles (most of which was accounted for by subpial lesions). Extensive demyelination observed in the cerebellar cortex in SPMS is speculated to be caused by a toxic cerebrospinal fluid (CSF) milieu, which is partly independent of detectable inflammatory infiltrates in the tight confines of the cerebellar subarachnoid space [59]. The patients with lymphoid follicles also show more cortical microglial activation, and lower numbers of cortical neurons, oligodendrocytes and astrocytes than patients who lack lymphoid follicles. While patients with meningeal lymphoid follicles seem more likely to have B-cells and plasma cells in the perivascular spaces of white matter lesions than patients who lack lymphoid follicles, they do not show any significant difference in their overall extent of white matter demyelination. Lymphoid follicles are almost always located within sulci, often at their deepest point [55, 58]. Similar structures suggestive of ectopic lymphoid follicles have been observed in one case of tuberculous meningitis but not in eight other cases of non-MS inflammatory neurological disease [58].

Interestingly, subpial demyelination may be specific to MS; patients with progressive multifocal leucoencephalopathy show intracortical and leucocortical lesions but no subpial lesions [46]. Another possible explanation for the stereotyped morphology of certain cortical lesions is their relationship to cortical veins. Kidd et al. found the majority of cortical lesions in the post mortem brains of 12 MS patients to arise within the territory of a principle vein [60].

The constituents of grey matter demyelinating lesions differ from those found in white matter. The main difference appears to be the relative hypocellularity of grey matter demyelinating lesions. Numerous authors document a higher degree of inflammatory infiltrates in white matter lesions versus the cortical lesions even when matched for levels of activity [42, 43, 50, 52], although in fulminant, early MS cases that required a biopsy profound perivascular inflammation in cortical lesions was found [61]. In the deep grey matter, inflammation appears to be intermediate between low inflammatory cortical lesions and active white matter lesions [48]. In addition, MHC class-II positive cells in grey matter lesions often exhibit the appearance of active microglia, in contrast to the predominance of lipid-laden macrophages in comparable white matter lesions [50, 52]. A consequence of the low cellularity of grey matter lesions is that they are difficult to detect macroscopically in autopsy specimens and are also not highlighted by routine histological stains such as hematoxylin and eosin [62]. The differences in cellularity of white matter and grey matter demyelinating lesions may arise because of regional differences in pathogenesis, or as a result of the same pathogenesis occurring in different microenvironments.

In line with studies of white matter lesion pathology, grey matter lesions have been shown to exhibit neuro-axonal loss compared with surrounding myelinated grey matter. Investigation of post mortem brains of seven patients (of whom six had progressive MS) revealed transected dendrites and axons within cortical demyelinated lesions [52]. The frequency of transected neurites correlates with the degree of inflammation with actively inflamed lesions demonstrating a 500-fold increase in transected neurites in comparison with myelinated MS cortex. Apoptotic neurons are also seen within demyelinating cortical lesions, predominantly in the large pyramidal cell layers III and V, with an incidence 100-fold higher than in myelinated MS cortex. The microglia in cortical lesions have an activated appearance and often extend processes, which encircle adjacent neurites and neurons though it is not clear whether this association is destructive or protective [52]. Subsequent studies have also found reductions in neuronal density within cerebral and cerebellar cortical lesions as well as spinal cord grey matter lesions compared with local myelinated grey matter [43, 44, 54, 63], although in the most common subpial (Type 3 lesions) that exhibited significant neurodegenerative changes, no significant difference in neuron and axon density was found compared to normally myelinated normal-appearing gray matter [64].

Even more striking is a recent observation of profound loss (more than 50%) of synapses in MS irrespective of the presence of cortical demyelination and axonal loss [65]. The pathophysiology of this important finding remains enigmatic.

As grey matter demyelination remains relatively difficult to detect using in vivo imaging methods, little can be said of the clinical implications of grey matter demyelination. Its higher prevalence in patients with progressive disease raises the possibility that it may relate to progressive disability. Limitations in clinical data that accompany most pathology studies have so far made it difficult to further address this hypothesis. However, one clinico-pathological study did find that patients with extensive cortical demyelination may have a higher incidence of cognitive impairment [42]. In another study, clinical signs suggestive of cerebellar involvement were found in medical records of patients who had extensive grey matter demyelination in the cerebellum regardless of the degree of white matter cerebellar disease [44].

3.5 Neuro-Axonal Pathology

The most convincing candidate as the pathological substrate underlying chronic disability in MS is neuronal and axonal loss. Indeed, if other pathological processes contribute to progressive disability in MS, it is likely that they do so by invoking a final common pathway of neuro-axonal dysfunction or death. Despite the fact that

MS is largely regarded as a demyelinating disease, the presence of neuronal and axonal damage is well established. Early neuropathological reports of neuro-axonal injury were largely descriptive whereas more recently authors have attempted to quantify the degree of axonal loss in MS, identify its location and its association with inflammatory demyelination.

Histological methods such as silver staining or alternatively immunostains targeting neurofilaments both allow comparison of axonal number between the CNS tissue of MS subjects and controls. An alternative method that has been used to quantify axonal injury is the identification of axonal transection or interruption of axonal transport. Axonal stains themselves can facilitate the identification of axonal transection by demonstrating swollen axonal end bulbs—so-called *spheroids* or *ovoids*. Immunohistochemical staining of beta-amyloid precursor protein (βAPP), a protein that is anterogradely transported along axons can also be used as a marker of axonal injury as it rapidly accumulates at sites of interrupted axonal transport. Positive staining for βAPP indicates *recent* damage but APP is thought to disappear some days after axonal injury so is only sensitive in areas where there is ongoing axonal injury. Furthermore, interruption of axonal transport is not synonymous with axonal death; it may be transient and followed by axonal recovery [66]. It is also possible to immunostain for the Neuropeptide Y receptor Y1 (NPY-Y1R), a marker of axons undergoing Wallerian degeneration [67]. Terminal deoxynucleotidyl Transferase Biotin-dUTP Nick End Labelling (TUNEL) is a method used to detect cells undergoing apoptosis. This technique labels fragments of DNA produced during apoptosis with biotin-dUTP; the biotin-dUTP can subsequently be visualised using standard IHC methods. Much like βAPP, TUNEL positive neurons are likely to be cleared from the tissue within a short time of formation (perhaps 24 h [68]) and therefore reflect evidence of recent apoptosis.

Several groups have shown extensive axonal loss within the white matter tracts of patients with MS versus non-neurological controls (Fig. 3.3) [30, 32,

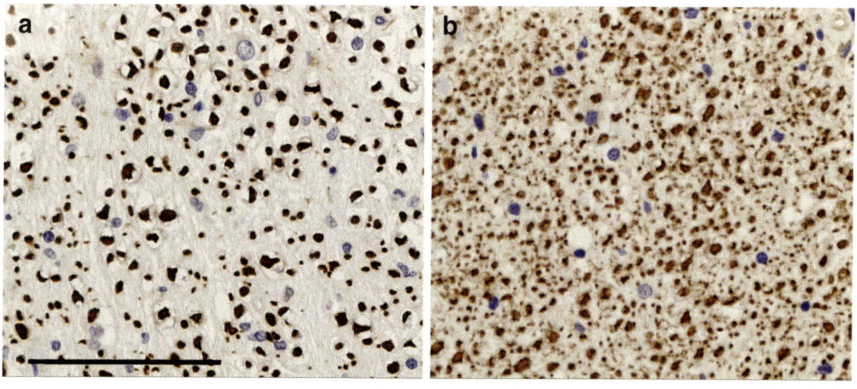

Fig. 3.3 Sections from the corticospinal tract of a patient with MS (**a**) and a non-neurological control (**b**) stained for neurofilament. Axonal loss is apparent in section (**a**), particularly the loss of small diameter axons. Scale bar represents 100 μm

69–72]. Estimates of the degree of axonal loss vary from around 25–65% depending on the region studied and the methods employed. Furthermore, there appears to be pathological evidence of considerable axonal dysfunction even prior to axonal degeneration in progressive MS, which may contribute to disability [73].

Using various methods mentioned above, several studies have demonstrated that neuro-axonal injury appears to be centred on demyelinating lesions compared with the same subject's non-demyelinated parenchyma [11, 26, 28–30, 43, 52, 54, 74–77]. Furthermore, there is substantial evidence that the degree of neuro-axonal damage relates to the amount of inflammation within demyelinating lesions [11, 29, 52, 58, 74, 77, 78]. Acute axonal injury has also been observed to occur, albeit at lower levels than in lesions, within the normal appearing white matter. This phenomenon appears particularly prevalent in progressive versus acute, relapsing MS [11, 33]. There is evidence that Wallerian degeneration is a major contributor to axonal pathology in the peri-lesional white matter in MS [79]. It is suspected that this process is driven by retrograde degeneration of axons once they are transected within white matter demyelinating lesions.

The suggestion of a causal association between inflammatory demyelination and axonal loss is also supported by the finding of a strong correlation between lesion load in cerebral white matter areas and axonal number in their relevant projection areas within the corpus callosum [45].

3.5.1 Possible Mechanisms for Neuro-Axonal Pathology in MS

The available evidence suggests some interplay between inflammatory demyelination in the white and grey matter and neuro-axonal injury raising several possibilities in terms of mechanism. Firstly, the correlation between the degree of inflammation in demyelinated lesions and the degree of axonal injury found by several authors, lends support to the theory that bystander effects of inflammation cause axonal damage. Possible mediators of damage include cytokines such as TNFα or IFNγ or compounds capable of inducing oxidative damage such as the nitric oxide released from activated macrophages [80, 81]. Other proposed mechanisms are neuronal excitotoxicity resulting from the production of glutamic acid at sites of inflammation [82], or alternatively the mechanical compression of axons due to local oedema.

A second possibility to explain the co-localisation of demyelination with axonal damage is that oligodendrocytes death occurring during inflammatory demyelination has repercussions on axonal viability. Oligodendrocytes have been recognised as fulfilling roles of axonal support above and beyond their contribution to CNS myelination [83]. It seems possible that they help to sustain local axons by means such as the production of trophic factors or the mediation of axonal metabolism. Oligodendrocyte precursor cells are known to exist in the adult CNS and represent a possible pool of cells capable of replenishing local oligodendrocyte population in demyelinated areas. However, evidence that OPCs have a limited capacity for repopulating demyelinated CNS lesions, particularly in older subjects [18, 19, 84], suggests that neurons and axons within demyelinated areas may become chronically depleted of trophic support.

Oligodendrocytes are not the only glial cell to be implicated in the mechanism of neuro-axonal damage in MS. Microglia and astrocytes may also play a role in neurodegeneration, either by invoking or sustaining a harmful inflammatory response or by failing to provide a reparative response. Microglial nodules are well recognised to occur in the peri-lesional white matter of individuals with MS, irrespective of the plaque activity [9, 85, 86]. Microglial nodules appear to co-localise with degenerative axons, in a similar way to the pattern observed in ischaemic or traumatic axonal injury. This finding may support the hypothesis that microglial inflammation within and outside of lesions has detrimental effects and contributes to axonal damage [87, 88]. However, not all axons undergoing Wallerian degeneration adjacent to MS lesions are surrounded by microglia, and some microglia within nodules exhibit anti-inflammatory phenotypes, raising the possibility that microglial nodule formation is a protective mechanism, driven by axonal degeneration in CNS white matter [85].

There is also growing evidence that astrocytes may play a role in neurodegeneration in MS, either by promoting lesion development or failing to provide anti-inflammatory support [89–91]. Astrocytes may contribute to axonal damage within lesions by expressing chemoattractant molecules and up-regulating adhesion molecules that recruit leucocytes to the lesion, by producing factors toxic to oligodendrocytes and neurons, by blocking the maturation of oligodendrocyte precursor cells or by forming a gliotic scar, which impedes remyelination [92]. Conversely, like microglia, astrocytes can adopt anti-inflammatory phenotypes and may contribute to neuroaxonal repair either directly, or by supporting and regulating neural progenitor cells and even by acting themselves as pluri- or unipotent progenitors. It is clear that astrocytes can be an early (perhaps even primary) target in the development of the MS lesion, and that the damage to astrocytes can be long lasting. Such damage to astrocytes could interfere with any of the reparative pathways above, thus promoting neuro-axonal pathology in MS [90].

An alternative theory to explain the co-localisation of demyelination and axonal damage is that demyelinated axons are more susceptible to autoimmune attack. The exposure of cryptic epitopes from previously privileged sites is known to be associated with the production of autoimmune attack in some circumstances. This mechanism would be compatible with exposure of antigens on the axolemma previously covered by myelin. The identification of intra-thecal antibodies against axonal proteins in patients with MS [93–96], along with the finding of ectopic lymphoid tissue in close proximity to cortical lesions [55], could support the concept of a humoral contribution to chronic neuroaxonal injury in MS. However, there is no evidence that the antibodies are pathogenic. Furthermore, small axons, which tend to lack a myelin sheath [97], are preferentially lost in MS [71, 72]. This implies that many of the axons that are lost in MS are unmyelinated to begin with and thus injury may not be attributed to loss of their myelin sheath per se.

A further theory that has been proposed to link demyelination to axonal degeneration is that of axonopathy due to energy deficiency [98–100]. Normally, sodium channels are clustered around the node of Ranvier, serving to facilitate saltatory conduction of action potentials. After demyelination, the conduction of action potentials is restored by redistribution of these sodium channels along the length of the denuded axon sheath. The redistribution of sodium channels resulting in a higher density of sodium channels than normal, or even an acquired channelopathy [101], may cause increased energy expenditure per action potential. The combination of high energy demand, axonal mitochondrial dysfunction which has been observed in MS, and increased neuronal excitation arising from compounds such as glutamate in inflammatory lesions, could result in energy failure of neurons [73, 98, 99, 102, 103]. The consequence would be failure to maintain Na^+/K^+ homeostasis ultimately resulting in Na^+/Ca^{2+} exchange and neuronal death [101]. This could explain the apparent length-dependent nature of the axonopathy in MS [73].

Some authors propose that exhaustion of neuroprotective processes [104, 105], or the compartmentalisation of inflammation [11, 106], may contribute to a shift from an inflammatory phenotype to a degenerative phenotype later in the course of MS. The clonal expansion of B-cells and formation of ectopic lymphoid tissue in the meninges, is one theory of compartmentalisation that has gained particular attention as a potential mechanism responsible for progressive MS.

While there is considerable evidence linking inflammation and demyelination to axonal injury, it cannot be proven beyond doubt that the relationship is causative. Some authors have proposed that progressive disability in MS may be attributed to a primary neurodegenerative process and that the inflammation that is the hallmark feature could be a secondary effect [62, 107, 108]. Those who adhere to the hypothesis of a primary neurodegenerative process occurring in MS suggest that an axonopathy independent of MS plaque location or burden would better explain the highly stereotyped clinical phenotype of progressive MS irrespective of varied relapsing disability earlier in the disease [109]. Similarly, this concept could explain why disability progressively worsens in many patients in the absence of ongoing episodes of inflammatory demyelination [62].

3.6 Comparison of Neuropathology Between Primary Progressive (PP) and Secondary Progressive (SP) MS

While there have been many post mortem neuropathological studies of neuro-axonal damage in MS, few studies have been dedicated towards discerning differences between PP and SP subjects. Uncertainty remains as to whether patients with PP and SP subtypes share a common pathogenesis for the progressive accumulation of disability. Patients with PPMS appear to possess certain distinctive demographic, radiological and pathological features when compared with other types of MS. On the other hand, the similar rate of accumulation of disability observed in patients with PP and SPMS after the onset of progression raises the possibility that these two disease subtypes share a common mechanism of neurodegeneration [109–113].

Patients with SPMS appear to have a higher overall burden of white matter demyelination [114]. The morphological and topographical distribution of lesions also differs between PPMS and SPMS cases. Lesions in patients with SPMS are most likely to be located in the hemispheres and brainstem whereas the lesions in PPMS cases were most often in the hemisphere or the spinal cord [12, 114]. Brain lesions in patients with SPMS are larger than those in patients with PPMS [114].

Post mortem studies comparing the pathological appearance of white matter demyelinated lesions within the brains and spinal cords of subjects with PP or SP MS show predominantly chronic inactive lesions in both groups [12, 30, 33, 114]. However, patients with SPMS do show significantly more lesions demonstrating evidence of ongoing active inflammation in the brain than patients with PPMS [114]. When classified as active, chronic active and chronic inactive, the proportions of white matter lesion types are similar in the two groups in the brainstem and the spinal cord. However, patients with SPMS have been found by one group to show a higher incidence of perivascular cuffs of inflammatory cell compared with PPMS cases in all three locations [12]. On the other hand, another, more extensive review of inflammation in white matter brain lesions in post mortem material from patients with MS found no significant difference between the density of inflammatory infiltrates of patients with SP and PP MS [11].

Interestingly, a subset of patients with progressive MS appear to have pathologically inactive disease, defined as an absence of any active or slowly expanding (chronically active) brain lesions. In line with low levels of active inflammation, this subgroup of patients has a correspondingly low level of acute axonal injury within their brain. These same patients appear to experience a less aggressive disease course as they have longer disease durations and older age at death [11]. Nevertheless they had accumulated high levels of disability before death (median EDSS 8.5, corresponding to an individual being essentially restricted to bed). However, there was a high incidence of Alzheimer or vascular cerebral pathology in this group, leading the authors to propose that in the absence of much active inflammation, ongoing neurodegeneration may be driven in this group by non-MS pathology [11].

Differences in the extent of remyelination of white matter lesions in patients with PP versus SP MS have been reported by one group [114]. In their study of post mortem material from 51 patients, extensive (more than 60%) remyelination was evident in 58% of brain lesions in patients with PPMS. On the other hand, patients with SPMS showed extensive remyelination in just 38% of brain lesions. Meanwhile, the degree of remyelination was reported to be similar in the two disease courses in the spinal cord. Interestingly, there were frequent observations of slowly expanding fronts of demyelination within white matter areas with evidence of previous remyelination. These "second hit" areas were particularly common in patients with SPMS versus PPMS and this was taken to imply that the incomplete remyelination that was common in SPMS, could be accounted for by persistent slow burning demyelination [114].

In contrast to these results, another group investigating the degree of remyelination of white matter lesions found similar levels within patients with PP and SP MS. Areas of interest identified by post mortem MRI were classified histologically in the brains of 36 patients as showing normal myelin, demyelination or remyelination. Remyelinated lesions were defined as focal abnormalities with decreased intensity of myelin staining, uniformly thin myelin sheaths (in relationship to axon diameter), and occurring either at the borders of a lesion or throughout an entire lesion. Overall, signs of remyelination were found in 42% of white matter lesions. Remyelination was similarly common in patients with PP and SP MS [17].

On the other hand, during a study performed by Lucchinetti et al. investigating active MS lesions derived from brain biopsy material, results suggested that OG recruitment and remyelination predominate in lesions of RRMS/SPMS patients whereas three out of eight patients with PPMS demonstrated signs of a primary oligodendrocyte dystrophy [14]. As mentioned earlier, however, evidence of homogeneity of the pathological appearances of longstanding MS lesions across different disease courses calls into question a difference in pathogenesis between these clinical groups [15].

The extent of cortical demyelination appears to be similarly high in patients with PP and SP MS, in contrast to patients with relapsing-remitting or acute MS [33, 42]. Subpial demyelination of the cerebral cortex appears to predominate in both patient groups (authors own unpublished observations). However, evidence of ectopic lymphoid follicles in the meninges has only been shown in patients with SPMS to date. Magliozzi et al. found evidence of ectopic lymphoid follicles in 12 out of 29 patients with SPMS but in none out of seven patients with PPMS [55]. In their cohort, the seven patients with PPMS showed a higher proportion of type 1 cortical lesions (leucocortical lesions) than type 3 cortical lesions (subpial lesions) whereas type 3 lesions predominated in the SPMS group.

Patients with both forms of progressive MS show similarly high numbers of normal appearing white matter axonal spheroids [11, 33], and a similar extent of acute axonal injury within white matter lesions [11, 74]. The overall degree of axonal loss within the corticospinal tract of the spinal cord also appears to be similar in patients with longstanding PP or SP MS [30]. However, our group found axonal loss within spinal cord white matter lesions to be more extensive in patients with PPMS versus SPMS. This could be a possible explanation for the similar magnitude of overall corticospinal axonal loss in PP and SP MS despite a lower burden of white matter demyelination in PPMS [30].

3.7 Summary

The neuropathological findings in progressive MS support the hypothesis that neuroaxonal loss is the major substrate of progressive disability. Neuroaxonal injury appears to be initiated within focal regions of inflammatory demyelination. However, it is possible that at a certain stage, other factors ensue which result in neurodegeneration persisting in the absence of ongoing demyelination. Such factors might include compartmentalised low grade inflammation, loss of trophic support provided by myelin, oligodendrocytes and astrocytes and an energy deficient state induced by sodium channel redistribution and mitochondrial depletion. Axonal degeneration may be paralleled by a declining capacity for repair; failure to remyelinate and ongoing gliosis. Ultimately, a shift in the balance between injury and repair is likely to result in the numbers of functioning axons falling below a required threshold, causing permanent disability.

References

1. Carswell R. Pathological anatomy: illustrations of the elementary forms of disease. London: Longman; 1838.
2. Charcot JM. Histologie de la sclérose en plaques. Gaz Hôpitaux. 1868;41:554–5.
3. Kornek B, Lassmann H. Axonal pathology in multiple sclerosis. A historical note. Brain Pathol. 1999;9:651–6.
4. Cox G. Theory and practice of histological techniques. New York: Churchill-Livingstone; 1977. p. 249–73.
5. Pittock SJ, et al. Clinical course, pathological correlations, and outcome of biopsy proved inflammatory demyelinating disease. J Neurol Neurosurg Psychiatry. 2005;76:1693–7.
6. Kolasinski J, et al. A combined post-mortem magnetic resonance imaging and quantitative histological study of multiple sclerosis pathology. Brain. 2012;135:2938–51.
7. Kuhlmann T, et al. An updated histological classification system for multiple sclerosis lesions. Acta Neuropathol. 2016;133:13–24.
8. Frischer JM, et al. Clinical and pathological insights into the dynamic nature of the white matter multiple sclerosis plaque. Ann Neurol. 2015;78:710–21.
9. Prineas JW, et al. Immunopathology of secondary-progressive multiple sclerosis. Ann Neurol. 2001;50:646–57.
10. Ozawa K, et al. Patterns of oligodendroglia pathology in multiple-sclerosis. Brain. 1994;117:1311–22.
11. Frischer JM, et al. The relation between inflammation and neurodegeneration in multiple sclerosis brains. Brain. 2009;132:1175–89.
12. Revesz T, Kidd D, Thompson AJ, Barnard RO, Mcdonald WI. A comparison of the pathology of primary and secondary progressive multiple-sclerosis. Brain. 1994;117:759–65.
13. Barnett MH, Parratt JDE, Cho E-S, Prineas JW. Immunoglobulins and complement in postmortem multiple sclerosis tissue. Ann Neurol. 2009;65:32–46.
14. Lucchinetti C, et al. Heterogeneity of multiple sclerosis lesions: implications for the pathogenesis of demyelination. Ann Neurol. 2000;47:707–17.
15. Breij ECW, et al. Homogeneity of active demyelinating lesions in established multiple sclerosis. Ann Neurol. 2008;63:16–25.
16. Prineas JW, Connell F. Remyelination in multiple-sclerosis. Ann Neurol. 1979;5:22–31.
17. Barkhof F, et al. Remyelinated lesions in multiple sclerosis—magnetic resonance image appearance. Arch Neurol. 2003;60:1073–81.
18. Wolswijk G. Oligodendrocyte precursor cells in the demyelinated multiple sclerosis spinal cord. Brain. 2002;125:338–49.
19. Wolswijk G. Oligodendrocyte survival, loss and birth in lesions of chronic-stage multiple sclerosis. Brain. 2000;123:105–15.
20. Kwon EE, Prineas JW. Blood-brain-barrier abnormalities in longstanding multiple-sclerosis lesions-an immunohistochemical study. J Neuropathol Exp Neurol. 1994;53:625–36.

21. Leech S, Kirk J, Plumb J, McQuaid S. Persistent endothelial abnormalities and blood-brain barrier leak in primary and secondary progressive multiple sclerosis. Neuropathol Appl Neurobiol. 2007;33:86–98.
22. Plumb J, McQuaid S, Mirakhur M, Kirk J. Abnormal endothelial tight junctions in active lesions and normal-appearing white matter in multiple sclerosis. Brain Pathol. 2002;12: 154–69.
23. Claudio L, Raine CS, Brosnan CF. Evidence of persistent blood-brain-barrier abnormalities in chronic-progressive multiple-sclerosis. Acta Neuropathol. 1995;90:228–38.
24. Adams RA, et al. The fibrin-derived gamma(377–395) peptide inhibits microglia activation and suppresses relapsing paralysis in central nervous system autoimmune disease. J Exp Med. 2007;204:571–82.
25. Hochmeister S, et al. Dysferlin is a new marker for leaky brain blood vessels in multiple sclerosis. J Neuropathol Exp Neurol. 2006;65:855–65.
26. Ferguson B, Matyszak MK, Esiri MM, Perry VH. Axonal damage in acute multiple sclerosis lesions. Brain. 1997;120:393–9.
27. Kuhlmann T, Lingfeld G, Bitsch A, Schuchardt J, Bruck W. Acute axonal damage in multiple sclerosis is most extensive in early disease stages and decreases over time. Brain. 2002;125:2202–12.
28. Kornek B, et al. Multiple sclerosis and chronic autoimmune encephalomyelitis—a comparative quantitative study of axonal injury in active, inactive, and remyelinated lesions. Am J Pathol. 2000;157:267–76.
29. Trapp BD, et al. Axonal transection in the lesions of multiple sclerosis. N Engl J Med. 1998; 338:278–85.
30. Tallantyre EC, et al. Greater loss of axons in primary progressive multiple sclerosis plaques compared to secondary progressive disease. Brain. 2009;132:1190–9.
31. Bjartmar C, Kidd G, Mork S, Rudick R, Trapp BD. Neurological disability correlates with spinal cord axonal loss and reduced N-acetyl aspartate in chronic multiple sclerosis patients. Ann Neurol. 2000;48:893–901.
32. Lovas G, Szilagyi N, Majtenyi K, Palkovits M, Komoly S. Axonal changes in chronic demyelinated cervical spinal cord plaques. Brain. 2000;123:308–17.
33. Kutzelnigg A, et al. Cortical demyelination and diffuse white matter injury in multiple sclerosis. Brain. 2005;128:2705–12.
34. Seewann A, et al. Diffusely abnormal white matter in chronic multiple sclerosis imaging and histopathologic analysis. Arch Neurol. 2009;66:601–9.
35. Dawson JW. The histology of disseminated sclerosis. Trans R Soc Edinburgh. 1916;50:517–740.
36. Dinkler M. Zur Kasuistik der multiplen Herdsklerose des Gehirns und Ruckenmarks. Dtsch Z Nervenheilkd. 1904;26:233–47.
37. Sander M. Hirnrindenbefunde bei multiper Sklerose. Monatsschr Psychiatr Neurol. 1898;IV:427–36.
38. Schob F. Ein Betrag zur patologischen Anatomie der multiplen Sklerose. Monatsschr Psychiatr Neurol. 1907;22:62–87.
39. Brownell B, Hughes JT. The distribution of plaques in the cerebrum in multiple sclerosis. J Neurol Neurosurg Psychiatry. 1962;25:315–20.
40. Lumsden CE. In: Vinken PJ, Bruyn GW, editors. Handbook of clinical neurology. Amsterdam: North-Holland; 1970. p. 217–309.
41. Itoyama Y, et al. Immuno-cytochemical observations on the distribution of myelin-associated glycoprotein and myelin basic-protein in multiple-sclerosis lesions. Ann Neurol. 1980;7: 167–77.
42. Bo L, Vedeler CA, Nyland HI, Trapp BD, Mork SJ. Subpial demyelination in the cerebral cortex of multiple sclerosis patients. J Neuropathol Exp Neurol. 2003;62:723–32.
43. Vercellino M, et al. Grey matter pathology in multiple sclerosis. J Neuropathol Exp Neurol. 2005;64:1101–7.
44. Kutzelnigg A, et al. Widespread demyelination in the cerebellar cortex in multiple sclerosis. Brain Pathol. 2007;17:38–44.

45. Gilmore CP, et al. Regional variations in the extent and pattern of grey matter demyelination in multiple sclerosis: a comparison between the cerebral cortex, cerebellar cortex, deep grey matter nuclei and the spinal cord. J Neurol Neurosurg Psychiatry. 2009;80:182–7.
46. Moll NM, et al. Cortical demyelination in PML and MS—similarities and differences. Neurology. 2008;70:336–43.
47. Papadopoulos D, et al. Substantial archaeocortical atrophy and neuronal loss in multiple sclerosis. Brain Pathol. 2009;19:238–53.
48. Haider L, et al. Multiple sclerosis deep grey matter: the relation between demyelination, neurodegeneration, inflammation and iron. J Neurol Neurosurg Psychiatry. 2014;85:1386–95.
49. Gilmore CP, et al. Spinal cord gray matter demyelination in multiple sclerosis—a novel pattern of residual plaque morphology. Brain Pathol. 2006;16:202–8.
50. Bo L, Vedeler CA, Nyland H, Trapp BD, Mork SJ. Intracortical multiple sclerosis lesions are not associated with increased lymphocyte infiltration. Mult Scler. 2003;9:323–31.
51. Bo L, Geurts JJG, van der Valk P, Polman C, Barkhof F. Lack of correlation between cortical demyelination and white matter pathologic changes in multiple sclerosis. Arch Neurol. 2007; 64:76–80.
52. Peterson JW, Bo L, Mork S, Chang A, Trapp BD. Transected neurites, apoptotic neurons, and reduced inflammation in cortical multiple sclerosis lesions. Ann Neurol. 2001;50:389–400.
53. Geurts JJG, et al. Cortical lesions in multiple sclerosis: combined postmortem MR imaging and histopathology. Am J Neuroradiol. 2005;26:572–7.
54. Wegner C, Esiri MM, Chance SA, Palace J, Matthews PM. Neocortical neuronal, synaptic, and glial loss in multiple sclerosis. Neurology. 2006;67:960–7.
55. Magliozzi R, et al. Meningeal B-cell follicles in secondary progressive multiple sclerosis associate with early onset of disease and severe cortical pathology. Brain. 2007;130:1089–104.
56. Serafini B, Rosicarelli B, Magliozzi R, Stigliano E, Aloisi F. Detection of ectopic B-cell follicles with germinal centers in the meninges of patients with secondary progressive multiple sclerosis. Brain Pathol. 2004;14:164–74.
57. Aloisi F, Pujol-Borrell R. Lymphoid neogenesis in chronic inflammatory diseases. Nat Rev Immunol. 2006;6:205–17.
58. Magliozzi R, et al. A Gradient of neuronal loss and meningeal inflammation in multiple sclerosis. Ann Neurol. 2010;68:477–93.
59. Howell OW, et al. Extensive grey matter pathology in the cerebellum in multiple sclerosis is linked to inflammation in the subarachnoid space. Neuropathol Appl Neurobiol. 2015;41:798–813.
60. Kidd D, et al. Cortical lesions in multiple sclerosis. Brain. 1999;122:17–26.
61. Lucchinetti CF, et al. Inflammatory cortical demyelination in early multiple sclerosis. N Engl J Med. 2011;365:2188–97.
62. Trapp BD, Nave K-A. Multiple sclerosis: an immune or neurodegenerative disorder? Annu Rev Neurosci. 2008;31:247–69.
63. Gilmore CP, et al. Spinal cord neuronal pathology in multiple sclerosis. Brain Pathol. 2009;19: 642–9.
64. Klaver R, et al. Neuronal and axonal loss in normal-appearing gray matter and subpial lesions in multiple sclerosis. J Neuropathol Exp Neurol. 2015;74:453–8.
65. Juergens T, et al. Reconstruction of single cortical projection neurons reveals primary spine loss in multiple sclerosis. Brain. 2016;139:39–46.
66. Bruck W. The pathology of multiple sclerosis is the result of focal inflammatory demyelination with axonal damage. J Neurol. 2005;252:V3–9.
67. Pesini P, et al. An immunohistochemical marker for Wallerian degeneration of fibers in the central and peripheral nervous system. Brain Res. 1999;828:41–59.
68. Al-Abdulla NA, Portera-Cailliau C, Martin LJ. Occipital cortex ablation in adult rat causes retrograde neuronal death in the lateral geniculate nucleus that resembles apoptosis. Neuroscience. 1998;86:191–209.
69. Bergers E, et al. Axonal damage in the spinal cord of MS patients occurs largely independent of T2 MRI lesions. Neurology. 2002;59:1766–71.

70. Evangelou N, Esiri MM, Smith S, Palace J, Matthews PM. Quantitative pathological evidence for axonal loss in normal appearing white matter in multiple sclerosis. Ann Neurol. 2000;47:391–5.
71. Ganter P, Prince C, Esiri MM. Spinal cord axonal loss in multiple sclerosis: a post-mortem study. Neuropathol Appl Neurobiol. 1999;25:459–67.
72. DeLuca GC, Ebers GC, Esiri MM. Axonal loss in multiple sclerosis: a pathological survey of the corticospinal and sensory tracts. Brain. 2004;127:1009–18.
73. Dutta R, et al. Mitochondrial dysfunction as a cause of axonal degeneration in multiple sclerosis patients. Ann Neurol. 2006;59:478–89.
74. Bitsch A, Schuchardt J, Bunkowski S, Kuhlmann T, Bruck W. Acute axonal injury in multiple sclerosis—correlation with demyelination and inflammation. Brain. 2000;123:1174–83.
75. Mews I, Bergmann M, Bunkowski S, Gullotta F, Bruck W. Oligodendrocyte and axon pathology in clinically silent multiple sclerosis lesions. Mult Scler. 1998;4:55–62.
76. Barnes D, Munro PMG, Youl BD, Prineas JW, Mcdonald WI. The longstanding MS lesion—a quantitative MRI and electron-microscopic study. Brain. 1991;114:1271–80.
77. Singh S, et al. Relationship of acute axonal damage, Wallerian degeneration, and clinical disability in multiple sclerosis. J Neuroinflammation. 2017;14(1):57.
78. Androdias G, et al. Meningeal T cells associate with diffuse axonal loss in multiple sclerosis spinal cords. Ann Neurol. 2010;68:465–76.
79. Dziedzic T, et al. Wallerian degeneration: a major component of early axonal pathology in multiple sclerosis. Brain Pathol. 2010;20:976–85.
80. Redford EJ, Kapoor R, Smith KJ. Nitric oxide donors reversibly block axonal conduction: demyelinated axons are especially susceptible. Brain. 1997;120:2149–57.
81. Sun D, Newman TA, Perry VH, Weller RO. Cytokine-induced enhancement of autoimmune inflammation in the brain and spinal cord: implications for multiple sclerosis. Neuropathol Appl Neurobiol. 2004;30:374–84.
82. Werner P, Pitt D, Raine CS. Multiple sclerosis: Altered glutamate homeostasis in lesions correlates with oligodendrocyte and axonal damage. Ann Neurol. 2001;50:169–80.
83. Lappe-Siefke C, et al. Disruption of Cnp1 uncouples oligodendroglial functions in axonal support and myelination. Nat Genet. 2003;33:366–74.
84. Chari DM, Crang AJ, Blakemore WF. Decline in rate of colonization of oligodendrocyte progenitor cell (OPC)-depleted tissue by adult OPCs with age. J Neuropathol Exp Neurol. 2003;62:908–16.
85. Singh S, et al. Microglial nodules in early multiple sclerosis white matter are associated with degenerating axons. Acta Neuropathol. 2013;125:595–608.
86. De Groot CJA, et al. Post-mortem MRI-guided sampling of multiple sclerosis brain lesions—increased yield of active demyelinating and (p)reactive lesions. Brain. 2001;124:1635–45.
87. Correale J. The role of microglial activation in disease progression. Mult Scler J. 2014;20:1288–95.
88. Fischer MT, et al. NADPH oxidase expression in active multiple sclerosis lesions in relation to oxidative tissue damage and mitochondrial injury. Brain. 2012;135:886–99.
89. Ponath G, et al. Myelin phagocytosis by astrocytes after myelin damage promotes lesion pathology. Brain. 2017;140:399–413.
90. Brosnan CF, Raine CS. The astrocyte in multiple sclerosis revisited. Glia. 2013;61:453–65.
91. Correale J, Farez MF. The role of astrocytes in multiple sclerosis progression. Front Neurol. 2015;6:180.
92. Rossi S, et al. Tumor necrosis factor is elevated in progressive multiple sclerosis and causes excitotoxic neurodegeneration. Mult Scler J. 2014;20:304–12.
93. Bartos A, et al. Elevated intrathecal antibodies against the medium neurofilament subunit in multiple sclerosis. J Neurol. 2007;254:20–5.
94. Rawes JA, Calabrese VP, Khan OA, DeVries GH. Antibodies to the axolemma-enriched fraction in the cerebrospinal fluid and serum of patients with multiple sclerosis and other neurological diseases. Mult Scler. 1997;3:363–9.

95. Lycke JN, Karlsson JE, Andersen O, Rosengren LE. Neurofilament protein in cerebrospinal fluid: a potential marker of activity in multiple sclerosis. J Neurol Neurosurg Psychiatry. 1998;64:402–4.
96. Silber E, Semra YK, Gregson NA, Sharief MK. Patients with progressive multiple sclerosis have elevated antibodies to neurofilament subunit. Neurology. 2002;58:1372–81.
97. Hirano A, Llena JF. Morphology of central nervous system axons. In: Waxman SG, Kocsis JD, Stys PK, editors. The axon: structure, function and pathophysiology. New York: Oxford University Press; 1995. p. 49–67.
98. Campbell GR, Worrall JT, Mahad DJ. The central role of mitochondria in axonal degeneration in multiple sclerosis. Mult Scler J. 2014;20:1806–13.
99. Campbell GR, et al. Mitochondrial DNA deletions and neurodegeneration in multiple sclerosis. Ann Neurol. 2011;69:481–92.
100. Friese MA, Schattling B, Fugger L. Mechanisms of neurodegeneration and axonal dysfunction in multiple sclerosis. Nat Rev Neurol. 2014;10:225–38.
101. Waxman SG. Acquired channelopathies in nerve injury and MS. Neurology. 2001;56:1621–7.
102. Smith KJ. Newly lesioned tissue in multiple sclerosis-a role for oxidative damage? Brain. 2011;134:1877–81.
103. Mahad DJ, et al. Mitochondrial changes within axons in multiple sclerosis. Brain. 2009;132: 1161–74.
104. Meuth SG, et al. CNS inflammation and neuronal degeneration is aggravated by impaired CD200-CD200R-mediated macrophage silencing. J Neuroimmunol. 2008;194:62–9.
105. Gnanapavan S, et al. Progression in multiple sclerosis is associated with low endogenous NCAM. J Neurochem. 2013;125:766–73.
106. Lovato L, et al. Related B cell clones populate the meninges and parenchyma of patients with multiple sclerosis. Brain. 2011;134:534–41.
107. Louapre C, Lubetzki C. Neurodegeneration in multiple sclerosis is a process separate from inflammation: yes. Mult Scler J. 2015;21:1626–8.
108. Kassmann CM, et al. Axonal loss and neuroinflammation caused by peroxisome-deficient oligodendrocytes. Nat Genet. 2007;39:969–76.
109. Kremenchutzky M, Rice GPA, Baskerville J, Wingerchuk DM, Ebers GC. The natural history of multiple sclerosis: a geographically based study—9: Observations on the progressive phase of the disease. Brain. 2006;129:584–94.
110. Confavreux C, Vukusic S, Moreau T, Adeleine P. Relapses and progression of disability in multiple sclerosis. N Engl J Med. 2000;343:1430–8.
111. Cottrell DA, et al. The natural history of multiple sclerosis: a geographically based study—5. The clinical features and natural history of primary progressive multiple sclerosis. Brain. 1999;122:625–39.
112. Runmarker B, Andersen O. Prognostic factors in a multiple-sclerosis incidence cohort with 25 years of follow-up. Brain. 1993;116:117–34.
113. Weinshenker BGEA. The natural-history of multiple-sclerosis—a geographically based study. Brain. 1989;112:133–46.
114. Bramow S, et al. Demyelination versus remyelination in progressive multiple sclerosis. Brain. 2010;133:2983–98.

Chapter 4
Mechanisms of Disease Progression

Alastair Wilkins

4.1 Introduction

Advances in therapeutics for relapsing and remitting MS (RRMS) have been a major success story in recent years. In contrast, there remains a paucity of therapies for progressive disease. Hopes that the drugs and strategies employed for RRMS may translate into progressive MS treatments have not, in general, been borne out. Despite this, the understanding of mechanisms of progressive MS have advanced significantly and a realisation that alternative strategies at this stage of the disease are required has been important.

Specifically, an increased recognition of the importance of axonal injury in progressive disease has emerged. Whereas relapses are the likely consequence of acute focal inflammatory lesions within the CNS (leading to demyelination, cytokine release and conduction block), axonal injury appears to account for much of the disability seen during the progressive phase and, importantly, may be irreversible once certain structural changes have appeared in axons. This is in contrast to myelin injury which is, to some extent, reparable [1]. Thus has emerged the recognition that strategies to protect axons early in the disease are required.

4.2 What Have Clinical Studies Told Us About the Likely Pathophysiology of Axonal Injury in MS?

The correlation between progressive disability and axonal degeneration has been studied predominantly by using clinical scales and magnetic resonance markers of axon injury, linked to tissue analysis. The inherent difficulties of studying tissue

A. Wilkins
Institute of Clinical Neurosciences, University of Bristol, Southmead Hospital, Bristol, UK
e-mail: Alastair.Wilkins@bris.ac.uk

A. Wilkins (ed.), *Progressive Multiple Sclerosis*,
https://doi.org/10.1007/978-3-319-65921-3_4

changes in any neurological disorder have led to the development of a number of biomarkers for disease progression. Whilst significant increases in our understanding of disease processes has occurred using biomarkers, there is an urgent need to develop further markers of disease progression, not least as a tool to guide future treatment trials for progressive disease (see Chap. 6).

Magnetic resonance spectroscopy (MRS) is a technique which allows quantification of certain tissue metabolites in the brains of patients with MS and has the advantage of being a non-invasive test which can be repeated at intervals during the course of the disease. N-acetyl aspartate (NAA) is found predominantly in neurons and the spectroscopic detection of the compound by MRS is a marker of axonal density in the nervous system [2]. Reductions in brain NAA levels have been detected in acute active lesions of MS, chronic active lesions and so-called normal appearing white matter (NAWM) of patients with the disease [3, 4]. Furthermore, persistent neurological disability correlates to reductions in NAA levels in MS (and in some other progressive neurological diseases, such as spinocerebellar ataxias) [2, 5]. Longitudinal MRS studies have shown that reductions in NAA levels correlate with higher disability scores in RRMS [6]. Whole brain NAA levels decline over the course of progressive MS [7]. Axonal metabolic function, independent of structural integrity, may be a major determinant of NAA measures in MS [8]. A further, cruder marker of tissue injury is whole brain atrophy. Whilst not cell specific, disability levels, perhaps not surprisingly, are linked to progressive cerebral atrophy [9]. Brain atrophy reflects generalised brain tissue loss, but may particularly reflect grey matter (cortical) atrophy. Cortical atrophy appears to correlate well with levels of disability [10].

The above studies have suggested that reductions in neuronal/axonal density or metabolic function may be the key determinant of progressive disability. However, since a variety of tissue changes occur over the course of MS disease course, the cellular substrate of disease progression may be complex and multifactorial. For instance, chronic demyelination, may have a major influence on axonal survival, but how the process influences disease progression *per se*, is unknown. Similarly, chronic gliosis may reduce intrinsic repair and thus add to progressive tissue injury. The remainder of this chapter will focus on the mechanisms of axonal injury and how they relate to progressive MS.

Post mortem tissue analysis and treatment trial data have been particularly informative in elucidating the causes of axonal injury in MS. Histopathological analyses of multiple sclerosis tissue have confirmed significant reductions in axon density compared to controls [11]. Attempts to correlate pathological markers of injury with disability levels are fraught with difficulty, since post mortem analysis offers only an end-stage 'snap shot' of a chronic disease. However, a higher Expanded Disability Status Scale (EDSS) ante-mortem is associated with lower axonal densities in spinal cord corticospinal tracts [12]. Loss of axons may be size-selective with a propensity for early loss of small calibre axons within specific axonal tracts [13]. Despite being noted in Charcot's early descriptions of MS pathology, research into axonal injury remained inactive until the late 1990s when two papers re-ignited interest in the field [14, 15]. Using markers of axonal injury these papers demonstrated axonal injury predominantly occurring in active lesions of MS. Amyloid precursor protein (APP) is transported in axons via fast axonal transport (FAT) and accumulation along the length of axons is reported as an early indicator of axon injury [16]. Ferguson et al. reported axonal APP accumulation within active lesions, co-localising with macrophages [14]. APP accumulation was also noted in active borders of less acute lesions with much lower levels in chronic lesions. From this, they concluded that acute inflammation may be a major cause of axonal damage in MS. In a similar way, Trapp et al. studied neurofilament dephosphorylation as a marker of axonal structural injury and found high levels of axons with dephosphorylated neurofilaments (and characteristic axonal 'spheroids' representing transected axons) within acute lesions [15]. The definition of an acute lesion used in this report was the presence of class-II positive lymphocytes in areas of demyelination. These areas were associated with myelin debris and phagocytic cells were demonstrated in close association with axonal spheroids within active lesions. Comparing the levels of axonal transection within active, chronic active and non-lesion white matter, the authors conclude that axonal transection in MS is closely linked to inflammation.

Further pathological studies have attempted to define more precisely the relationship between inflammation and axonal pathology. Within acute lesions of MS (analysed from brain biopsy specimens) it has been reported that there is a correlation between density of CD8+ve cells and APP expression within axons; and a correlation between density of macrophages/microglia and APP expression within axons [17]. The presence of axonal pathology (marked by APP accumulation) may be more marked early in the disease course and decrease over time [18]. Again this study showed a correlation between inflammatory cell infiltrate (CD8+ve cells) and axonal injury, but also suggested that lesions studied (either by biopsy or post mortem) early in the disease course (less than 1 year since onset of disease) showed higher levels of inflammatory activity. However, the 'early' lesions were often from biopsied tissue, so may represent an atypical or fulminant variant of MS lesion.

Interestingly, all pathological studies show markers of axonal injury outside of acute lesions (albeit at lower levels). From this has arisen the question of how much axonal injury is non-inflammatory. Another important consideration is to what extent demyelination rather than inflammation is driving axonal loss in acute lesions. Demyelination in acute lesions results from inflammatory and immunological attack, so dissecting out the relative contribution of demyelination and inflammation in axonal injury is difficult [17]. Distinct disease mechanisms are likely to be responsible for particular clinical manifestations of MS. Demyelination causes several functional effects, notably reduction in saltatory conduction, but also exposes denuded axons to the harmful effects of circulating cytokines and may result in conduction block [19]. These neurophysiological changes are closely linked to relapses and remission may occur via reduction in cytokine-mediated conduction block or, over a longer time period, remyelination. Remyelination does occur to a variable degree, although the process ultimately fails or is insufficient in the vast majority of cases [1]. The reasons for remyelination failure and strategies to enhance remyelination have been the subject of active research for several decades [20].

Inflammation alone, however, cannot explain the whole spectrum of disease mechanisms of MS. Both epidemiological studies of the relationship between relapses and disease progression and trials of anti-inflammatory treatments in MS have indicated a likely non-inflammatory aetiology (at least in part) for chronic disease progression. The epidemiology of progressive disease has suggested that once disease progression has 'set-in' (Kurtzke Disability Score (DSS) > 4) subsequent relapses do not have much effect on the rate of progression; and that once disease progression has set-in (DSS > 4) the history and severity of prior relapses has little bearing on subsequent progression rates [21–23]. These observations suggest that once a certain threshold of disability has been reached disease progression is uninfluenced by relapses, either those that have occurred previously or those which have occurred subsequently. Epidemiological studies of disease progression have also looked at the influence of age. Interestingly, although primary progressive patients present at an older age, there appears little difference in the age of entering the progressive phase between different subtypes of patients (primary progressive, those with a single relapse followed by progression and secondary progression) [21, 22, 24]. Patients whose MS starts at a younger age reach disability milestones at a younger age, but take longer to reach those milestones from the onset of their disease and young-onset patients take longer to convert from relapsing and remitting to secondary progressive disease [25]. Thus it would appear from the epidemiological studies that progression in MS may be an age-dependent process occurring in a predefined schedule and uninfluenced by current or past relapses. Indeed some authors have concluded that relapsing and remitting disease to be MS in which 'insufficient time has elapsed for the conversion to secondary progression; secondary progressive forms as relapsing-remitting MS that has 'grown older'; and progressive from onset cases as MS 'amputated' from the usual preceding relapsing-remitting phase' [24].

Similarly treatment trials have provided important observations on the aetiology of disease progression [26–29]. The failure of the 'first-wave' of disease modifying therapies (DMTs), such as β-interferon and glatiramer acetate, to impact significantly on disease progression, despite being disappointing, has been informative from a neurobiological perspective. The observation that these drugs reduce relapse rates (albeit by a moderate amount) but have little impact on disease progression implies a dissociation of inflammatory relapses from disease progression [30, 31]. The use of a more powerful agent, alemtuzumab (formerly CAMPATH-1H), has allowed for this phenomenon to be elucidated in more detail [32]. Almost complete suppression of relapses in patients that have already entered the progressive phase of MS had little effect on subsequent disease progression [33]. Importantly use of the drug at earlier disease stages (before onset of progressive disease) has demonstrated that the drug may have effects on preventing or delaying onset of disease progression [34]. Indeed, more recent studies of the drug have demonstrated that administration of the drug to patients with RRMS may reduce levels of sustained accumulation of disability (relative to β-interferon) [35, 36]. These observations have suggested a 'window of opportunity' for anti-inflammatory/anti-immune therapies for MS and that once a clinical level of disability has been reached these therapies become less effective.

4.3 What Are the Possible Mechanisms of Axonal Injury in MS?

Mechanisms of axonal injury in MS may be multiple and dependent on a variety of factors. Here the role of inflammation, chronic demyelination, induced changes to axonal structure and function and the influence of grey matter inflammation will be discussed (Fig. 4.1).

4.3.1 Inflammation and Immunological Injury

Inflammatory mediators have long been implicated in the pathophysiology of MS [37, 38]. Immune mechanisms involved in myelin injury include both cellular, with T cells directed against myelin and oligodendrocyte components with subsequent macrophage and microglial recruitment; and humoral immunity, with secretion of antibodies by B cells and subsequent complement involvement in opsonisation and phagocytosis of myelin debris [39]. Common mechanisms are likely to operate in the pathogenesis of inflammatory axonal injury.

Although the initial immunological cascade in MS is thought to be a T cell dependent process, multiple cellular effectors are involved in tissue damage and specifically axonal injury. T lymphocytes play an important role in the generation and propagation of immune changes in MS through autoimmune activation via as yet unknown antigen stimulation [40]. In EAE CD4$^+$ T cells polarized to a T_h (T-helper; and specifically T_h1) phenotype induce much of the immunological damage and indeed these cells are prominent within active MS lesions [41]. Dysregulated T_h1 responses have been implicated in much of the organ specific autoimmunity of MS through actions of cytokines, such as γIFN, and through the activation of macrophages and microglia. MHC class 1-restricted, CD8$^+$ T cells are also prominent in active MS lesions and T_h17 cells (producing IL-17) are also likely to play an

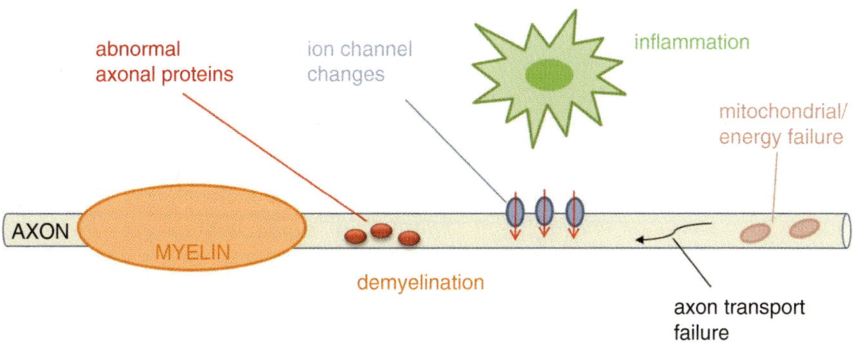

Fig. 4.1 Potential mechanisms of axonal injury in progressive MS

important role in MS [42]. T-reg (FOXp3$^+$) cells are involved in the process of tolerance and immunosuppression and other cells such as invariant natural killer (NK) cells, CD56$^+$ NK cells and possibly stem cells have roles in immunological injury and immunomodulation [43].

With regards to cell-mediated axonal injury in MS, CD8$^+$ T cells and microglia are currently thought to be a major cell type. Interestingly class 1 MHC molecules, which are required for antigen presentation to CD8$^+$ T cells, are rarely expressed in electrically active neurons but are expressed during prolonged electrical silence and when neurons are exposed to γIFN [44]. Neurites expressing class 1 MHC molecules are then susceptible to damage from CD8$^+$ T cells [45]. Thus a combination of the inflammatory milieu and the electrical state of the neuron may combine to induce axon injury. CD8$^+$ T cells are prominent in active MS plaques and their numbers have been shown to correlate with axonal injury within lesions [17, 18]. The relative contribution of CD8$^+$ T cells versus CD4$^+$ T cells to axonal injury in MS is unknown, but common mechanisms involving cytokine release (see below) are implicated. Levels of acute axonal transection correlate well with microglial numbers in human post mortem tissue are thought to be axonotoxic through mechanisms including oxidative stress (see below) [14].

The study of auto-antibodies in CNS inflammatory disorders has been rejuvenated by the discovery of anti-aquaporin-4 antibodies in neuromyelitis optica which are directed against astrocyte water channels [46]. Using a proteomics-based approach, antibodies to neurofascin were identified in a subset of patients with MS [47]. Neurofascin is a neuronal protein which is concentrated at the node of Ranvier of myelinated fibres. Co-transferring anti-neurofascin antibodies with oligodendrocyte glycoprotein-specific encephalitogenic T cells into rodents led to specific antibody targeting of the nodes of Ranvier with subsequent axonal injury. Interestingly, changes in neurofascin staining patterns have been documented in human *post mortem* tissue from patients with MS, which is associated with axonal loss [48]. Similarly antibodies against neurofilaments have been detected in spinal fluid samples of patients with MS [49, 50]. Determining whether the presence of these antibodies represents primary and specific antibody-mediated targeting of axons or whether they occur in response to widespread tissue injury with exposure of previously sequestered antigens (and thus are effectively epiphenomena), remains a challenge.

The role of B cells and antibody production in progressive MS has, however, come to the fore in recent years with the discovery of ectopic B cell follicles in the meninges of patients with progressive MS [51, 52]. The follicles have been associated with early onset of secondary progressive disease and severe cortical pathology [53]. Recent trials of the B cell depleting anti-CD20 monoclonal antibody ocrelizumab have indicated reductions in confirmed disability after 12 and 24 weeks treatment PPMS [54]. Similarly, ocrelizumab has also shown effects on disability progression markers in trials of RRMS [55]. These trials will be discussed in more detail in subsequent chapters.

In vitro and *in vivo* studies have revealed potential mechanisms by which reactive oxygen and reactive nitrogen species (ROS/RNS) may damage central nervous system axons. Nitric oxide (NO), which serves many physiological functions within the nervous system, has been implicated as a likely mediator of axonal injury and at sites of central nervous system inflammation (both MS itself and experimental models of MS) high concentrations of NO are found [56]. Pathological studies have also shown activity of the enzyme responsible for production of NO (inducible nitric oxide sythetase (iNOS)) within MS lesions [57, 58]. Microglia produce NO which is a major mechanism by which these cells induce axonal injury [59, 60]. *In vivo* application of nitric oxide donors to rat dorsal root axons causes degeneration when electrically stimulated [61]. Interestingly, blockade of the electrical activity by sodium channel blockers or inhibitors of sodium/calcium exchange his process may attenuate axon destruction [62]. A potential explanation for these observations are that NO inhibits mitochondrial respiration, causing failure of sodium/potassium ATPase, which, in turn, leads to increased levels of sodium within the axon causing a reversal in the sodium/calcium exchanger allowing excess levels of calcium to mediate axonal degeneration [56]. *In vitro* studies have shown NO causes dose-dependent neurotoxicitiy via a number of intracellular pathways, ultimately leading to inhibition of mitochondrial respiration and cell death [63–66]. NO also has specific axonotoxic effects *in vitro* and high concentrations of NO reduce neurofilament phosphorylation levels within axons, leading to axonal destruction [67, 68]. A number of other reactive oxygen and reactive nitrogen species (ROS/RNS) may also be important in the pathogenesis of axonal injury in MS [69].

Cytokine mediated tissue damage has also been extensively studied in relation to MS and indeed there have been trials of anti-cytokine therapies for the disease. Two cytokines in particular have attracted attention—γIFN and TNFα. The cytokine profile classically associated with T_h1 cells, γIFN, TNFα and IL-2, are found in acute lesions and these cytokines (as well as mRNA transcripts of these cytokines) can be detected in tissue and CSF derived from patients with MS [70, 71]. The deleterious effect of γIFN on axonal survival in neuroinflammatory conditions may be via activation of microglia (see above) [65]. Circulating TNFα levels are raised in MS relapses and the role of TNFα in oligodendrocyte injury and demyelination has been extensively studied [72, 73]. Whilst much evidence exists for a pro-inflammatory function for TNFα, the function of TNFα in MS is likely to be complex. For instance, some reports have demonstrated a likely anti-inflammatory effect of TNFα [74]. The probable explanation for the variability in effects in animal models is the pleiotropic effect of TNFα on different cell types, acting through different receptors. The complexity of the role of TNFα in MS was highlighted by the disappointing trials of TNFα-blocking agents in the disease which caused exacerbation of disease activity [75, 76].

Whether inflammation plays any protective role in neuroinflammatory conditions is an important question, since the rationale for almost all therapies for multiple sclerosis has been to reduce inflammation. Trying to elucidate any potential beneficial effects of inflammation may help to tailor anti-inflammatory therapies to be more specific. The inherent repair that occurs in the early stages of MS (remission) suggests a powerful beneficial effect of certain mediators involved in the immune response. Inflammatory cells, notably T lymphocytes produce growth factors and cytokines which may be beneficial in promoting repair [77]. Specifically brain-derived neurotrophic factor (BDNF) immunoreactivity within lymphocytes in multiple sclerosis lesions has been demonstrated [78]. Intriguingly following alemtuzumab therapy, lymphocytes may show increased expression of a number of neurotrophic factors, including BDNF, platelet-derived growth factor (PDGF) and ciliary neurotrophic factor (CNTF), which may be a partial explanation of some of the improvements seen in disability following therapy with the drug [79]. In experimental models of demyelination inflammation may encourage remyelination which, in turn, may have beneficial protective effects on the axon [80]. The recognition that immune cells may contribute to neuroprotection implies non-specific immunosuppression may not always be beneficial at all stages of the disease.

4.3.2 Chronic White Matter Demyelination

Neurodegenerative processes are thought to contribute to disease progression, particularly in established disease. The respective contributions to disease progression of inflammatory and non-inflammatory mechanisms are unknown and may vary as the disease become more chronic, with inflammation contributing less as the disease course progresses. Chronic demyelination of normally myelinated axons has been suggested as a possible mechanism for non-inflammatory axon injury and a number of experimental models have shown that myelin and oligodendrocytes have trophic properties towards axons.

CNS myelin contains a number of proteins and glycoproteins, which are involved in the development and maintenance of the axon-myelin unit. These include proteolipid protein (PLP) and DM20 (an alternate spliced isoform), myelin basic protein (MBP), myelin associated glycoprotein (MAG), myelin-oligodendrocyte glycoprotein (MOG) and 2′,3′-cyclic nucleotide 3′-phosphodiesterase (CNPase). A number of myelin mutants have been generated experimentally (or exist naturally) which have demonstrated the importance of myelin to axon development. For example, *shiverer* mice have an absence of compact CNS myelin (caused by a deletion in the MBP gene) and exhibit multiple axonal abnormalities, including an increase in slow axonal transport, alterations in microtubule density and number, and altered neurofilament assembly and phosphorylation [81–83].

Similarly myelin components are thought to be involved in long term axon maintenance. Studies have shown that PLP may have a major role in axonal maintenance, since mice lacking the *plp* gene are able to synthesise large amounts of myelin, yet show late onset axonal degeneration with ‘ovoid’ formation and impairment of axonal transport mechanisms [84, 85]. Indeed, axons may become dependent on oligodendrocyte support sometime after myelination has been completed, as non-myelinated axons within optic nerves from chimeric females (which show patches of normally myelinated and non-myelinated axons) never develop axonal swellings over the expected time course. Mice which are engineered to express the peripheral myelin component P_0 instead of PLP within the CNS show a structure and periodicity of myelin which resembled peripheral myelin, yet had severe disability and degeneration of myelinated axons, indicating a specific central neuroprotective role of CNS myelin [86]. Other components of myelin also provide trophic support to axons. For instance, mice lacking CNPase have morphologically normal myelin, but show delayed axonal swelling and degeneration [87]. A problem with the study of myelin mutants is that axons are never exposed to 'normal' myelin and thus, it may be argued, may develop abnormal axon-glial interactions and axon degeneration in these models may not be relevant to diseases in which myelin contain a full complement of components. A study of a non-inflammatory model of demyelination has shown that chronic loss of axons occurs even in the absence of a significant primary immunological event and in the presence of myelin containing all the necessary components of compact CNS myelin [88]. Importantly, replacement of myelin experimentally has been shown to protect axons from chronic axon loss induced by demyelination [89].

The relevance of myelin components to axon maintenance in humans may be studied in related white matter disorders. Pelizaeus–Merzbacher disease (PMD) is caused by disturbances in the function of the PLP gene [90]. Whilst most cases of PMD are caused by PLP duplication, some are caused by a null mutation in the PLP gene, which is associated with a milder clinical phenotype and a relative preservation of myelin [91]. Axonal abnormalities occur in these patients, even in areas where myelin levels appear normal and MRS imaging data in PMD has shown a decrease in NAA levels in the CNS when compared to control, consistent with decrease axonal densities [92]. These observations indicate the importance of myelin to maintenance of human axons within the CNS.

Impairments in the arrangement of myelin at the nodes of Ranvier has attracted recent interest in the peripheral nervous system. So called nodopathies are predominantly immune-mediated and lead to impaired saltatory conduction [93]. How disruption of the node of Ranvier is implicated in multiple sclerosis is not known, but loss of the node leads to rearrangement of ion channels along the length of the axon which is discussed below.

4.3.3 *Ion Channel Disruptions*

A number of distinct pathological changes occur in axons which may predispose to chronic degeneration. Many of these occur as a consequence of disturbance of the axon-glial subunit. For instance, alterations in ion channel composition and distribution occur along the length of demyelinated axons. Clustering of sodium channels (particularly $Na_v1.6$) at the node of Ranvier is a physiological principle that underpins saltatory conduction and demyelination causes redistribution of ion channels [94]. Sodium channel clustering is dependent on oligodendrocyte signalling since *md* (myelin deficient) mice (which lack oligodendrocytes but not astrocytes) show almost no sodium channel clustering along axons at postnatal day 16, an age at which the phenomenon is prominent in wild type mice [95, 96]. Reduction in clustering and expression of $Na_v1.6$ along the length of demyelinated axons occurs in EAE [94]. This process is thought to serve as a physiological adaptive response to preserve propagation of the action potential, but may also have chronic deleterious effects on axonal stability. Expression of $Na_v1.6$ along the length of demyelinated axons is accompanied by increased expression of the Na^+/Ca^{2+} exchanger [97]. Increased levels of sodium within axons may cause reversal in the sodium/calcium exchanger which allows excess levels of calcium to mediate axonal degeneration [62]. Furthermore, electrical activity in axons exposed to inflammatory mediators may further dysregulate ion flow within axons leading to degeneration [61]. These observations have formed the basis for trials of sodium channel blockers in MS [98, 99].

4.3.4 Mitochondrial Dysfunction and Energy Failure

Disrupted mitochondrial function may contribute to axonal degeneration in MS. Interest was first generated in the field with the observation that an MS-like illness occurs in some patients with Leber's Hereditary optic neuropathy (LHON), which is caused by mutations in mitochondrial DNA [100]. One mechanism by which mitochondrial dysfunction might link into axonal degeneration in MS is through blocking of respiratory chain enzymes by inflammatory mediators.

Mitochondria and mitochondrial DNA (mtDNA) are susceptible to oxidative stress injury from reactive oxygen and nitrogen species. Substances such as NO, produced as part of the inflammatory cascade in the disease, cause damage to mitochondrial DNA and decrease oxidative phosphorylation [101]. Changes in mitochondrial complex I, III and IV occur within axons and neurons of MS tissue, either representing an adaptive response or potentially a pathogenic mechanism [102, 103]. Mitochondrial gene deletions and clonal expansion of abnormal mitochondria have been demonstrated in neurons derived from patients with progressive MS [104]. In addition, it has been shown that nuclear export of histone deacetylase 1 (HDAC1) into the cytoplasm is necessary for the onset of axonal damage in an experimental model of MS [105]. Cytosolic HDAC1 may impair mitochondrial transport mechanism within axons and thus contribute to reduced energy production.

Reduced mitochondrial oxidative phosphorylation in mitochondria (leading to reduced ATP formation) may contribute to energy deficiency states within axons. The energy requirements of demyelinated axons are greatly increased due to the diffuse spreading of voltage gated sodium channels along the axolemma and the inefficiency of action potential propagation [106]. Furthermore increase in intra-axonal sodium ion levels mentioned above may be caused by reduced mitochondrial ATP production leading to failure of the Na^+/K^+ ATPase pump [94]. The combination of increased energy demand within the axon, impaired mitochondrial function resulting from ROS/RNS and inflammation induced mtDNA deletions within axons are postulated to set up a vicious cycle of progressive energy failure in progressive disease.

4.3.5 Axon Transport Deficits

Transport of cellular organelles and proteins throughout the neuron, including along the axon and dendrites, is crucial for maintenance of neuronal function. Proteins and organelles are transported throughout cells via a number of well characterised motor proteins, many of which are also involved in maintenance of axonal structure. Deficits in motor protein-mediated neuronal transport mechanisms have been implicated in a number of neurodegenerative disorders including hereditary spastic paraplegia, Charcot–Marie–Tooth disease [107]. In MS, a combination both inflammation-driven and neurodegenerative processes may impact of axon transport, but increasing evidence suggests a role for disturbed axonal transport in contributing to axonal injury in the disease. Potential mechanisms relating to this are summarised in Fig. 4.2.

Perturbation in axonal transport leads to mislocalisation of proteins and organelles within the axon, which, in turn, can result in accumulation of abnormal protein within the cell and impaired distribution of mitochondria, with subsequent energy failure (see above).

Kinesin superfamily proteins (KIFs) are a family of motor proteins whose primary role is to facilitate anterograde axonal transport (from the cell body where the majority of proteins are translated along the axon and dendrites) of various protein cargoes, through association with microtubule 'rails'. KIFs have an NH_2-terminal

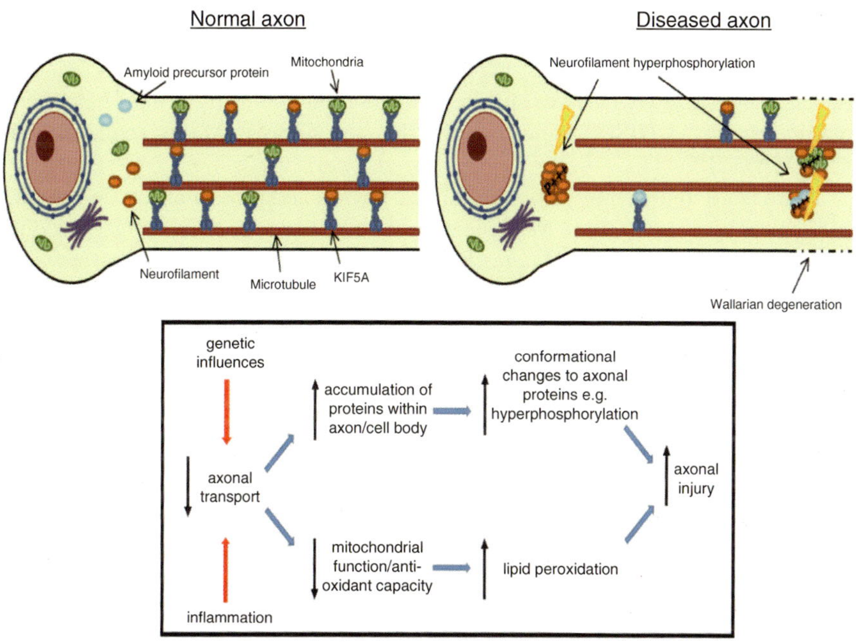

Fig. 4.2 Schematic representation of the relevance of axonal transport deficits to MS

(head) comprising a microtubule binding domain and a conserved globular motor domain which hydrolyses ATP to produce the energy required for movement of cargoes along the microtubule and through the axon. The head is attached by an α-helical stalk to a COOH-terminal (tail) where cargoes can bind. Cargoes bind directly or indirectly, through kinesin light chain (KLC) associations and protein adaptor complexes, to the tail domain. KIFs transport numerous essential cargoes including: cellular organelles, such as mitochondria; pre- and post- synaptic membrane proteins; and a range of structural proteins such as neurofilaments (NFs) [108].

Certain KIFs, including KIF5A, KIF1B and KIF21B, may have particular relevance to disease processes in MS. Reduced transport of proteins and accumulation of substances such as APP within axonal tracts indicates dysfunction of axonal transport mechanisms and precedes axon fragmentation. In addition, phosphorylated NF proteins, which are integral to axon structure and integrity, are susceptible to hyperphosphorylation in disease states, including MS. Therefore, abnormal accumulation of insoluble proteins in both the cell body and axon may cause structural instability to the axon and toxic effects on the neuronal cell body, both of which may contribute to neuronal and axonal loss in MS. Furthermore, reduced trafficking of mitochondria may contribute to inadequate energy supply to axons and a reduction in defence against ROS.

KIF5A plays an important role in the transport of axonal components. KIF5A is the main kinesin subtype involved in anterograde transport of NF [109]. Postnatal targeted knockout of the *kif5a* gene in mice causes NF accumulation in cell bodies, reduced axonal calibre, eventual axon loss and hind limb paralysis. In addition to NF, KIF5A is known to transport amyloid precursor protein (APP), mitochondria, pre-synaptic membrane proteins (SNAP-25 and syntaxin-1); and synaptic vesicle precursors (synaptotagmin and synaptobrevin). KIF5A mutations are found in various neurodegenerative diseases such as an autosomal dominant form of hereditary spastic paraplegia (HSP), known as SPG10, and Charcot–Marie–Tooth disease (CMT-2A) [110].

There is a significant reduction in KIF5A mRNA and protein expression in MS non-lesional grey matter; and MS lesional and normal-appearing white matter, compared to control [111, 112]. Interestingly, there is a positive correlation between KIF5A protein expression and MS patient disease duration, suggesting that reduced expression of KIF5A may have particular relevance to the severity of axonal pathology in MS. Additionally, several single nucleotide polymorphisms (SNP) within the KIF5A-CYP27B1-METTL1-FAM119B gene locus (rs12368653, rs703842, rs1678536, rs1678542 and rs775322) have been linked to MS susceptibility [113, 114]. There is a significant reduction in KIF5A protein expression in MS patients who are homozygous carriers (AA) of the rs12368653 and rs703842 SNP, compared to MS patients who are not (GG); in non-lesional cerebral cortex and combined lesional and normal appearing white matter, suggesting some link between MS susceptibility genotype and the degree of axon dysfunction [111, 112].

In addition, a SNP in the region of KIF21B has been shown to be a susceptibility locus for MS [115]. A recent study suggested that levels of KIF21B correlate with grey matter demyelination in MS [116]. There are also reductions in KIF21B mRNA in MS grey matter compared to control [111]. KIF1B was originally thought to be a susceptibility gene in MS, with a SNP identified at intron 5 of the gene locus rs10492972, though subsequent studies did not replicate this observation [117]. Studies have highlighted a role for KIF1B in oligodendrocyte intracellular transport mechanisms and MBP localisation [118]. Therefore, changes in KIF1B gene expression may hinder remyelination occurring in MS or possibly cause mislocalisation of MBP that could trigger auto-immune attack [119].

Axon transport defects are likely to precede irreversible axon degeneration. A mouse MS model study using in vivo imaging assays has demonstrated widespread transport deficits which preceded structural alterations of axons and could be reversed by anti-inflammatory interventions [120]. Identifying potential therapeutic targets to improve axonal transport or reduce the consequences of impaired axonal transport before the onset of irreversible axonal loss may help prevent progressive disability.

4.3.6 Defects in Axonal Structure

Structural changes to axons include disturbance in axonal continuity (transection), alterations in structural components of the axon cytoskeleton and accumulation of substances within the axon [14, 15]. Axonal transection and spheroid formation most likely represent irreversible axonal destruction. These features are seen within white matter tracts and higher numbers of axonal spheroids appear within acute inflammatory lesions [15, 17, 121]. However, significant numbers of axonal spheroids are also seen within chronic active, chronic inactive and normal appearing white matter.

In addition to these well-defined pathological changes, neurofilament (NF) defects are the next most studied structural abnormality in MS axons. In particular, alterations in NF phosphorylation represent a crucial step in the development of structural instability [122]. Neuronal and axonal cytoskeletons are composed of variably phosphorylated neurofilaments of low, medium and high molecular weight (MW) that perform many diverse cellular functions, but are predominantly involved in providing structural stability [123, 124]. Typically axonal NFs are highly phosphorylated and have a particular phospho-epitope staining pattern. NF phosphorylation improves structural stability by increasing the charge-based repulsion of neighbouring NFs (which maximises spacing and determines axonal calibre) and protects against proteolytic injury [125]. Dephosphorylation of axonal NFs is commonly seen in MS white matter (both lesional and non-lesional) [15, 126, 127]. In addition, hyperphosphorylated NF (NF-heavy chains) are also seen both with the white matter and within grey matter neuronal cell bodies [126, 128]. Hyperphosphorylation of cytoskeletal components, including NFs, are observed in a number of neurodegenerative disorders and aggregates of these substances may contribute to neurodegeneration [129, 130]. Accumulation of phosphorylated neurofilament in motor neurons are found in ALS [131]. Neurofilament levels are altered also in AD [132] and neurofilaments found in neurofibrillary tangles are extensively phosphorylated [133]. Furthermore, β-amyloid plaques from patients in a preclinical stage of the disease are associated with abnormal accumulation of NF in the absence of tau abnormalities, suggesting that neurofilament changes may represent the earliest cytoskeleton alteration associated with dystrophic neurite formation [134, 135]. Understanding how build-up of these substances occurs and therapies to reduce aggregate formation are key areas of drug development.

Since NFs are major structural components of neurons, their presence in spinal fluid has been studied as a potential biomarker for numerous neurodegenerative conditions. The correlation of clinical disability with elevated neurofilament phosphoisoforms in cerebrospinal fluid (CSF) of MS patients highlights its importance as a potential biomarker for axonal and neuronal injury [136]. However, there is marked elevation of phosphorylated NF heavy subunit levels (pNFH) in the CSF of patients with ALS, supporting the use of pNFH as a new diagnostic biomarker of widespread neuronal degeneration, rather than as a specific marker of MS [137].

4.3.7 Grey Matter Disease

Grey matter pathology, predominantly occurring in the cerebral cortex is now a well-recognised phenomenon in multiple sclerosis [138]. Cortical demyelination, injury to cortical neuronal cell bodies and, more recently, meningeal inflammation are found in pathological specimens derived from patients with MS. The degree of grey matter damage correlates well with physical disability and particularly cognitive impairment in MS [10]. Indeed, rate of disease progression appears to correlate with the severity of cortical inflammation [53].

Cortical lesions have been classified into various types dependent on their location within the cortex. Leucocortical lesions involve both white and grey matter (type 1); intracortical (type 2) are lesions located solely within the cortex distributed around cortical blood vessels; subpial lesions (type 3) occur superficially along the surface of one or more gyri; and type 4 lesions span the whole of the cortex. The latter two lesion types are particularly associated with progressive MS [139]. Interesting recent observations on the relationship between subpial demyelination and inflammation of the overlying meninges in progressive MS has been the driver for novel therapeutic targets for the disease. Interestingly in MS, cortical inflammation appears different to white matter inflammation. Cortical lesions have reduced levels of inflammatory cellular infiltrate and pure intracortical lesions typically have low levels of inflammation [140]. In both SPMS and PPMS there appears to be a correlation between the degree of subpial demyelination and leptomeningeal inflammation, suggesting a potent driver for the process [51, 52]. How these are linked is not entirely clear, but the meninges are a site of ectopic B cell follicles in progressive MS [53]. The presence of meningeal inflammation and ectopic B cell follicles adjacent to cortical lesions has suggested a role for these aberrant B cell follicles in the propagation of cortical lesions and potentially a driver for disease progression [141]. However, the association between meningeal inflammation and cortical demyelination remains unclear [142]. The observation of these B cell containing follicles has, however, been one of the driving forces behind novels trials of B cell depleting agents in progressive MS, which has led to a successful trial of ocrelizumab in PPMS [54]. Interestingly, previous Epstein Barr virus (EBV) infection correlates with the presence of B cells, plasma cells and ectopic follicles in meningeal infiltrates of patients with MS [141]. The link between EBV and MS pathogenesis has been postulated for some time and EBV remains one of the strongest candidates as an environmental risk factor for the disease [143]. The work on EBV and B cell follicles has suggested that viral latency within the CNS of those with MS may contribute to on-going pathology.

Further understanding of the aetiology and pathogenesis of cortical lesions and particularly mechanisms of neuronal cell body injury, will help to further understand disease mechanisms in progressive disease [128].

4.4 How Does the Understanding of Disease Mechanisms in Progressive MS Inform Future Therapies?

How then might advances in our understanding of the mechanisms of progressive disease translate into the development of new therapies?

A major component of axonal injury, particularly in the acute lesion, appears to be inflammation-driven. Anti-inflammatory therapies thus undoubtedly have a role in preventing axonal injury early in the disease course. We know that if anti-inflammatory therapies are instituted after the onset of disease progression, however, their efficacy in preventing subsequent disease progression is poor [32]. However, recent and emerging evidence suggests that early treatment with powerful immunosuppressant drugs such as alemtuzumab and natalizumab, prior to onset of established disease progression, may reduce progressive disability over time [35, 36]. The interesting data emerging from ocrelizumab in PPMS indicates further that modulation of the immune system may yield important therapeutic advances in this subset of patients [54]. It may be that as we learn more about the inflammatory process in MS that specific components of axon damage induced by inflammation can be targeted. For instance, understanding more the role of specific auto-antibodies or other cellular effectors in axonal injury may allow targeted immunomodulation [48]. Nitric oxide may also be a potential therapeutic target, although iNOS inhibition may lead to a broad range of cellular responses which are not always beneficial to survival [56]. 'Blanket' immunosuppression is at best ineffective in progressive disease, and may possibly hinder intrinsic repair mechanisms, as discussed.

4.4.1 Neuroprotection in MS?

There is a major global drive to develop neuroprotective therapies for a range of chronic neurodegenerative diseases. MS has its own specific issues which need to be addressed in the development of neuroprotective strategies: the diffuse, rather multi-focal nature of the disease; prolonged time phase of disease progression; and difficulties of delivering the treatment to a disease disseminated in time and space within the nervous system.

Neuroprotectants may act in a variety of ways, for example: preventing build-up or action of toxic material within the neuron/axon; directly influencing intracellular signalling pathways within neurons/axons to reverse signalling effects that cause neurotoxicity; or stabilising axon structure. Initial breakthroughs in neuroprotectant research focused on inhibition of excitotoxic compounds, such as inhibition of glutamate transmission. For instance, riluzole was developed as an agent to slow down progression in amyotrophic lateral sclerosis (ALS). The drug has shown beneficial effects in EAE, an observation that has yet to be systematically replicated in multiple sclerosis [144]. Similarly, the observation that excess intra-axonal sodium results in toxic levels of intra-axonal calcium, has been the rationale for trials of sodium channel blockade in MS. Sodium channel blockade using agents including flecainide and phenytoin have reduced axonal injury in models of multiple sclerosis [62, 145]. Initial trials have been performed and are underway to test the hypothesis in MS [98, 99]. Other drugs may have general neuroprotective effects via a number of signalling pathways. Cannabinoids have rather broad-spectrum effects in experimental models, including modulation of immune responses and direct neuroprotectant properties via specific cannabinoid receptors [146]. Trials so far have, however, been disappointing [147]. Similarly, statins have broad neuroprotective and immunomodulatory properties and have been trialled in MS with encouraging early results [148].

The range of other drugs which are being developed specifically for progressive MS will be discussed in later chapters.

4.5 Conclusions

Neuronal injury and axon loss, occurring through a number of mechanisms is the major substrate for progressive disability in MS. Tailoring therapies to address specific disease mechanisms and relating these to the precise temporal course of neuronal and axonal injury is the next major step in MS therapeutics.

References

1. Patani R, et al. Remyelination can be extensive in multiple sclerosis despite a long disease course. Neuropathol Appl Neurobiol. 2007;33(3):277–87.
2. Bjartmar C, et al. Neurological disability correlates with spinal cord axonal loss and reduced N-acetyl aspartate in chronic multiple sclerosis patients. Ann Neurol. 2000;48(6):893–901.
3. Davie CA, et al. 1H magnetic resonance spectroscopy of chronic cerebral white matter lesions and normal appearing white matter in multiple sclerosis. J Neurol Neurosurg Psychiatry. 1997;63(6):736–42.

4. Leary SM, et al. 1H magnetic resonance spectroscopy of normal appearing white matter in primary progressive multiple sclerosis. J Neurol. 1999;246(11):1023–6.
5. Davie CA, et al. Persistent functional deficit in multiple sclerosis and autosomal dominant cerebellar ataxia is associated with axon loss. Brain. 1995;118(Pt 6):1583–92.
6. De Stefano N, et al. Axonal damage correlates with disability in patients with relapsing-remitting multiple sclerosis. Results of a longitudinal magnetic resonance spectroscopy study. Brain. 1998;121(Pt 8):1469–77.
7. Gonen O, et al. Total brain N-acetylaspartate: a new measure of disease load in MS. Neurology. 2000;54(1):15–9.
8. Cader S, et al. Discordant white matter N-acetylasparate and diffusion MRI measures suggest that chronic metabolic dysfunction contributes to axonal pathology in multiple sclerosis. Neuroimage. 2007;36(1):19–27.
9. Bermel RA, Bakshi R. The measurement and clinical relevance of brain atrophy in multiple sclerosis. Lancet Neurol. 2006;5(2):158–70.
10. Amato MP, et al. Neocortical volume decrease in relapsing-remitting MS patients with mild cognitive impairment. Neurology. 2004;63(1):89–93.
11. Lovas G, et al. Axonal changes in chronic demyelinated cervical spinal cord plaques. Brain. 2000;123(Pt 2):308–17.
12. Tallantyre EC, et al. Clinico-pathological evidence that axonal loss underlies disability in progressive multiple sclerosis. Mult Scler. 2010;16(4):406–11.
13. DeLuca GC, Ebers GC, Esiri MM. Axonal loss in multiple sclerosis: a pathological survey of the corticospinal and sensory tracts. Brain. 2004;127(Pt 5):1009–18.
14. Ferguson B, et al. Axonal damage in acute multiple sclerosis lesions. Brain. 1997;120(Pt 3): 393–9.
15. Trapp BD, et al. Axonal transection in the lesions of multiple sclerosis. N Engl J Med. 1998;338(5):278–85.
16. Sherriff FE, et al. Markers of axonal injury in post mortem human brain. Acta Neuropathol. 1994;88(5):433–9.
17. Bitsch A, et al. Acute axonal injury in multiple sclerosis. Correlation with demyelination and inflammation. Brain. 2000;123(Pt 6):1174–83.
18. Kuhlmann T, et al. Acute axonal damage in multiple sclerosis is most extensive in early disease stages and decreases over time. Brain. 2002;125(Pt 10):2202–12.
19. Redford EJ, Kapoor R, Smith KJ. Nitric oxide donors reversibly block axonal conduction: demyelinated axons are especially susceptible. Brain. 1997;120(Pt 12):2149–57.
20. Franklin RJ, Ffrench-Constant C. Remyelination in the CNS: from biology to therapy. Nat Rev Neurosci. 2008;9(11):839–55.
21. Kremenchutzky M, et al. The natural history of multiple sclerosis: a geographically based study 9: observations on the progressive phase of the disease. Brain. 2006;129(Pt 3):584–94.
22. Confavreux C, et al. Relapses and progression of disability in multiple sclerosis. N Engl J Med. 2000;343(20):1430–8.
23. Scalfari A, et al. The natural history of multiple sclerosis: a geographically based study 10: relapses and long-term disability. Brain. 2010;133(Pt 7):1914–29.
24. Confavreux C, Vukusic S. Age at disability milestones in multiple sclerosis. Brain. 2006;129(Pt 3):595–605.
25. Vukusic S, Confavreux C. Prognostic factors for progression of disability in the secondary progressive phase of multiple sclerosis. J Neurol Sci. 2003;206(2):135–7.
26. Jacobs LD, et al. Intramuscular interferon beta-1a for disease progression in relapsing multiple sclerosis. The Multiple Sclerosis Collaborative Research Group (MSCRG). Ann Neurol. 1996;39(3):285–94.
27. Randomised double-blind placebo-controlled study of interferon beta-1a in relapsing/remitting multiple sclerosis. PRISMS (Prevention of Relapses and Disability by Interferon beta-1a Subcutaneously in Multiple Sclerosis) Study Group. Lancet. 1998;352(9139): 1498–504.

28. Interferon beta-1b is effective in relapsing-remitting multiple sclerosis. I. Clinical results of a multicenter, randomized, double-blind, placebo-controlled trial. The IFNB Multiple Sclerosis Study Group. Neurology. 1993;43(4):655–61.
29. Johnson KP, et al. Copolymer 1 reduces relapse rate and improves disability in relapsing-remitting multiple sclerosis: results of a phase III multicenter, double-blind placebo-controlled trial. The Copolymer 1 Multiple Sclerosis Study Group. Neurology. 1995;45(7): 1268–76.
30. Rojas JI, et al. Interferon Beta for primary progressive multiple sclerosis. Cochrane Database Syst Rev. 2010;1:CD006643.
31. La Mantia L, Munari LM, Lovati R. Glatiramer acetate for multiple sclerosis. Cochrane Database Syst Rev. 2010;5:CD004678.
32. Coles AJ, et al. The window of therapeutic opportunity in multiple sclerosis: evidence from monoclonal antibody therapy. J Neurol. 2006;253(1):98–108.
33. Moreau T, et al. CAMPATH-IH in multiple sclerosis. Mult Scler. 1996;1(6):357–65.
34. Coles AJ, et al. Alemtuzumab vs. interferon beta-1a in early multiple sclerosis. N Engl J Med. 2008;359(17):1786–801.
35. Coles AJ, et al. Alemtuzumab for patients with relapsing multiple sclerosis after disease-modifying therapy: a randomised controlled phase 3 trial. Lancet. 2012;380(9856): 1829–39.
36. Kalincik T, et al. Treatment effectiveness of alemtuzumab compared with natalizumab, fingolimod, and interferon beta in relapsing-remitting multiple sclerosis: a cohort study. Lancet Neurol. 2017;16(4):271–81.
37. Bruck W. The pathology of multiple sclerosis is the result of focal inflammatory demyelination with axonal damage. J Neurol. 2005;252(Suppl 5):v3–9.
38. Lucchinetti C, et al. Heterogeneity of multiple sclerosis lesions: implications for the pathogenesis of demyelination. Ann Neurol. 2000;47(6):707–17.
39. Hohlfeld R, Wekerle H. Immunological update on multiple sclerosis. Curr Opin Neurol. 2001;14(3):299–304.
40. Hohlfeld R, Wekerle H. Autoimmune concepts of multiple sclerosis as a basis for selective immunotherapy: from pipe dreams to (therapeutic) pipelines. Proc Natl Acad Sci U S A. 2004;101(Suppl 2):14599–606.
41. Gold R, Linington C, Lassmann H. Understanding pathogenesis and therapy of multiple sclerosis via animal models: 70 years of merits and culprits in experimental autoimmune encephalomyelitis research. Brain. 2006;129(Pt 8):1953–71.
42. Matusevicius D, et al. Interleukin-17 mRNA expression in blood and CSF mononuclear cells is augmented in multiple sclerosis. Mult Scler. 1999;5(2):101–4.
43. Bettini M, Vignali DA. Regulatory T cells and inhibitory cytokines in autoimmunity. Curr Opin Immunol. 2009;21(6):612–8.
44. Neumann H, et al. Induction of MHC class I genes in neurons. Science. 1995;269(5223):549–52.
45. Medana I, et al. Transection of major histocompatibility complex class I-induced neurites by cytotoxic T lymphocytes. Am J Pathol. 2001;159(3):809–15.
46. Lennon VA, et al. A serum autoantibody marker of neuromyelitis optica: distinction from multiple sclerosis. Lancet. 2004;364(9451):2106–12.
47. Mathey EK, et al. Neurofascin as a novel target for autoantibody-mediated axonal injury. J Exp Med. 2007;204(10):2363–72.
48. Howell OW, et al. Disruption of neurofascin localization reveals early changes preceding demyelination and remyelination in multiple sclerosis. Brain. 2006;129(Pt 12):3173–85.
49. Bartos A, et al. Elevated intrathecal antibodies against the medium neurofilament subunit in multiple sclerosis. J Neurol. 2007;254(1):20–5.
50. Teunissen CE, Dijkstra C, Polman C. Biological markers in CSF and blood for axonal degeneration in multiple sclerosis. Lancet Neurol. 2005;4(1):32–41.
51. Choi SR, et al. Meningeal inflammation plays a role in the pathology of primary progressive multiple sclerosis. Brain. 2012;135(Pt 10):2925–37.
52. Howell OW, et al. Meningeal inflammation is widespread and linked to cortical pathology in multiple sclerosis. Brain. 2011;134(Pt 9):2755–71.

53. Magliozzi R, et al. Meningeal B-cell follicles in secondary progressive multiple sclerosis associate with early onset of disease and severe cortical pathology. Brain. 2007;130(Pt 4):1089–104.
54. Montalban X, et al. Ocrelizumab versus placebo in primary progressive multiple sclerosis. N Engl J Med. 2017;376(3):209–20.
55. Hauser SL, et al. Ocrelizumab versus interferon beta-1a in relapsing multiple sclerosis. N Engl J Med. 2017;376(3):221–34.
56. Smith KJ, Lassmann H. The role of nitric oxide in multiple sclerosis. Lancet Neurol. 2002;1(4):232–41.
57. Bagasra O, et al. Activation of the inducible form of nitric oxide synthase in the brains of patients with multiple sclerosis. Proc Natl Acad Sci U S A. 1995;92(26):12041–5.
58. Hill KE, et al. Inducible nitric oxide synthase in chronic active multiple sclerosis plaques: distribution, cellular expression and association with myelin damage. J Neuroimmunol. 2004;151(1–2):171–9.
59. Gray E, et al. Peroxisome proliferator-activated receptor-alpha agonists protect cortical neurons from inflammatory mediators and improve peroxisomal function. Eur J Neurosci. 2011;33(8):1421–32.
60. Gibbons HM, Dragunow M. Microglia induce neural cell death via a proximity-dependent mechanism involving nitric oxide. Brain Res. 2006;1084(1):1–15.
61. Smith KJ, et al. Electrically active axons degenerate when exposed to nitric oxide. Ann Neurol. 2001;49(4):470–6.
62. Kapoor R, et al. Blockers of sodium and calcium entry protect axons from nitric oxide-mediated degeneration. Ann Neurol. 2003;53(2):174–80.
63. Ghatan S, et al. p38 MAP kinase mediates bax translocation in nitric oxide-induced apoptosis in neurons. J Cell Biol. 2000;150(2):335–47.
64. Bal-Price A, Brown GC. Inflammatory neurodegeneration mediated by nitric oxide from activated glia-inhibiting neuronal respiration, causing glutamate release and excitotoxicity. J Neurosci. 2001;21(17):6480–91.
65. Golde S, et al. Different pathways for iNOS-mediated toxicity in vitro dependent on neuronal maturation and NMDA receptor expression. J Neurochem. 2002;82(2):269–82.
66. Brown GC, Borutaite V. Nitric oxide inhibition of mitochondrial respiration and its role in cell death. Free Radic Biol Med. 2002;33(11):1440–50.
67. Wilkins A, Compston A. Trophic factors attenuate nitric oxide mediated neuronal and axonal injury in vitro: roles and interactions of mitogen-activated protein kinase signalling pathways. J Neurochem. 2005;92(6):1487–96.
68. Hares K, et al. Neurofilament dot blot assays: novel means of assessing axon viability in culture. J Neurosci Methods. 2011;198(2):195–203.
69. Calabrese V, et al. Nitric oxide synthase is present in the cerebrospinal fluid of patients with active multiple sclerosis and is associated with increases in cerebrospinal fluid protein nitrotyrosine and S-nitrosothiols and with changes in glutathione levels. J Neurosci Res. 2002;70(4):580–7.
70. Calabresi PA, et al. Cytokine gene expression in cells derived from CSF of multiple sclerosis patients. J Neuroimmunol. 1998;89(1–2):198–205.
71. Hofman FM, et al. Tumor necrosis factor identified in multiple sclerosis brain. J Exp Med. 1989;170(2):607–12.
72. Rieckmann P, et al. Tumor necrosis factor-alpha messenger RNA expression in patients with relapsing-remitting multiple sclerosis is associated with disease activity. Ann Neurol. 1995;37(1):82–8.
73. Jurewicz A, et al. Tumour necrosis factor-induced death of adult human oligodendrocytes is mediated by apoptosis inducing factor. Brain. 2005;128(Pt 11):2675–88.
74. Liu J, et al. TNF is a potent anti-inflammatory cytokine in autoimmune-mediated demyelination. Nat Med. 1998;4(1):78–83.
75. TNF neutralization in MS: results of a randomized, placebo-controlled multicenter study. The Lenercept Multiple Sclerosis Study Group and The University of British Columbia MS/MRI Analysis Group. Neurology. 1999;53(3):457–65.

76. van Oosten BW, et al. Increased MRI activity and immune activation in two multiple sclerosis patients treated with the monoclonal anti-tumor necrosis factor antibody cA2. Neurology. 1996;47(6):1531–4.
77. Hohlfeld R, et al. The neuroprotective effect of inflammation: implications for the therapy of multiple sclerosis. Neurol Sci. 2006;27(Suppl 1):S1–7.
78. Stadelmann C, et al. BDNF and gp145trkB in multiple sclerosis brain lesions: neuroprotective interactions between immune and neuronal cells? Brain. 2002;125(Pt 1):75–85.
79. Jones JL, et al. Improvement in disability after alemtuzumab treatment of multiple sclerosis is associated with neuroprotective autoimmunity. Brain. 2010;133(Pt 8):2232–47.
80. Foote AK, Blakemore WF. Inflammation stimulates remyelination in areas of chronic demyelination. Brain. 2005;128(Pt 3):528–39.
81. Brady ST, et al. Formation of compact myelin is required for maturation of the axonal cytoskeleton. J Neurosci. 1999;19(17):7278–88.
82. Sanchez I, et al. Local control of neurofilament accumulation during radial growth of myelinating axons in vivo. Selective role of site-specific phosphorylation. J Cell Biol. 2000;151(5):1013–24.
83. Kirkpatrick LL, et al. Changes in microtubule stability and density in myelin-deficient shiverer mouse CNS axons. J Neurosci. 2001;21(7):2288–97.
84. Griffiths I, et al. Axonal swellings and degeneration in mice lacking the major proteolipid of myelin. Science. 1998;280(5369):1610–3.
85. Edgar JM, et al. Age-related axonal and myelin changes in the rumpshaker mutation of the Plp gene. Acta Neuropathol. 2004;107(4):331–5.
86. Yin X, et al. Evolution of a neuroprotective function of central nervous system myelin. J Cell Biol. 2006;172(3):469–78.
87. Lappe-Siefke C, et al. Disruption of Cnp1 uncouples oligodendroglial functions in axonal support and myelination. Nat Genet. 2003;33(3):366–74.
88. Wilkins A, et al. Slowly progressive axonal degeneration in a rat model of chronic, nonimmune-mediated demyelination. J Neuropathol Exp Neurol. 2010;69(12):1256–69.
89. Irvine KA, Blakemore WF. Remyelination protects axons from demyelination-associated axon degeneration. Brain. 2008;131(Pt 6):1464–77.
90. Yool DA, et al. The proteolipid protein gene and myelin disorders in man and animal models. Hum Mol Genet. 2000;9(6):987–92.
91. Garbern JY, et al. Patients lacking the major CNS myelin protein, proteolipid protein 1, develop length-dependent axonal degeneration in the absence of demyelination and inflammation. Brain. 2002;125(Pt 3):551–61.
92. Bonavita S, et al. Evidence for neuroaxonal injury in patients with proteolipid protein gene mutations. Neurology. 2001;56(6):785–8.
93. Uncini A, Kuwabara S. Nodopathies of the peripheral nerve: an emerging concept. J Neurol Neurosurg Psychiatry. 2015;86(11):1186–95.
94. Craner MJ, et al. Co-localization of sodium channel Nav1.6 and the sodium-calcium exchanger at sites of axonal injury in the spinal cord in EAE. Brain. 2004;127(Pt 2):294–303.
95. Kaplan MR, et al. Induction of sodium channel clustering by oligodendrocytes. Nature. 1997;386(6626):724–8.
96. Rasband MN, et al. Dysregulation of axonal sodium channel isoforms after adult-onset chronic demyelination. J Neurosci Res. 2003;73(4):465–70.
97. Craner MJ, et al. Molecular changes in neurons in multiple sclerosis: altered axonal expression of Nav1.2 and Nav1.6 sodium channels and Na^+/Ca^{2+} exchanger. Proc Natl Acad Sci U S A. 2004;101(21):8168–73.
98. Kapoor R, et al. Lamotrigine for neuroprotection in secondary progressive multiple sclerosis: a randomised, double-blind, placebo-controlled, parallel-group trial. Lancet Neurol. 2010;9(7):681–8.
99. Raftopoulos R, et al. Phenytoin for neuroprotection in patients with acute optic neuritis: a randomised, placebo-controlled, phase 2 trial. Lancet Neurol. 2016;15(3):259–69.

100. Olsen NK, et al. Leber's hereditary optic neuropathy associated with a disorder indistinguishable from multiple sclerosis in a male harbouring the mitochondrial DNA 11778 mutation. Acta Neurol Scand. 1995;91(5):326–9.
101. Lu F, et al. Oxidative damage to mitochondrial DNA and activity of mitochondrial enzymes in chronic active lesions of multiple sclerosis. J Neurol Sci. 2000;177(2):95–103.
102. Mahad DJ, et al. Mitochondrial changes within axons in multiple sclerosis. Brain. 2009;132(Pt 5):1161–74.
103. Dutta R, et al. Mitochondrial dysfunction as a cause of axonal degeneration in multiple sclerosis patients. Ann Neurol. 2006;59(3):478–89.
104. Campbell GR, et al. Mitochondrial DNA deletions and neurodegeneration in multiple sclerosis. Ann Neurol. 2011;69(3):481–92.
105. Kim JY, et al. HDAC1 nuclear export induced by pathological conditions is essential for the onset of axonal damage. Nat Neurosci. 2010;13(2):180–9.
106. Stys PK. White matter injury mechanisms. Curr Mol Med. 2004;4(2):113–30.
107. McDermott CJ, et al. Hereditary spastic paraparesis: disrupted intracellular transport associated with spastin mutation. Ann Neurol. 2003;54(6):748–59.
108. Hirokawa N, Niwa S, Tanaka Y. Molecular motors in neurons: transport mechanisms and roles in brain function, development, and disease. Neuron. 2010;68(4):610–38.
109. Xia CH, et al. Abnormal neurofilament transport caused by targeted disruption of neuronal kinesin heavy chain KIF5A. J Cell Biol. 2003;161(1):55–66.
110. Crimella C, et al. Mutations in the motor and stalk domains of KIF5A in spastic paraplegia type 10 and in axonal Charcot-Marie-Tooth type 2. Clin Genet. 2012;82(2):157–64.
111. Hares K, et al. Reduced axonal motor protein expression in non-lesional grey matter in multiple sclerosis. Mult Scler. 2014;20(7):812–21.
112. Hares K, et al. Axonal motor protein KIF5A and associated cargo deficits in multiple sclerosis lesional and normal-appearing white matter. Neuropathol Appl Neurobiol. 2017;43(3):227–41.
113. International Multiple Sclerosis Genetics Consortium, et al. Analysis of immune-related loci identifies 48 new susceptibility variants for multiple sclerosis. Nat Genet. 2013;45(11):1353–60.
114. Alcina A, et al. Identification of a functional variant in the KIF5A-CYP27B1-METTL1-FAM119B locus associated with multiple sclerosis. J Med Genet. 2013;50(1):25–33.
115. Goris A, et al. Replication of KIF21B as a susceptibility locus for multiple sclerosis. J Med Genet. 2010;47(11):775–6.
116. Kreft KL, et al. Abundant kif21b is associated with accelerated progression in neurodegenerative diseases. Acta Neuropathol Commun. 2014;2:144.
117. Booth DR, et al. Lack of support for association between the KIF1B rs10492972[C] variant and multiple sclerosis. Nat Genet. 2010;42(6):469–70. author reply 470-1
118. Lyons DA, et al. Kif1b is essential for mRNA localization in oligodendrocytes and development of myelinated axons. Nat Genet. 2009;41(7):854–8.
119. Meinl E, Hohlfeld R. Immunopathogenesis of multiple sclerosis: MBP and beyond. Clin Exp Immunol. 2002;128(3):395–7.
120. Sorbara CD, et al. Pervasive axonal transport deficits in multiple sclerosis models. Neuron. 2014;84(6):1183–90.
121. Redondo J, et al. Purkinje cell pathology and loss in multiple sclerosis cerebellum. Brain Pathol. 2014;25(6):692–700.
122. Holmgren A, Bouhy D, Timmerman V. Neurofilament phosphorylation and their proline-directed kinases in health and disease. J Peripher Nerv Syst. 2012;17(4):365–76.
123. Lariviere RC, Julien JP. Functions of intermediate filaments in neuronal development and disease. J Neurobiol. 2004;58(1):131–48.
124. Shea TB, Jung C, Pant HC. Does neurofilament phosphorylation regulate axonal transport? Trends Neurosci. 2003;26(8):397–400.
125. Goldstein ME, et al. Phosphorylation of neurofilament proteins and chromatolysis following transection of rat sciatic nerve. J Neurosci. 1987;7(5):1586–94.

126. Petzold A, et al. Phosphorylation and compactness of neurofilaments in multiple sclerosis: indicators of axonal pathology. Exp Neurol. 2008;213(2):326–35.
127. Schirmer L, et al. Axonal loss and neurofilament phosphorylation changes accompany lesion development and clinical progression in multiple sclerosis. Brain Pathol. 2011;21(4):428–40.
128. Gray E, et al. Accumulation of cortical hyperphosphorylated neurofilaments as a marker of neurodegeneration in multiple sclerosis. Mult Scler. 2013;19(2):153–61.
129. Rudrabhatla P. Regulation of neuronal cytoskeletal protein phosphorylation in neurodegenerative diseases. J Alzheimers Dis. 2014;41(3):671–84.
130. Liu Q, et al. Neurofilamentopathy in neurodegenerative diseases. Open Neurol J. 2011;5: 58–62.
131. Strong MJ, et al. Phosphorylation state of the native high-molecular-weight neurofilament subunit protein from cervical spinal cord in sporadic amyotrophic lateral sclerosis. J Neurochem. 2001;76(5):1315–25.
132. Vickers JC, et al. Alterations in neurofilament protein immunoreactivity in human hippocampal neurons related to normal aging and Alzheimer's disease. Neuroscience. 1994;62(1):1–13.
133. Maccioni RB, et al. The protein kinase Cdk5. Structural aspects, roles in neurogenesis and involvement in Alzheimer's pathology. Eur J Biochem. 2001;268(6):1518–27.
134. Vickers JC, et al. Dystrophic neurite formation associated with age-related beta amyloid deposition in the neocortex: clues to the genesis of neurofibrillary pathology. Exp Neurol. 1996;141(1):1–11.
135. Dickson TC, et al. Neurochemical diversity of dystrophic neurites in the early and late stages of Alzheimer's disease. Exp Neurol. 1999;156(1):100–10.
136. Petzold A. Neurofilament phosphoforms: surrogate markers for axonal injury, degeneration and loss. J Neurol Sci. 2005;233(1–2):183–98.
137. Ganesalingam J, et al. pNfH is a promising biomarker for ALS. Amyotroph Lateral Scler Frontotemporal Degener. 2013;14(2):146–9.
138. Stadelmann C, et al. Cortical pathology in multiple sclerosis. Curr Opin Neurol. 2008;21(3):229–34.
139. Kutzelnigg A, et al. Cortical demyelination and diffuse white matter injury in multiple sclerosis. Brain. 2005;128(Pt 11):2705–12.
140. Peterson JW, et al. Transected neurites, apoptotic neurons, and reduced inflammation in cortical multiple sclerosis lesions. Ann Neurol. 2001;50(3):389–400.
141. Serafini B, et al. Detection of ectopic B-cell follicles with germinal centers in the meninges of patients with secondary progressive multiple sclerosis. Brain Pathol. 2004;14(2):164–74.
142. Kooi EJ, et al. Meningeal inflammation is not associated with cortical demyelination in chronic multiple sclerosis. J Neuropathol Exp Neurol. 2009;68(9):1021–8.
143. Ascherio A, Munger KL. Epstein-barr virus infection and multiple sclerosis: a review. J Neuroimmune Pharmacol. 2010;5(3):271–7.
144. Gilgun-Sherki Y, et al. Riluzole suppresses experimental autoimmune encephalomyelitis: implications for the treatment of multiple sclerosis. Brain Res. 2003;989(2):196–204.
145. Black JA, et al. Long-term protection of central axons with phenytoin in monophasic and chronic-relapsing EAE. Brain. 2006;129(Pt 12):3196–208.
146. Zajicek JP, Apostu VI. Role of cannabinoids in multiple sclerosis. CNS Drugs. 2011;25(3):187–201.
147. Zajicek J, et al. Effect of dronabinol on progression in progressive multiple sclerosis (CUPID): a randomised, placebo-controlled trial. Lancet Neurol. 2013;12(9):857–65.
148. Chataway J, et al. Effect of high-dose simvastatin on brain atrophy and disability in secondary progressive multiple sclerosis (MS-STAT): a randomised, placebo-controlled, phase 2 trial. Lancet. 2014;383(9936):2213–21.

Chapter 5
Imaging Disease Progression

Declan Chard and Olga Ciccarelli

5.1 Introduction

In this chapter we will consider how imaging techniques can be used to assess disease progression in progressive multiple sclerosis (MS). Given its dominance in the field our main focus will be on magnetic resonance imaging (MRI), but we will also touch on optical coherence tomography (OCT), a technique that continues to develop potentially useful measures of neurodegeneration.

MRI already has an established role in the diagnosis of MS [1], helping to exclude other causes of neurological symptoms whilst demonstrating the dissemination in space and time of typical MS lesions. Additionally, MRI is routinely used to assess disease activity and treatment response in patients treated with disease modifying-treatments (DMTs) [2]. This assessment focuses on the counting of the brain T2 lesions. Other important MRI features, which may reflect pathological changes contributing to disease progression, such as brain and spinal cord atrophy, are not routinely assessed in clinical practice.

While obtaining the high-resolution scans needed for atrophy measures is achievable on clinical MRI scanners, the complex image processing required to extract brain and spinal cord volume measurements (in addition to the variability in the measurements related to MRI hardware and acquisition protocol) limit their application beyond research and treatment trials. Although brain volume measurements are not ready for use in clinical practice, in light of recent and

D. Chard (✉) • O. Ciccarelli
Queen Square MS Centre, Department of Neuroinflammation, UCL Institute of Neurology, University College London (UCL), London, UK

National Institute for Health Research (NIHR), University College London Hospitals (UCLH), Biomedical Research Centre, London, UK
e-mail: d.chard@ucl.ac.uk

A. Wilkins (ed.), *Progressive Multiple Sclerosis*,
https://doi.org/10.1007/978-3-319-65921-3_5

encouraging results from treatment trials in progressive MS, it is likely that longitudinal atrophy assessments will increasingly be used as a marker of progression. Two phase III trials (siponimod in secondary progressive [SP] MS [3] and ocrelizumab in primary progressive [PP] MS [4]) have proven positive, and there have been further promising phase II results (simvastatin [5] and lipoic acid [6]) which have shown significant reductions in the rate of brain atrophy measure using MRI. Together, these findings provide good clinical reasons to more reliably identify progressive MS early on and to more sensitively monitor progression, and MRI may have a role to play in this.

5.2 Background

5.2.1 What Is Progressive MS?

When considering how to image disease progression in MS, it is useful to first understand what we mean by progressive MS, how this relates to relapsing-remitting (RR) disease, and progressive neurological disability.

While this book focuses on progressive MS, it is not so straightforward to separate it from relapsing remitting (RR) disease either clinically or pathologically. The transition from RR to secondary progressive (SP) MS is not clear-cut, with a gradual reduction in relapse rates and background clinical progression often taking several years to become apparent. This is reflected in the Lublin and Reingold [7] consensus criteria for SPMS that explicitly allow for on-going relapses. Comparing primary progressive (PP) MS with SPMS, other than the preceding RR phase seen in the latter, clinically they are similar: the age of onset of progression does not differ greatly between them [8], and people with an SP or PP course reach disability milestones at only marginally different ages [9]. However, people with PPMS do appear to have lower brain lesion loads when compared with people with other forms of MS [10]. This suggests that brain lesions, as seen on conventional MRI scans such as T2-weighted (T2w) images, play a lesser role determining longer-term disease progression in PP compared with RR or SPMS, but also serves to highlight the relatively weak association between lesion accrual and disability. Even in RR and SP disease lesion load seems to be less closely related to disability than brain or cord atrophy [11–14]. Since the differences in imaging measures and clinical progression between SPMS and PPMS appear to be relative rather than absolute, the two progressive forms of MS may be considered together, as suggested by Lublin et al. [15].

Diagnosing progressive MS relies on what a patient notices and clinician can readily detect, and is therefore biased towards impairment of limb function. The expanded disability status scale (EDSS [16]) pragmatically recognises this, and is heavily weighted towards walking deficits, particularly in the upper two thirds of the scale. However, there is no agreed definition of what constitutes progressive MS, or MS progression, based on EDSS scores. Recently Lorschieder and colleagues [17] looked at defining SPMS using data from over 17,000 people with MS. They tested

576 definitions of SPMS, based on combinations of EDSS and functional scores, against consensus diagnoses reached by independent raters. The best performing required a minimum EDSS score of 4 and pyramidal functional score of 2 and (in the absence of a relapse) progression of 1 EDSS point in those with an EDSS score at or below 5.5, of 0.5 EDSS points in those with a score above this, confirmed over at least 3 months. This definition achieved 87% accuracy. Lowering the minimum EDSS score to 3 required confirmation of progression over 2 years in order to achieve the same accuracy. This highlights the complexity of trying to define progressive MS, and that the threshold for doing so accurately is higher in people with lower levels of disability. In addition, it is clear the effects of MS are not limited the domains that mostly drive progression through the EDSS, for example there are extensive cognitive abnormalities in people with MS [18], and these may be detected early in the course of the disease and are more marked in progressive MS [19]. Defining how much cognitive disability is related to relapses and how much to background progression is difficult, as cognitive relapses are not commonly reported and are difficult to characterise. It is also interesting to note that relapses that are not primarily cognitive in nature may be associated with cognitive changes [20].

Pathologically, the processes observed in RRMS appear to be present in progressive disease, albeit perhaps with different weighting. However, there have been few histopathology studies comparing different phases of the disease, given that *post mortem* material is usually obtained from people long-standing progressive disease or biopsy material from people with unusual MS presentations. With regard to demyelination, while active lesions (and associated acute axonal injury) appear more prominent in early (mostly RR) MS, both have been seen in longer duration progressive disease [21]. Grey matter (GM) demyelination is increasingly recognised as a pathologically important element of MS, and is also seen in both RR and progressive MS: Bo et al. found the extent of GM appearing to be demyelinated in PPMS was about 37%, SP 23% and RR 16%; in contrast WM demyelination in PP was about 3%, SP 8% and RR 8% respectively [22]. In the same study, Bo et al. also noted that lesions did not occur consistently throughout the cortex, but instead nearly 70% occurred in the subpial layers (adjacent to the outer surface of the brain). Interestingly, subpial lesions have been linked with overlying meningeal inflammation [23], and this too is seen in both progressive MS [23] and RRMS [24]. Neurodegeneration is thought to be a, if not the, major substrate of irreversible disability in MS. Axonal transection is seen in WM [25] and GM lesions [26], and neuronal loss has been observed in lesional and extra-lesional cortical GM [27].

MRI markers of pathology also seem broadly consistent with this. WM lesion accrual does not necessarily stop in people who develop SPMS [11], and is seen in progressive onset MS [28]. Similarly, while GM lesion accrual may be greater in progressive MS, it is seen in RRMS [29]. Brain atrophy (and GM in particular) can also be readily seen in people with progressive MS, may [30] or may not [31] accelerate in those with SP compared with RRMS, and is already detectable from the earliest stages of the disease [32, 33]. Considered overall, these studies suggest that differentiating clinical subtypes of MS on histopathological or MRI grounds alone is not possible (or at least unlikely to be reliable) using currently available techniques, and that pathological progression on MRI does not directly equate to a progressive clinical course.

5.2.2 When Does Progression Start?

There is the potential for a significant latent period between the first occurrence of pathology and its ultimate effect on function. For example, while the formation of an MS lesion in a clinically eloquent location may be closely associated with symptom onset, subsequent axonal loss within the lesion and the neurological impairments it causes may take months or years to occur. Frischer et al. noted that axonal loss occurred mostly in the context of active inflammation even in progressive disease [34], however on-going axonal loss still occurs in chronically demyelinated plaques [35]. From MRI it has been noted that brain atrophy, a putative marker of neurodegeneration [36], occurs throughout the course of the disease, is only partly related to white matter (WM) lesion loads (for example [33, 37, 38]), and that there may be a delay of several years between WM lesion formation and subsequent brain atrophy [39]. This raises the possibility that inflammatory activity can have a rapidly apparent clinical effect early on but its greatest overall impact on neurological function in the longer term.

The potential for a significant interval between a pathological event and its ultimate consequences is important when considering the use of MRI as a tool for assessing disease progression. For example, MRI brain scans will show lesions of different ages: in some of these lesions inflammatory activity and healing may not yet have finished, and in other apparently inactive lesions on-going axonal degeneration may be gradually progressing. As such, looking at cross-sectional or short-term longitudinal associations between MRI measures and clinical outcomes may give a falsely pessimistic assessment of the strength of link between them.

5.2.3 Purpose of an Imaging Marker

MRI can broadly be used in four ways in MS: As an aid to diagnosis; as a marker of current disease activity; as a predictor of future clinical outcomes; and as an indicator of treatment effectiveness. We will not consider its role in diagnosis further here, as this aspect is covered elsewhere in this book. As a marker of current activity, MRI has a firmly established place in clinical trials. New brain lesion accrual is often used as a measure of MS disease activity, particularly in RRMS trials, and the suppression of lesion formation used as evidence of efficacy in treatment trials (for example [40]). More recently, MRI measures of brain atrophy have been included as endpoints in treatment trials, and primary outcomes in early phase trials, for example, in the lamotrigine, simvastatin and multi-arm MS SMART studies in SPMS [41, 5, 42] and ocrelizumab in PPMS [4]. As a predictor of longer-term outcomes, there is some evidence to suggest that brain WM lesion loads and atrophy are relevant, however MRI measures of these are only partly related to long-term clinical outcomes [11, 12], and are not currently able to offer robust patient specific prognostic information. We explore this in greater detail below.

5.2.4 *Cross-Sectional and Serial Studies*

While cross-sectional work cannot directly assess progression, it can do so indirectly by looking for correlations with disease duration. When compared with longitudinal studies, cross-sectional work is intrinsically less time consuming, less vulnerable to measurement drift (i.e. the variation measures due to changes in instrument performance), and more likely to be achieved with the same clinical team and equipment. However, when compared with longitudinal studies, in situations where the measurement of interest varies significantly between people, as for example may brain tissue volumes, cross-sectional studies can be less sensitive to progressive disease effects as inter-subject variability overwhelms them (Fig. 5.1).

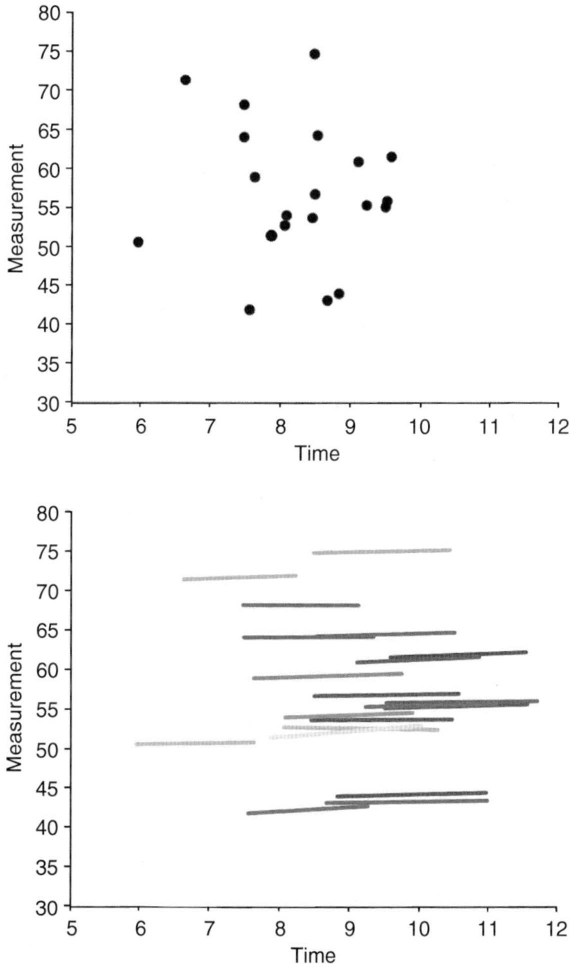

Fig. 5.1 Simulated data demonstrating how cross-sectional data (*top*) may not reveal an association (in this case positive) with time that is clearly seen with longitudinal data (*bottom*). Measurement values are simulated to represent a normal distribution with a positive disease duration effect in both cross-sectional and longitudinal data

5.2.5 *Pathological Specificity of MRI Measures*

Current MRI measures are not pathologically specific. They may be regarded as being weighted towards one process more than another, but they are not absolute measures. This is due to a combination of factors, some imaging and others tissue related.

Firstly, the imaging methods themselves are tuned to produce scans with good contrast, high resolution and limited artefacts, rather than quantifying a particular tissue characteristic. So T2w scans are not usually described as T2-scans, because they are also influenced by other factors such as T1 relaxation times (RT), proton density (PD), scanner magnetic and radiofrequency field homogeneity. There is a move within research to use MRI techniques that measure a particular feature and generate a quantitative image, so for example, T2 RT maps can be produced that provide a measure of the T2 RT at a given point; in contrast a T2w scan produces an image where the brightness of a point gives an indication of its relative, but not its actual, T2 RT.

Secondly, multiple pathological processes can affect the same MRI parameter. For example T2 RT are related to axonal and myelin densities (sharing ~60% variability) [43], although as axonal and myelin densities are also correlated (also sharing ~60% variability), it is not possible to determine if T2 RT are determined by axonal or myelin densities, or both. Similarly, magnetisation transfer ratio (MTR) measures, while sensitive to myelin density in WM (and so a leading contender as an imaging outcome measure in trials of agents that may promote remyelination [44]), are also correlated with axonal counts and gliosis (myelin density ~70% shared variability, axonal counts ~45% and gliosis ~10%) [45].

5.3 The MRI Toolkit

MRI relies on the properties of atoms in magnetic fields and how they react when disturbed by electromagnetic (radiofrequency) pulses. While most images obtained in clinical practice are based on the signal from hydrogen in water, using proton spectroscopy other molecules can be assessed, for example N-acetyl-aspartate which is found mostly in neurons and their axonal projections [46]. It is also possible to use other atoms as the basis of MRI, such as phosphorus and sodium, but due to their much lower abundance in tissues, the signal they produce is far weaker than that from protons in water, and the resultant images therefore have much lower signal to noise.

There are a variety of MRI methods available to image the brain and spinal cord. These may be broadly divided into four categories: macrostructural, i.e. those that generate anatomical images and allow localisation of lesions, or enable tissue volumes to be measured; microstructural, i.e. those that yield measures of cellular physical features, such as the degree of myelination, or density of axons; molecular, which assess the amount a given molecule within a tissue for example glutamate and glutamine, or lactate; and metabolic (including functional MRI), which assess features such as tissue blood flow and oxygen extraction. There has been some cross-sectional work demonstrating functional MRI [47–50] and perfusion [51–53] abnormalities in progressive MS, and the few longitudinal MRI studies in MS that have been undertaken have been in RRMS [54], and so the dynamics and prognostic significance of these measures in progressive MS is unknown. As such, it is not possible to determine their role predicting or monitoring progressive MS, and we will not consider them further in this chapter.

5.3.1 Conventional Structural Scans

Conventional MRI scans generate anatomical images and are tuned to maximise tissue contrast and make abnormalities obvious. In the case of brain and spinal cord imaging in MS, routine clinical and research scans include T1w and T2w images, and fluid-attenuated inversion recovery (FLAIR, which only provides useable images in the brain, not the spinal cord) sequences which suppress signal from CSF (Fig. 5.2). Lesions can be counted and their volume measured. Lesion counts are usually achieved manually, while lesion volumes are most often measured using a semi-automated lesion contouring method, for example [55], although automated methods have been developed [56].

In the cerebral hemispheres hyperintense WM lesions are more visible on FLAIR than T2w scans [57], while only a subset of lesions seen on T2w images are also apparent as hypointensities on T1w images (for example [58]). Interestingly, lesions seen on T1w scans may be more destructive than those observed on T2w scans alone [59], although correlations with EDSS scores are not markedly different [60]. Gadolinium (Gd) contrast can be given intravenously to demonstrate areas where there is breakdown in the blood brain barrier, and on monthly scans identifies about twice as many active (new or enlarging) lesions than does FLAIR or T2w imaging [57]. There is some uncertainty as to the frequency of Gd-enhancing lesions in PP when compared with RR and SPMS, as both disease subtype and disease duration may be relevant (discussed below).

GM is extensively demyelinated in MS, but until recently it has proven very difficult to see this using MRI. Conventional MRI techniques such as PD/T2w and FLAIR imaging are able to detect the majority of WM lesions (about 70% prospectively) but only a minority of GM lesions (on FLAIR about 5% of those confined to the cortex (intracortical), and 40% of those that also involve adjacent WM) [61]. This considerable difference has led to a search for other MRI methods optimised to image GM lesions, with double inversion recovery (DIR) currently (as of 2017) the most widely accepted technique. DIR is similar to FLAIR, suppressing signal from CSF, but in addition nulls signal from the WM, leaving GM most visible. GM lesions appear bright on such a scan (Fig. 5.3). However, while improving on FLAIR, DIR increases the detection intracortical GM lesions by about 150% and mixed GM-WM lesions by 30% [62], implying that it still does not identify the majority of such plaques. A combined histopathological MRI study has confirmed

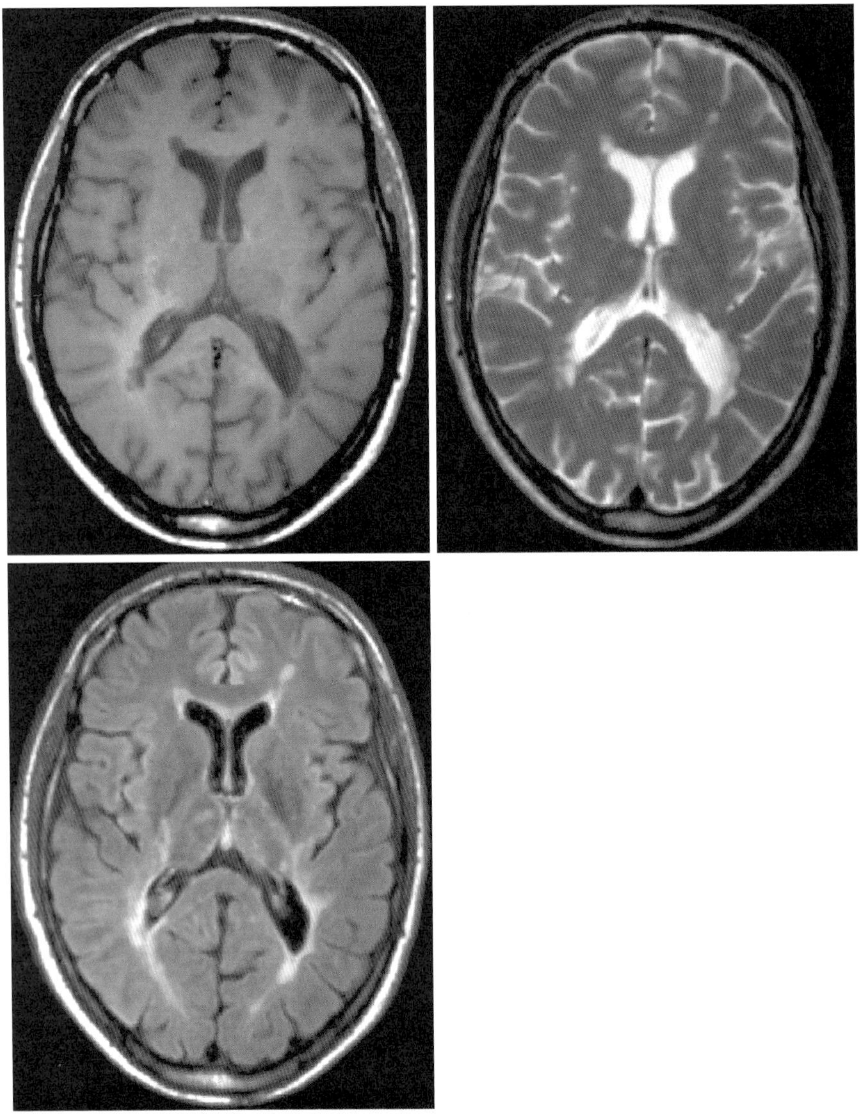

Fig. 5.2 Matched axial slices through the cerebrum on (from *top left* clockwise) T1-weighted, T2-weighted and FLAIR scans. While MS lesions are more conspicuous on FLAIR, they are usually also seen on T2-weighted scans. In contrast, not all lesions seen on the FLAIR or T2-weighted scan are visible on the T1-weighted images

the relatively low sensitivity of DIR for intracortical GM lesions, with about 10% detected prospectively, while in contrast about ~80% of mixed GM-WM lesions were seen [63]. To improve on this further, phase sensitive inversion recovery (PSIR) imaging was first used to increase the confidence of GM lesion detection on

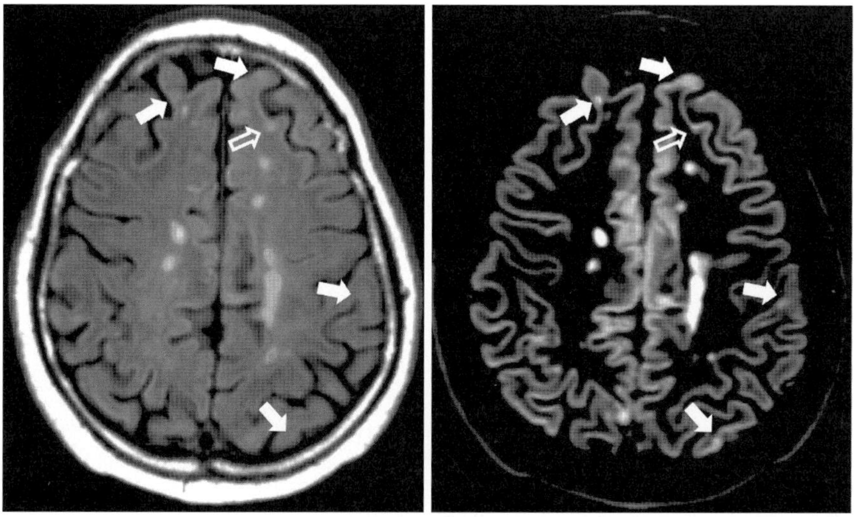

Fig. 5.3 Matched axial slices through the cerebrum on FLAIR (*left*) and DIR (*right*). While some cortical lesions are seen on FLAIR, about 40% more are detected on DIR. The *open arrow* marks a cortical lesion seen on both scans, the *full arrows* lesions clearly seen on DIR, but less readily so on FLAIR

DIR [64], and more recently on its own [65]. Despite the limited sensitivity of MRI to cortical lesions, they are still usually seen in people with SPMS using DIR, with higher cortical lesion loads found in people with SP when compared with RRMS (mean 11.3 compared with 5.4) [66]. We discuss this further below.

5.3.2 Atrophy Measures

Measures of brain and spinal cord volumes have proven of great interest in MS as they appear to be more closely related to long-term disability than WM lesion loads [12, 13].

Techniques for assessing brain atrophy can be divided in to those that measure tissue volumes and those that directly assess change without first estimating volumes. Both approaches rely on high-resolution structural imaging (usually a 3D T1-weighted scan with 1 mm^3 resolution). Several brain segmentation techniques have been developed, including SIENA and SIENAX [67], SPM [68, 69], and FreeSurfer [70]. Brain volumes are frequently assessed as fractions of total intracranial volume, usually defined as the sum of GM, WM and CSF. Such measures are less vulnerable to the effects of scanner scaling drift over time, with intra-cranial volume acting as a subject specific reference. Scaling to intracranial volume also reduces inter-subject variability, which in cross-sectional work allows more subtle disease effects to be observed when compared with absolute tissue volumes [36].

Change measures rely on warping one scan to match another, and measuring the amount of distortion required to achieve this [67, 71]. A significant issue in MS brain atrophy measurement is the effect WM lesions have on segmentation. On T1-weighted volumetric images, lesions appear darker than normal-appearing WM, and may be classified as GM or CSF instead. In addition, their presence may subtly distort segmentation of GM and WM boundaries throughout the brain, by making WM appear darker than is truly is. These effects can both be significantly reduced by filling WM lesions with normal-appearing WM [72], and several techniques have now been developed to achieve this either by simulating normal-appearing WM (e.g. [72, 73])or by patch-based sampling of similar but lesion free regions [74]. However, at present this still requires time consuming manual or semi-automated contouring of the lesions on volumetric scans.

Spinal cord atrophy is usually assessed by measuring the cord cross-sectional area rather than volume with segmentation-based methods. There are several reasons for this. Firstly, there is marked inter-subject variability cord segmental lengths, but less noticeable variation in cross-sectional area [75], which means that inter-subject variability in segmental volumes will be greater than segmental areas. Secondly, and more importantly, it is difficult to consistently identify spinal cord segmental levels using MRI, as there are few cord landmarks conspicuous enough to allow this. In comparison, it is relatively easy to locate the boundary between CSF and cord to measure cross-sectional area. Until recently, the most frequently used technique to achieve this relied on semi-automated contouring of a series of axial T1-weighted slices through the cervical cord (centred on C2/3) [76]. More recently, a nearly fully automated method has been developed to shrink wrap the cord in a computer defined mesh, and from this extract measures of cross-sectional area [77, 78]. This active surface method is not only less user-dependent, it also appears to be more reproducible than the established semi-automated technique, and this should translate into greater sensitivity to disease effects. Applying this active surface segmentation method to PSIR, rather than conventional T1-weighted scans, appears to further improve reproducibility [79], and this technique can also be used to measure cord cross sectional area on the cervical cord that is often included in brain scans [80]. Another segmentation-based method fits a Gaussian mixed model to the histogram of the upper cervical cord region to segment the cord and takes partial volume into account; the mean upper cervical cord area (MUCCA) is obtained by dividing the resulting volume by the length of the cord [81]. Further work is needed to develop registration-based methods, which will allow automated calculation of percentage spinal cord area change, similar to the calculation of brain volume change.

5.3.3 Microstructural Imaging

There are currently two main MRI techniques that assess tissue microstructure, magnetisation transfer imaging (MTI) and diffusion tensor imaging (DTI).

MTI uses an indirect method to image protons associated closely with cell membranes. MTI usually takes the form of a magnetisation transfer ratio (MTR) scan, generated from paired T2w scans, one of which has been prepared with a magnetisation transfer pulse that excites bound protons such as those associated with cell membranes. The difference between the paired images provides a measure of the density of bound protons, and so an indication of the density of cell membranes. MTI is of particular interest in MS because it has been found to correlate with myelination [45], albeit with the caveat that it may also be significantly influenced by axonal density (the independence of this is difficult to determine as axonal density and myelination are also correlated [43]).

DTI uses the molecular movement of water in a tissue to determine structural characteristics. It relies upon the principle that water will diffuse more rapidly along cell membranes than through them. A DTI dataset comprises multiple images sensitised to water movement in many directions, and from this information about the direction and extent of water movement at a given location can be extracted. Asymmetry of water diffusion is often measured as fractional anisotropy (FA), i.e. the proportion of molecular water movement along rather than across the main diffusion axis. The magnitude of water diffusion, regardless of direction, is estimated as the mean diffusivity (MD). FA is relatively higher in WM than GM, while MD may be marginally higher in GM than WM (for example [82]), and this reflects underlying tissue architectures: in WM tracts, with their highly ordered myelinated tracts, water diffusion will tend to occur along their axis; in contrast the layered and columnar arrangement of neurons and their dendritic arbour will result in a more complicated diffusion profile, with relatively less directionally consistent diffusion.

5.3.4 MR Spectroscopy

MR Spectroscopy is perhaps the most challenging of the methods described here. It requires careful calibration of a scanner, and given the low concentrations of metabolites when compared with water, obtains data with low signal to noise. As such it is only possible to obtain reliable measurements in large regions (cm^3 compared with mm^3 for the imaging methods outlined above). However, it enables the measurement of brain molecule concentrations in vivo, as such offers a unique perspective on pathology. It relies upon each molecule having a unique fingerprint that can be identified by looking at an MR spectrum (Fig. 5.4). Spectroscopy is not confined to molecules containing protons alone, for example phosphorous spectroscopy is also possible, but to date work in progressive MS has focused on proton spectra.

Only some molecules are present at sufficiently high concentrations to be able to discern spectroscopically. The main peaks visible on proton spectra are creatine and phosphocreatine (Cr), choline containing compounds (Cho), N-acetyl-aspartate (NAA), myo-inositol (Ins), and glutamate with glutamine. Of these Cr is often used as an internal standard, with other molecular concentrations presented as a ratio to it, i.e. Cho/Cr or NAA/Cr ratios. However, this assumes that Cr is unaffected by disease, which may not be the case in MS, and as such there is a move towards

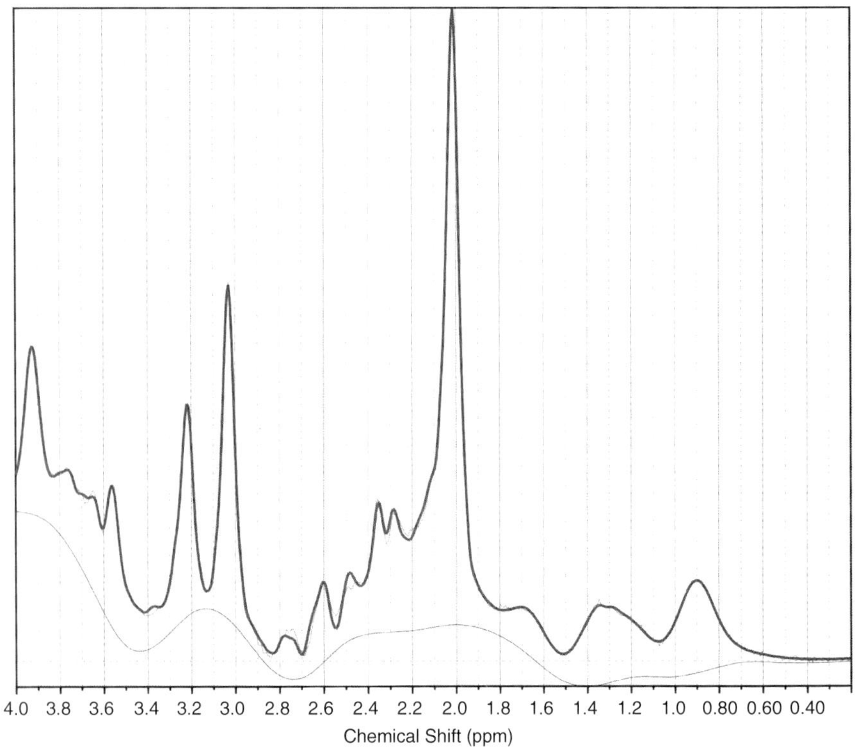

Fig. 5.4 A proton spectrum from a 35 mm^3 PRESS voxel acquired with a echo time of 35 ms and repetition time of 3 s. Overlying this (*solid black line*) are the fitted metabolite peaks from LCModel [91]. The main peak at about 2.0 ppm is N-acetyl-aspartate (found mostly in neurons and their axons), at 3.0 ppm creatine and 3.2 ppm choline. Courtesy of Dr. Bhavana Solanky

absolute quantification of metabolite concentrations, i.e. measures in mmol/L. Of the metabolite mentioned, two are of particular interest as they appear to be relatively cell-specific: NAA, found mostly in neurons and their axonal projections [58], and Ins present in astroglia [83, 84].

5.3.5 *Sodium Imaging*

Most current MRI scans rely on signal from water, but it is possible to obtain images based on other atoms such as sodium. Sodium concentrations are of interest in MS, as it has been proposed the sodium accumulation may in part underly neurodegeneration [85]. Sodium is much less abundant in the tissues than water, and so difficult to use as the basis for an MRI scan, but despite this it has proven possible to obtain sodium images in people with RRMS [86], and more recently it has been shown that sodium concentrations are higher in the brain tissues of people with progressive MS compared with RRMS [87]. However, it is not currently possible to reliably determine if this sodium accumulation is intra- or extra-cellular using clinical scanners, but novel methods at 7T that separate intra- and extra-cellular sodium signals are emerging [88].

5.4 Observing Progression Using MRI

5.4.1 Lesions

While new and contrast enhancing lesions are seen in progressive MS, particularly in SP when compared with PPMS, they appear to be less clinically relevant than in RRMS.

Before looking at this further, it is worth flagging the caveat that estimates of lesion load change vary quite widely between studies even in the same subtype of MS. Taking SPMS as an example: over 1 year Dalton et al. estimated that on average there was a 1.0 mL increase in T2w lesion load in 23 people with SPMS (and a 0.7 mL increase in T2—in 41 people with RRMS, using data from the placebo arm of a Natalizumab trial) [89]; while Ge et al. [90] estimated a median *decrease* of 0.02 mL over a year in nine people with SPMS (and 0.35 mL increase in 27 with RRMS); and Kapoor et al. observed an average yearly increase of 3.6 mL per year in 57 people with SPMS (data from the placebo arm of a trial of lamotrigine) [41]. From this, it can be seen than factors other than the disease subtype may be important determinants of lesion accrual.

Firstly, comparing progressive MS with RR disease, the transition from RR to SP appears to be marked by a deceleration in WM lesion formation. Fisher et al. [30], in a 4 year follow-up study observed an average 1.34 mL increase in T2 lesion load in people with RRMS, 1.06 mL in those in transition to SPMS during this time, and 0.64 mL in people with established SPMS. Interestingly, there was a less clear cut negative gradient for T1 lesions, with mean changes over 4 years of 0.84, 1.88 and 1.01 mL respectively, perhaps hinting at a shift toward lower but more destructive inflammatory activity, or maturation within lesions that have already formed. These observations contrast most starkly with brain atrophy that seems to be at least similar [31], and perhaps accelerates (particularly in GM) [30], from RR through to SPMS (discussed further below).

Turning to differences in new T2-lesion formation in PP and SPMS, Kidd et al. [28] followed up a group of 10 people with PPMS and nine with SPMS over 1 year. They found that while change in expanded disability status scale (EDSS) [16] was similar in both groups (about 1 EDSS point), there were noticeably more new brain T2 lesions in SP compared with PP patients (median 12.4 and 2.0 respectively). Interestingly in this study 95% of the lesions seen in people with SPMS enhanced, compared with 70% in PPMS, although the latter was almost entirely attributable to a single very active PPMS patient, and as such may not be typical (see below). Changes in lesions loads were not found to correlate with change in EDSS, although this is perhaps not surprising given the small cohort and limited progression observed over the year. Over 2 years lesion accrual in 56 people with SPMS was also not found to correlate with EDSS change: when comparing those who clinically progressed (17 subjects, mean EDSS change ~1) with those who did not, increases in lesion load did not significantly differ between groups (4.8 mL versus 6.4 mL respectively) [91]. Similarly, in 41 PPMS patients followed up for 5 years, no associations between T2 lesion accumulation and increasing EDSS were seen, although the increase in disability was small (median 0.5 of an EDSS point) as was lesion accrual (about 1 mL per year) [92].

Considering contrast enhancement with Gd, an early serial study comparing people with established SP and PPMS (mean disease duration 7.8 and 7.0 y respectively), found that over 6 months enhancing lesions were much more common in SP than PPMS patients (mean about 18 new lesions per SPMS patient per year, of which ~80% enhanced, compared with about 3 new lesions per PPMS patient per year, of which ~5% enhanced) [93]. Similarly Silver et al. [94] found that Gd-enhancement was more frequent in SP (~56%, mean disease duration 12 years) than in PPMS (~13%, 9 years). The enhancing lesion rates were found to be similar in another study of people with SPMS (60 patients, enhancing lesions at baseline in 53% and over 3 months new enhancing lesions in 70%) [95]. However in a study of people with early PPMS (mean disease duration 3.3 years from clinical onset) using triple dose Gd dosage, enhancing lesions appeared to be more frequent (~42%) [96]. Overall, this suggests that contrast enhancement is relatively common in SPMS, less frequent in PPMS, and that in PPMS it may be more noticeable earlier rather than later in the course of the disease.

There have now been several studies looking at GM lesion accrual with DIR, and one that has compared this in all MS subtypes over 5 years [29]. In their study, Calabrese and colleagues assessed changes in cortical GM lesion numbers and volumes over 5 years in 157 people with RRMS, 44 with PPMS and 31 with SPMS. They found similar rates of cortical lesion formation (3.3 in RRMS, 3.6 and 3.2 in PP and SPMS respectively, with no significant difference between them) while WM lesion accrual was noticeably lower in PP and SPMS (1.3 and 1.5) compared with RRMS (4.2) over the same period. In the same groups they also found that baseline cortical GM lesion volumes predicted ~28% of the subsequent change in EDSS scores, while WM lesion volumes predicted ~13%, although new lesion accrual was not significantly associated with change in EDSS scores.

Overall, these studies suggest that WM lesion formation has limited use as a marker of progression in progressive MS, but they also flag a potential role for GM lesions at least as predictors of progression.

5.4.2 *Atrophy*

CNS tissue volume loss is emerging as a key marker of clinically relevant pathology in MS. It is thought mostly to reflect neurodegeneration, albeit with qualification that loss of other cell types can also lead to volume loss [97]. Early work sought to measure ventricular or whole brain volumes, but with the advent of technology allowing separate GM and WM volume estimates, it appears that progressive brain atrophy occurs predominantly in the GM [30].

Due to the complexities of segmenting brain tissues, early work simplified this by measuring distances between structures, such a ventricular width, or cross-sectional areas of the brain over a limited number of slices [36]. One such technique estimated ventricular volumes by contouring them on axial slices through the brain [89], and using this technique Dalton et al. demonstrated greater ventricular enlargement over a year in people with SPMS compared with RRMS (mean increase 1.1 mL in 23 people with SPMS and 0.5 mL in 41 with RRMS). Similarly, progressive ventricular enlargement has been observed in PPMS: in the placebo arm of an exploratory trial of interferon in PPMS [98], over 2 years in 20 people ventricular volumes were observed to increase by 2.8 mL, which per year is close the rate noted for SPMS. Ventricular enlargement has been found to correlate with whole brain volumes ($r = -0.65$ in a mixed cohort of 86 people with MS [22 with RRMS, 32 with PP and SPMS]) [99].

Whole brain atrophy has also been seen in progressive sub-types of MS, but in most recent serial studies has been measured alongside tissue specific GM and WM volume estimates. In primary progressive MS, Sastre-Garriga et al. [100] found in a group of 31 people with early PPMS (within 5 years of symptom onset) ~1% decrease in brain parenchymal fractional (BPF; the total volume of brain tissue divided by total intracranial volume) over 1 year, but a ~1.5% reduction in GM fraction (GMF) and non-significant change in WM fraction (WMF). Tissue volume changes did not correlate with changes in EDSS or MSFC scores. BPF correlated with baseline PD-weighted and contrast enhancing lesion loads, albeit modestly ($r = -0.36$ and -0.42 respectively), and this appeared to be driven by subtle associations with WMF rather than GMF. Similar results have been obtained in SPMS, with a 2 year follow-up study of 56 patients revealing ~0.6% reduction in whole brain volume, this being mostly attributable to GM (~1.2%) rather than WM (~0.1%) loss [91]. While WM atrophy did not correlate with change in EDSS, whole brain and GM atrophy and spinal cord area did correlate with MSFC scores ($r = 0.35$, 0.42 and 0.34 respectively). Calabrese et al. in their longitudinal (5 year) study of cortical lesions, also measured tissue volumes, and observed ~2.3% reduction in GMF in SPMS, ~3.0% in PPMS, compared with ~1.8% in RRMS [29]. In the serial study undertaken by Fisher et al. [30] (discussed above), in the same cohort they noted an acceleration of GMF but not WMF loss: in healthy controls GMF declined by 0.03% per year, in RRMS 0.23%, those converting to SPMS 0.35% and those with established SPMS 0.39%; in contrast the corresponding figures for WMF were 0.08%, 0.24%, 0.33% and 0.25% respectively. They also observed greater GMF but not WMF loss associated with increased EDSS scores, but did not explore this relationship in the RR and SP sub-groups separately. In the SPMS group, baseline contrast enhancing lesion loads, lesion and normal-appearing brain tissue MTR did not predict subsequent brain atrophy, while in RRMS they did. Calabrese et al., in their 5 year study, found that GMF was correlated with new cortical GM lesions ($r = 0.41$), although this still leaves the majority of GM atrophy unexplained by cortical lesions.

In this regard, it is interesting to note that Wegner et al. found no clear difference in cortical neuronal cell loss in lesional and extra-lesional tissues, although synaptic loss was more apparent in lesions [27]. This suggests that WM lesion formation is a less important factor determining GM atrophy in SPMS when compared with RRMS, and that GM lesions also have a limited direct role in this. There is also evidence suggesting that GM atrophy is not evenly distributed throughout GM in progressive MS. Sepulcre and colleagues [101], studying the same PPMS cohort as Sastre-Garriga et al. [100], observed over 1 year preferential loss in deep GM and some cortical areas, and using different methods Eshaghi et al. observed regional variation in atrophy which also changed over time [102].

There continues to be increasing interest in spinal cord atrophy with the recognition that it may have an important, and at least partly independent, role to play determining long-term disability [5, 6]. Earlier work had already shown that it was clinically relevant, but there have been very few serial studies. Stevenson et al. [103] observed progressive cervical cord atrophy in people with progressive MS. Over 1 year mean upper cervical cord area decreased in 12 people with PPMS by $-3.53\ mm^3$, compared with $-0.26\ mm^3$ in six people with SPMS (although due caution should be exercised given the small sample size). In a larger group including six people with RR and four with benign MS, they did not find an association between change in EDSS and cord atrophy, although only 8 of the 28 people studied were found to have progressed over this period. More recently Agosta et al. [104] reported that cervical cord area decreased by 3.1 mL (4%) in 15 people with PPMS over a mean of 2.4 years, compared with 2.2 mL in 14 people with SPMS (3%) and 5.4 mL in 13 people with RRMS (6%), but did not undertake comparisons between groups. That cord atrophy is at least semi-independent of brain volume loss has been noted in mixed cohorts [13, 14, 105], and the absence of a correlation between cord area and partial brain volume in PPMS reinforces this [92]. Cross-sectional studies have shown that the highest degree of spinal cord atrophy is observed in progressive MS, although not significantly different between SPMS and PPMS, and that a relationship between cord cross-sectional area and concurrent disability in both single-centre [106] and multi-centre studies [107]. Longitudinal studies have shown that the rate of spinal cord atrophy is at least 1% across MS subtypes, but the highest rates are seen in progressive MS [108].

Considered together, these longitudinal studies suggest that in progressive MS brain atrophy occurs more rapidly in GM than WM. Tissue specific atrophy rates in PP and SPMS have not been systematically compared, but it does appear that brain atrophy is at least as, if not more, rapid in PPMS as in SPMS. In contrast to brain WM lesion load, brain and spinal cord atrophy have been found to be more consistently associated with clinical progression. A recent study of 131 CIS patients with non-spinal MS has shown that baseline spinal cord lesion number, change in cord lesion number and change in upper cervical cord area were independently associated with EDSS at 5 years follow-up [109]; including brain T2 lesion load and brain atrophy only modestly increased the predictive power of the model, suggesting that spinal cord MRI reflects pathological changes that contribute to disability accumulation.

5.4.3 Microstructural and Metabolic Studies

There has been very little serial work using MTR, DTI or proton spectroscopy in progressive MS.

Considering first MT imaging, in an early study looking at whole brain and normal appearing brain MTR values, changes over 1 year were apparent in SP but not PP or RRMS [110]. While the RRMS cohort was quite large (39 subjects), the progressive cohorts were smaller (19 SP and 9 PP). Subsequently, in the placebo arm (n = 40) of an SPMS interferon trial a decrease in whole brain MTR was seen over 3 years, and NAWM MTR over the first 2 years, although this did not correlate with EDSS [111]. However, in contrast, in the placebo arm of a trial of lamotrigine, no significant change in MTR histogram measures in NAWM, NAGM or lesions was found in 56 people over 2 years [112]. Work in early PPMS (within 5 years of symptom onset) has found more rapid changes in GM rather than WM. Khaleeli et al. [113], studied 30 people with PPMS, following them up clinically and radiologically over 1 year. Fifteen healthy controls were also scanned. They observed a greater reduction in mean MTR in normal-appearing GM (NAGM; mean 0.9% in the year) in patients compared with controls, but no significant difference in normal-appearing WM (NAWM; 0.6% in the year). They did not report on associations between change in clinical and MTR measures, but did note that baseline mean NAWM MTR predicted change in EDSS and MSFC over the subsequent year, while NAGM MTR parameters did not. They also found that changes in MTR values correlated with atrophy, although sharing less than 50% variability. In a mixed cohort (40 RRMS, 24 SPMS and 14 SPMS), Harrison and colleagues noted that changes in MTR were not evenly distributed over the brain. In the whole cohort they noted a decline in MTR of −0.3% per year in the supratentorial brain tissues, which was faster in SPMS (−0.7% per year) than RRMS (−0.1%) but not PPMS (−0.6%), but regionally they found that MTR decline was faster in the corpus callosum in PPMS (−1.8% per year) compared with RRMS (−0.6%) but not SPMS (−0.9%) [114]. While it is difficult to fully reconcile these study results, they do suggest that a decline in brain MTR may be greater in progressive compared with RRMS, and highlight potentially significant regional differences in MTR decline.

Turning to DTI, a longitudinal assessment of this has been undertaken by Agosta et al. in a mixed cohort of people with MS (13 RR, 14 SP and 15 PP, followed up on average for 2.4 years) [104]. In their study, they assessed both brain and cervical cord measures. Brain NAWM MD was observed to increase, NAWM FA decline (only in people with SPMS), but brain GM MD did not change. Concurrent with this, cervical cord area was noted to decline, and cervical cord mean MD increase and FA decrease. Cord and brain DTI, and cord atrophy measures did not correlate with change in EDSS scores, although progression over the year was limited in all the MS sub-groups (on average between 0.5 and 1 EDSS points), limiting the scope to detect associations. Harrison et al. [115] along with MTR also assessed DTI measures, and in the whole brain noted no significant difference between MS subtypes, but did find that FA declined faster in the optic radiations of the PPMS group when compared with the RRMS group (PPMS −1.2% per year, SPMS −0.2%, RRMS 0%). Interestingly, in a study evaluating the predictive value of DTI in PPMS, Rovaris et al. [116] found that in a multivariate analysis GM MD, but not NAWM MD or FA, was an independent predictor of clinical deterioration over the next 5 years, suggesting that even if diffusion changes are less dynamic in GM than WM, they may be of greater clinical consequence.

Proton spectroscopy has been used in one serial PPMS study of glatiramer acetate. Sajja et al. [117] studied 37 people with PPMS (9 in the placebo arm) patients over 1 year, and 19 people to 3 years. The work was undertaken at four centres, and this was found to have a significant effect in metabolite ratios. They estimated NAA/Cr and Cho/Cr ratios, and noted no change over time, and no difference between people receiving the active agent or placebo. More recently, Obert et al. assessed metabolite concentrations in 22 people with RRMS, 15 SPMS and 12 healthy controls, and over 2 years they noted a decline in NAWM NAA/Cr ratio in SPMS only [118]. In 13 people with MS and 12 controls, Choi et al. assessed glutathione (interpreted as a marker of oxidative damage) over an average of 3.7 years, they noted a decline in the frontal and fronto-parietal regions in those who MS clinical progressed over the course of the study [119].

Given the limited scope of these studies, it is difficult to draw clear conclusions from them. DTI and MTR abnormalities are present, but do not seem to be equally evident in GM and WM. The discrepancy in the DTI data, suggesting more rapid short term changes in WM than GM MD, but in the longer term that GM MD is a better predictor of disability, also reinforces the concept that there may be a considerable delay between the first appearance of pathology and its ultimate clinical impact.

5.5 Predicting Progression Using MRI

For many people with MS, knowing what the future holds for them is important. Robust prognostic markers would aid decisions about treatments, particularly when balancing the pros and cons of increasingly powerful and potentially harmful agents. We currently have no reliable clinical or MRI marker that allows us to predict the transition from RR to SPMS, or the rate of progression in SP or PPMS.

Considering conversion from RR to SPMS, there are few studies exploring the predictive value of MRI markers. In one study that followed people up clinically and radiologically for 20 years after a clinically isolated syndrome, baseline lesion loads and early lesion accrual, particularly in the first five years, appeared to be higher in people who developed SPMS when compared with those who had RRMS or no further events [11]. Similarly, Mostert et al. assessed the predictive value of baseline brain lesion load and linear measures of the brain (bicaudate ratio and third ventricular width) for conversion from RR to SPMS over 10 years, and found that more than 10 lesions visible on T2w scan conferred an increased risk of conversion (hazard ratio 2.36), increasing with greater lesion loads [120]. In a later study, this group also found that while early T2w lesion loads partly predicted progression of disability in RRMS, it did not in PP or SPMS [121]. This would seem to mirror finding from large scale cohort observational work suggesting the relapses do not ultimately affect the rate of progression once progression is established [122]. With regard to GM lesions, Calabrese and colleagues, in a 3 year study, found that baseline cortical lesion volumes (but not counts) significantly correlated with subsequent change in EDSS (SPMS $r = 0.43$, RRMS $r = 0.55$) [66].

Returning to Mostert et al. [120], in their study linear measures of brain atrophy did not predict conversion, although this result should be regarded with caution as the method used did not sample the whole brain, and has been superseded by tissue specific brain atrophy measures. Also, this should not be taken to mean that atrophy is not relevant in the conversion from RR to SPMS for, as noted above, brain atrophy may accelerate into the progressive phase of MS [30]. Recalling that there may be a delay of many years between lesion formation and associated brain atrophy [39], these data would appear consistent with a predictive model where lesion loads provide a warning of progression to come, while brain atrophy more closely tracks actual clinical progression.

Turning to prediction of progression in established progressive MS, there is similarly little data to draw firm conclusions from. In one MTR study in early PPMS, baseline NAWM MTR was found to predict change in EDSS and MSFC scores over 1 year [113]. The same group found that in PPMS baseline T2w and Gd-enhancing lesion load correlated with EDSS 5 years later [123], although in a multivariate analysis only T2w lesion loads were retained in the model, and the effect size was modest (odds ratio 1.03. In a study of people with PPMS followed up for 10 years, reductions in brain volume and change in EDSS over the initial 2 years, both appear to predict EDSS 10 years later [124]. Rovaris et al. found in a multivariate analysis in PPMS, baseline EDSS and GM MD, but not WM MD or FA, or T2w lesion load, predicted an increase in EDSS over the next 5 years [116]. Considering the spinal cord, in a mixed cohort (13 RRMS, 14 SPMS, and 15 PPMS) baseline cervical cord cross-sectional area and cord FA were found to associate with subsequent EDSS changes over an average of 2.4 years follow-up [104].

While it is difficult to unify these results, given differences in the cohorts, duration of follow-up and methods used, they highlight that features from both brain GM and WM, and the spinal cord, are relevant. They also suggest that the MRI measure best able to predict outcomes may differ dependent on how well-established progression is (i.e. the same MRI marker may not be equally useful in early and later progressive disease).

5.6 Measuring Treatment Response

As noted above, and considered elsewhere in this book, the sensitivity of clinical outcomes measures is limited and it may take several years for progression to be confirmed. In comparison, brain atrophy measures (used as a marker of the neurodegeneration thought to underlie a substantial proportion of clinical progression), are much more sensitive to change. For example, over 2 years to detect a 50%

treatment effect on clinical progression (using disease status scale scores) a total cohort of nearly 500 people would be needed [125], while for MRI measures of brain atrophy (using SIENA) about one tenth of this number would be needed [126]. Given this, it is unsurprising the MRI now has an established role in early phase treatment trials in progressive MS. For example, the primary outcome in the (positive) phase II simvastatin trial in SPMS was brain atrophy [5], subsequently slowing of brain atrophy in SPMS been reported with biotin [127], and for MS SMART (a multi-arm adaptive trial in SPMS (42) brain atrophy is the primary outcome measure (ClinicalTrials.gov Identifier: NCT01910259). However, a (negative) trial of lamotrigine in SPMS highlighted the potential for treatments to transiently accelerate atrophy [41], termed psuedo-atrophy [128], which may confound an otherwise positive treatment response. This may be overcome by obtaining baseline measures for brain atrophy a few months after treatment has started, although it has yet to be established what is the optimal time for this, and whether or not this is similar for SPMS and PPMS, dependent on the degree of inflammatory activity apparent at treatment initiation, or consistent between treatments.

While the role of MRI measures of brain atrophy in early phase treatment trials is clear, their role measuring treatment responses in clinical practice is not [129]. In clinical practice we are interested in an outcome measure relevant to an individual, and so need to be able to determine not only if brain atrophy is more rapid than normal [130], but if a treatment has slowed this. Currently, we are only able to achieve this reliably at a group level [126].

5.7 Optical Coherence Tomography

Given that neurodegeneration is likely to be a significant determinant of irreversible disability in MS, there has been growing interest in OCT as it allows us to directly observe neurons and their axonal projections in the retina [131]. Since the first edition of this book, OCT technology has continued to advance with, for example, spectral domain OCT offering more rapid and higher resolution scans when compared with time domain OCT, so allowing three rather than two dimensional imaging [132]. Similarly, since the first edition, there have now been several large cross-sectional, and a few longitudinal, OCT studies in MS. Retinal nerve fibre layer (RNFL) thickness has been most studied in MS, although it is possible to extract other measures, for example the depth of the ganglion cell layer (for example [133] and total macular volume (TMV; for example [134]). When considering OCT studies in MS, it is important to recall the effects an episode of optic neuritis has on measures, and that in progressive MS OCT measures are likely to represent a composite of neurodegeneration arising from optic nerve demyelinating lesions (particularly in SPMS) and neurodegeneration resulting from other processes. Following an episode of optic neuritis, RFNL thickness [135, 136] and macular volume both appear to decrease [136] and so studies in unaffected eyes may be more informative of the processes underlying progression in progressive MS.

In progressive MS, early OCT studies yielded slightly differing results. In part this may have reflected study sensitivity (increasing with cohort size and more recent technology), confounding by previous optic neuritis, and (in particular for RR and SPMS, and the clinical continuity between them) potentially divisions between subgroups based on course rather than other features such as disease duration or clinical outcomes. However, there have now been several large (more than 100 participant) spectral domain OCT studies in MS, and while themes have emerged these are still not entirely consistent.

Gelfand et al. in their cross-sectional study of 403 people with RRMS, 60 with SPMS and 33 PPMS, compared with 53 controls, found that in eyes clinically unaffected by optic neuritis, controlling for age and disease duration, RFNL thickness and TMV were reduced in all types of MS, RFNL was similar in SP and PPMS, while TMV was slightly lower in PPMS [137]. Oberwahrenbrock et al., in their study (RRMS n = 308, SPMS n = 65, PPMS n = 41) also showed a reduction RFNL thickness and TMV, with significantly thinner RFNL in SPMS compared with RRMS, and total macular volume in SPMS and PPMS compared with RRMS [134]. They also found a disease duration effect on RFNL in the RRMS and SPMS group, and TMV for the RRMS group only. Balk and colleagues, in their study of 140 people with RRMS, 61 SPMS, 29 PPMS and 63 controls, again in eyes clinically unaffected by optic neuritis, found that RFNL was thinner and in addition ganglion cell complex volume lower in SPMS compared with RRMS, but in PPMS these were relatively preserved [138]. From this it appears that RFNL is consistently thinner, and TMV lower, in progressive MS, but differences between PPMS and SPMS are less definite. This discord between RFNL and TMV is interesting, as it implies that different mechanisms may influence them. In this regard, Burkholder et al. found—in a large mixed MS cohort (n = 541, of whom 82% had RRMS)—that RFNL and macular volume measures were partly correlated, marginally more so in eyes affected by optic neuritis ($r = 0.68$ compared with 0.62), although about half of the variation in macular volume was not explained by RFNL thickness, again suggesting at least partly independent mechanisms may be at work [139]. Practically, this means that in OCT studies, no single measure can be considered a comprehensive assessment of the effects progressive MS has on the retina.

Given that OCT enables a more direct assessment of neurodegeneration than brain tissue volumes measures, and that extracting measures is currently much less time consuming than assessing brain atrophy using MRI, there has been interest in using OCT as a proxy for MRI derived brain atrophy measures. Saidha et al. over about 4 years in a mixed cohort of people with MS (71 RRMS, 24 SPMS and 12 PPMS) found that faster rates of peripapillary (p) RNFL and combined ganglion cell and inner plexiform layer (GCIP) thinning were associated with faster rates of cerebral volume fraction (CVF), cortical GM, thalamic, and brainstem atrophy [140]. After adjustment for multiple comparisons, pRFNL thinning correlated with caudate ($r = 0.44$) and brainstem ($r = 0.33$) atrophy, while GCIP thinning correlated with CVF ($r = 0.45$), cortical GM($r = 0.37$), and thalamic atrophy ($r = 0.38$). However, as with correlations between OCT measures, correlations of OCT with brain atrophy measures were limited (with OCT measures at best explaining about a quarter of the variation in brain atrophy measures) and no single OCT measure emerged as being most representative of all aspects of brain atrophy, suggesting that multiple mechanisms may link OCT and brain atrophy measures. A more recent study in PPMS has further highlighted the complex relationship between MRI-detectable brain pathology and OCT measures, finding that while RFNL, macular volume, and GCIP are associated with brain volumes measures (RFNL with thalamic and visual cortex volume, GCIP and macular volume with thalamic volume), they may also be linked with cortical lesion loads (GCIP and macular volume) [141].

Considering sensitivity to change, there have been very few studies that have looked at progressive MS specifically. Tallman et al. studied 299 people with MS followed up for a mean of 18 months (subtypes not specified), and found progressive reductions in RFNL thickness with the proportion of people whose changed exceeded measurement error increasing from 11% from baseline to 1 year to 44% at 3–4.5 years ($p < 0.001$) [142]. However, this study did not include a control group, and in a mixed cohort (clinically isolated syndrome n = 8, RRMS 116, SPMS 24 and PPMS 16) over a median of 21 months follow up, when compared with controls (n = 59), Ratchford and colleagues found that RFNL thinning was similar in the MS and control groups, but the GCIP thinning was 46% faster [143]. They did not specifically look at MS subgroups in their study. Similarly, Serbecic et al. found in their study of 27 people with RRMS and 10 with SPMS over a median of 22 months RNFL thickness [144] and TMV [145] did not significantly change. Using time domain OCT, Henderson et al., in 16 people with PP and 18 with SPMS found no clear change in RFNL over ~1.6 years [146]. Taken together, these findings suggest that over about 2 years, current OCT measures do not reveal rapid changes over time, in the absence of an episode of optic neuritis, and therefore a potentially limited role for OCT measures as a generic marker of progression. However, after optic neuritis, and in particular in trials of putative neuroprotective agents, OCT may play a useful role [147].

While OCT measures in MS may not be sufficiently dynamic to monitor progression reliably over 2 years, interestingly they may predict clinical change. Martinez-Lapiscina et al. (IMSVISUAL consortium) in their multicentre study of 664 people with RRMS, 83 SPMS and 58 PPMS, over a median 2 years of follow-up found that a lower baseline pRFNL thickness was associated with greater risk of EDSS-measured disability progression, after allowing for age, previous optic neuritis, disease duration and baseline EDSS [148]. Given this, RFNL measures could potentially aid the identification of people for progressive MS treatment trials, and help inform decisions about treatments to slow progression (when they become available) in clinical practice.

5.8 Conclusions

Imaging disease progression in MS is far from straightforward. Markers that may be relevant in the prediction of conversion from RRMS to SPMS may not be of such use when trying to anticipate disability. MRI features that best correlate with current disability may change as the disease advances, and the optimal combination of measures may also differ between sub-types of MS. As such it seems likely that a combination of clinical and imaging markers will be required to characterise the impact of MS at any given time and optimally predict its future course. Of the currently available MRI markers, brain and spinal cord atrophy measures still seem most relevant in progressive MS.

References

1. Polman CH, Reingold SC, Banwell B, et al. Diagnostic criteria for multiple sclerosis: 2010 revisions to the McDonald criteria. Ann Neurol. 2011;69(2):292–302.
2. Wattjes MP, Rovira À, Miller D, et al. MAGNIMS study group. Evidence-based guidelines: MAGNIMS consensus guidelines on the use of MRI in multiple sclerosis—establishing disease prognosis and monitoring patients. Nat Rev Neurol. 2015;11(10):597–606.
3. https://www.novartis.com/news/media-releases/novartis-baf312-reduces-risk-disability-progression-pivotal-phase-iii-study
4. Montalbán X, Hauser SL, Kappos L, et al. Ocrelizumab versus placebo in primary progressive multiple sclerosis. N Engl J Med. 2017;376(3):209–20.
5. Chataway J, Schuerer N, Alsanousi A, et al. Effect of high-dose simvastatin on brain atrophy and disability in secondary progressive multiple sclerosis (MS-STAT): a randomised, placebo-controlled, phase 2 trial. Lancet. 2014;383(9936):2213–21.
6. https://clinicaltrials.gov/ct2/show/results/NCT01188811
7. Lublin FD, Reingold SC. Defining the clinical course of multiple sclerosis: results of an international survey. National Multiple Sclerosis Society (USA) Advisory Committee on Clinical Trials of New Agents in Multiple Sclerosis. Neurology. 1996;46(4):907–11.
8. Miller DH, Leary SM. Primary-progressive multiple sclerosis. Lancet Neurol. 2007;6(10): 903–12.
9. Confavreux C, Vukusic S. Accumulation of irreversible disability in multiple sclerosis: from epidemiology to treatment. Clin Neurol Neurosurg. 2006;108(3):327–32.
10. Thompson AJ, Kermode AG, MacManus DG, et al. Patterns of disease activity in multiple sclerosis: clinical and magnetic resonance imaging study. BMJ. 1990;300(6725):631–4.
11. Fisniku LK, Brex PA, Altmann DR, et al. Disability and T2 MRI lesions: a 20-year follow-up of patients with relapse onset of multiple sclerosis. Brain. 2008;131(Pt 3):808–17.
12. Fisniku LK, Chard DT, Jackson JS, et al. Gray matter atrophy is related to long-term disability in multiple sclerosis. Ann Neurol. 2008;64(3):247–54.
13. Bonati U, Fisniku LK, Altmann DR, et al. Cervical cord and brain grey matter atrophy independently associate with long-term MS disability. J Neurol Neurosurg Psychiatry. 2011;82(4):471–2.
14. Cohen AB, Neema M, Arora A, et al. The relationships among MRI-defined spinal cord involvement, brain involvement, and disability in multiple sclerosis. J Neuroimaging. 2012;22(2):122–8.
15. Lublin FD. Defining the clinical course of multiple sclerosis: the 2013 revisions. Neurology. 2014;83(3):278–86.
16. Kurtzke JF. Rating neurologic impairment in multiple sclerosis: an expanded disability status scale (EDSS). Neurology. 1983;33(11):1444–52.
17. Lorscheider J, Buzzard K, Jokubaitis V, et al. Defining secondary progressive multiple sclerosis. Brain. 2016;139(Pt 9):2395–405.
18. Benedict RHB, Zivadinov R. Risk factors for and management of cognitive dysfunction in multiple sclerosis. Nat Rev Neurol. 2011;7(6):332–42.
19. Ron MA, Callanan MM, Warrington EK. Cognitive abnormalities in multiple sclerosis: a psychometric and MRI study. Psychol Med. 1991;21(1):59–68.

20. Morrow SA, Jurgensen S, Forrestal F, Munchauer FE, Benedict RHB. Effects of acute relapses on neuropsychological status in multiple sclerosis patients. J Neurol. 2011 Sep; 258(9):1603–8.
21. Kuhlmann T, Lingfeld G, Bitsch A, Schuchardt J, Brück W. Acute axonal damage in multiple sclerosis is most extensive in early disease stages and decreases over time. Brain. 2002; 125(Pt 10):2202–12.
22. Bø L, Vedeler CA, Nyland HI, Trapp BD, Mørk SJ. Subpial demyelination in the cerebral cortex of multiple sclerosis patients. J Neuropathol Exp Neurol. 2003;62(7):723–32.
23. Magliozzi R, Howell O, Vora A, et al. Meningeal B-cell follicles in secondary progressive multiple sclerosis associate with early onset of disease and severe cortical pathology. Brain. 2006;130(4):1089–104.
24. Lucchinetti CF, Popescu BFG, Bunyan RF, et al. Inflammatory cortical demyelination in early multiple sclerosis. N Engl J Med. 2011;365(23):2188–97.
25. Trapp BD, Peterson J, Ransohoff RM, et al. Axonal transection in the lesions of multiple sclerosis. N Engl J Med. 1998;338(5):278–85.
26. Peterson JW, Bö L, Mörk S, Chang A, Trapp BD. Transected neurites, apoptotic neurons, and reduced inflammation in cortical multiple sclerosis lesions. Ann Neurol. 2001;50(3):389–400.
27. Wegner C, Esiri MM, Chance SA, Palace J, Matthews PM. Neocortical neuronal, synaptic, and glial loss in multiple sclerosis. Neurology. 2006;67(6):960–7.
28. Kidd D, Thorpe JW, Kendall BE, et al. MRI dynamics of brain and spinal cord in progressive multiple sclerosis. J Neurol Neurosurg Psychiatry. 1996;60(1):15–9.
29. Calabrese M, Poretto V, Favaretto A, et al. Cortical lesion load associates with progression of disability in multiple sclerosis. Brain. 2012;135(Pt 10):2952–61.
30. Fisher E, Lee J-C, Nakamura K, Rudick RA. Gray matter atrophy in multiple sclerosis: a longitudinal study. Ann Neurol. 2008;64(3):255–65.
31. De Stefano N, Giorgio A, Battaglini M, et al. Assessing brain atrophy rates in a large population of untreated multiple sclerosis subtypes. Neurology. 2010;74(23):1868–76.
32. Dalton CM, Chard DT, Davies GR, et al. Early development of multiple sclerosis is associated with progressive grey matter atrophy in patients presenting with clinically isolated syndromes. Brain. 2004;127(Pt 5):1101–7.
33. Chard DT, Griffin CM, Parker GJM, et al. Brain atrophy in clinically early relapsing-remitting multiple sclerosis. Brain. 2002;125(Pt 2):327–37.
34. Frischer JM, Bramow S, Dal-Bianco A, et al. The relation between inflammation and neurodegeneration in multiple sclerosis brains. Brain. 2009;132(Pt 5):1175–89.
35. Kornek B, Storch MK, Weissert R, et al. Multiple sclerosis and chronic autoimmune encephalomyelitis. Am J Pathol. 2000;157(1):267–76.
36. Miller DH, Barkhof F, Frank JA, Parker GJM, Thompson AJ. Measurement of atrophy in multiple sclerosis: pathological basis, methodological aspects and clinical relevance. Brain. 2002;125(Pt 8):1676–95.
37. Quarantelli M. Brain tissue volume changes in relapsing-remitting multiple sclerosis: correlation with lesion load. Neuroimage. 2003;18(2):360–6.
38. Tedeschi G, Lavorgna L, Russo P, et al. Brain atrophy and lesion load in a large population of patients with multiple sclerosis. Neurology. 2005;65(2):280–5.
39. Chard DT, Brex PA, Ciccarelli O, et al. The longitudinal relation between brain lesion load and atrophy in multiple sclerosis: a 14 year follow up study. J Neurol Neurosurg Psychiatry. 2003;74(11):1551–4.
40. Giovannoni G, Comi G, Cook S, et al. A placebo-controlled trial of oral cladribine for relapsing multiple sclerosis. N Engl J Med. 2010;362(5):416–26.
41. Kapoor R, Furby J, Hayton T, et al. Lamotrigine for neuroprotection in secondary progressive multiple sclerosis: a randomised, double-blind, placebo-controlled, parallel-group trial. Lancet Neurol. 2010;9(7):681–8.
42. Chataway J, Nicholas R, Todd S, et al. A novel adaptive design strategy increases the efficiency of clinical trials in secondary progressive multiple sclerosis. Mult Scler. 2011;17(1):81–8.

43. Schmierer K, Wheeler-Kingshott CAM, Tozer DJ, et al. Quantitative magnetic resonance of postmortem multiple sclerosis brain before and after fixation. Magn Reson Med. 2008;59(2):268–77.
44. Mallik S, Samson RS, Wheeler-Kingshott CAM, Miller DH. Imaging outcomes for trials of remyelination in multiple sclerosis. J Neurol Neurosurg Psychiatry. 2014;85(12):1396–404.
45. Schmierer K, Tozer DJ, Scaravilli F, et al. Quantitative magnetization transfer imaging in postmortem multiple sclerosis brain. J Magn Reson Imaging. 2007;26(1):41–51.
46. Bjartmar C, Battistuta J, Terada N, Dupree E, Trapp BD. N-acetylaspartate is an axon-specific marker of mature white matter in vivo: a biochemical and immunohistochemical study on the rat optic nerve. Ann Neurol. 2002;51(1):51–8.
47. Rocca MA, Valsasina P, Absinta M, et al. Default-mode network dysfunction and cognitive impairment in progressive MS. Neurology. 2010;74(16):1252–9.
48. Ceccarelli A, Rocca MA, Valsasina P, et al. Structural and functional magnetic resonance imaging correlates of motor network dysfunction in primary progressive multiple sclerosis. Eur J Neurosci. 2010;31(7):1273–80.
49. Ciccarelli O, Toosy AT, Marsden JF, et al. Functional response to active and passive ankle movements with clinical correlations in patients with primary progressive multiple sclerosis. J Neurol. 2006;253(7):882–91.
50. Rocca MA, Pagani E, Ghezzi A, et al. Functional cortical changes in patients with multiple sclerosis and nonspecific findings on conventional magnetic resonance imaging scans of the brain. Neuroimage. 2003;19(3):826–36.
51. Inglese M, Park S-J, Johnson G, et al. Deep gray matter perfusion in multiple sclerosis: dynamic susceptibility contrast perfusion magnetic resonance imaging at 3 T. Arch Neurol. 2007;64(2):196–202.
52. Adhya S, Johnson G, Herbert J, et al. Pattern of hemodynamic impairment in multiple sclerosis: dynamic susceptibility contrast perfusion MR imaging at 3.0 T. Neuroimage. 2006;33(4):1029–35.
53. Rashid W, Parkes LM, Ingle GT, et al. Abnormalities of cerebral perfusion in multiple sclerosis. J Neurol Neurosurg Psychiatry. 2004;75(9):1288–93.
54. Enzinger C, Pinter D, Rocca MA, et al. Longitudinal fMRI studies: exploring brain plasticity and repair in MS. Mult Scler. 2016;22(3):269–78.
55. Grimaud J, Lai M, Thorpe J, et al. Quantification of MRI lesion load in multiple sclerosis: a comparison of three computer-assisted techniques. Magn Reson Imaging. 1996;14(5):495–505.
56. Carass A, Roy S, Jog A, et al. Longitudinal multiple sclerosis lesion segmentation—resource and challenge. Neuroimage. 2017;148(C):77–102.
57. Tubridy N, Molyneux PD, Moseley IF, Miller DH. The sensitivity of thin-slice fast spin echo, fast FLAIR and gadolinium-enhanced T1-weighted MRI sequences in detecting new lesion activity in multiple sclerosis. J Neurol. 1999;246(12):1181–5.
58. Stevenson VL, Miller DH, Rovaris M, et al. Primary and transitional progressive MS: a clinical and MRI cross-sectional study. Neurology. 1999;52(4):839–45.
59. van Walderveen MA, Barkhof F, Pouwels PJ, van Schijndel RA, Polman CH, Castelijns JA. Neuronal damage in T1-hypointense multiple sclerosis lesions demonstrated in vivo using proton magnetic resonance spectroscopy. Ann Neurol. 1999;46(1):79–87.
60. Grimaud J, Barker GJ, Wang L, et al. Correlation of magnetic resonance imaging parameters with clinical disability in multiple sclerosis: a preliminary study. J Neurol. 1999;246(10):961–7.
61. Geurts JJG, Bö L, Pouwels PJW, et al. Cortical lesions in multiple sclerosis: combined postmortem MR imaging and histopathology. AJNR Am J Neuroradiol. 2005;26(3):572–7.
62. Geurts JJG, Pouwels PJW, Uitdehaag BMJ, et al. Intracortical lesions in multiple sclerosis: improved detection with 3D double inversion-recovery MR imaging. Radiology. 2005;236(1):254–60.
63. Seewann A, Kooi E-J, Roosendaal SD, et al. Postmortem verification of MS cortical lesion detection with 3D DIR. Neurology. 2012;78(5):302–8.

64. Nelson F, Poonawalla AH, Hou P, et al. Improved identification of intracortical lesions in multiple sclerosis with phase-sensitive inversion recovery in combination with fast double inversion recovery MR imaging. AJNR Am J Neuroradiol. 2007;28(9):1645–9.
65. Sethi V, Yousry TA, Muhlert N, et al. Improved detection of cortical MS lesions with phase-sensitive inversion recovery MRI. J Neurol Neurosurg Psychiatry. 2012;83(9):877–82.
66. Calabrese M, Rocca MA, Atzori M, et al. A 3-year magnetic resonance imaging study of cortical lesions in relapse-onset multiple sclerosis. Ann Neurol. 2010;67(3):376–83.
67. Smith SM, Zhang Y, Jenkinson M, et al. Accurate, robust, and automated longitudinal and cross-sectional brain change analysis. Neuroimage. 2002;17(1):479–89.
68. Ashburner J, Friston KJ. Voxel-based morphometry--the methods. Neuroimage. 2000;11(6 Pt 1):805–21.
69. Ashburner J, Friston KJ. Unified segmentation. Neuroimage. 2005;26(3):839–51.
70. Fischl B, Sereno MI, Dale AM. Cortical surface-based analysis. II: Inflation, flattening, and a surface-based coordinate system. Neuroimage. 1999;9(2):195–207.
71. Anderson VM, Fox NC, Miller DH. Magnetic resonance imaging measures of brain atrophy in multiple sclerosis. J Magn Reson Imaging. 2006;23(5):605–18.
72. Chard DT, Jackson JS, Miller DH, Wheeler-Kingshott CAM. Reducing the impact of white matter lesions on automated measures of brain gray and white matter volumes. J Magn Reson Imaging. 2010;32(1):223–8.
73. Battaglini M, Jenkinson M, De Stefano N. Evaluating and reducing the impact of white matter lesions on brain volume measurements. Hum Brain Mapp. 2012;33:2062–71.
74. Prados F, Cardoso MJ, Kanber B, et al. A multi-time-point modality-agnostic patch-based method for lesion filling in multiple sclerosis. Neuroimage. 2016;139(C):376–84.
75. Ko H-Y, Park JH, Shin YB, Baek SY. Gross quantitative measurements of spinal cord segments in human. Spinal Cord. 2004;42(1):35–40.
76. Losseff NA, Webb SL, O'Riordan JI, et al. Spinal cord atrophy and disability in multiple sclerosis. A new reproducible and sensitive MRI method with potential to monitor disease progression. Brain. 1996;119(Pt 3):701–8.
77. Coulon O, Hickman SJ, Parker GJ, et al. Quantification of spinal cord atrophy from magnetic resonance images via a B-spline active surface model. Magn Reson Med. 2002;47(6):1176–85.
78. Horsfield MA, Sala S, Neema M, et al. Rapid semi-automatic segmentation of the spinal cord from magnetic resonance images: application in multiple sclerosis. Neuroimage. 2010;50(2):446–55.
79. Kearney H, Yiannakas MC, Abdel-Aziz K, et al. Improved MRI quantification of spinal cord atrophy in multiple sclerosis. J Magn Reson Imaging. 2014;39(3):617–23.
80. Liu Z, Yaldizli Ö, Pardini M, et al. Cervical cord area measurement using volumetric brain magnetic resonance imaging in multiple sclerosis. Mult Scler Relat Disord. 2015;4(1):52–7.
81. Lukas C, Sombekke MH, Bellenberg B, et al. Relevance of spinal cord abnormalities to clinical disability in multiple sclerosis: MR imaging findings in a large cohort of patients. Radiology. 2013;269:542–52.
82. Griffin CM, Chard DT, Ciccarelli O, et al. Diffusion tensor imaging in early relapsing-remitting multiple sclerosis. Mult Scler. 2001;7(5):290–7.
83. Bitsch A, Bruhn H, Vougioukas V, et al. Inflammatory CNS demyelination: histopathologic correlation with in vivo quantitative proton MR spectroscopy. AJNR Am J Neuroradiol. 1999;20(9):1619–27.
84. Wolfson M, Bersudsky Y, Hertz E, et al. A model of inositol compartmentation in astrocytes based upon efflux kinetics and slow inositol depletion after uptake inhibition. Neurochem Res. 2000;25(7):977–82.
85. Friese MA, Schattling B, Fugger L. Mechanisms of neurodegeneration and axonal dysfunction in multiple sclerosis. Nat Rev Neurol. 2014;10(4):225–38.
86. Inglese M, Madelin G, Oesingmann N, et al. Brain tissue sodium concentration in multiple sclerosis: a sodium imaging study at 3 tesla. Brain. 2010;133(Pt 3):847–57.
87. Paling D, Solanky BS, Riemer F, et al. Sodium accumulation is associated with disability and a progressive course in multiple sclerosis. Brain. 2013;136(Pt 7):2305–17.

88. Fleysher L, Oesingmann N, Brown R, et al. Noninvasive quantification of intracellular sodium in human brain using ultrahigh-field MRI. NMR Biomed. 2013;26(1):9–19.
89. Dalton CM, Miszkiel KA, O'Connor PW, et al. Ventricular enlargement in MS: one-year change at various stages of disease. Neurology. 2006;66(5):693–8.
90. Ge Y, Grossman RI, Udupa JK, et al. Brain atrophy in relapsing-remitting multiple sclerosis and secondary progressive multiple sclerosis: longitudinal quantitative analysis. Radiology. 2000;214(3):665–70.
91. Furby J, Hayton T, Altmann D, et al. A longitudinal study of MRI-detected atrophy in secondary progressive multiple sclerosis. J Neurol. 2010;257(9):1508–16.
92. Ingle GT, Stevenson VL, Miller DH, Thompson AJ. Primary progressive multiple sclerosis: a 5-year clinical and MR study. Brain. 2003;126(Pt 11):2528–36.
93. Thompson AJ, Kermode AG, Wicks D, et al. Major differences in the dynamics of primary and secondary progressive multiple sclerosis. Ann Neurol. 1991;29(1):53–62.
94. Silver NC, Good CD, Barker GJ, et al. Sensitivity of contrast enhanced MRI in multiple sclerosis. Effects of gadolinium dose, magnetization transfer contrast and delayed imaging. Brain. 1997;120(Pt 7):1149–61.
95. Tubridy N, Coles AJ, Molyneux P, et al. Secondary progressive multiple sclerosis: the relationship between short-term MRI activity and clinical features. Brain. 1998;121(Pt 2):225–31.
96. Ingle GT, Sastre-Garriga J, Miller DH, Thompson AJI. inflammation important in early PPMS? a longitudinal MRI study. J Neurol Neurosurg Psychiatry. 2005;76(9):1255–8.
97. Chard D, Miller D. Grey matter pathology in clinically early multiple sclerosis: evidence from magnetic resonance imaging. J Neurol Sci. 2009;282(1–2):5–11.
98. Leary SM, Miller DH, Stevenson VL, Brex PA, Chard DT, Thompson AJ. Interferon beta-1a in primary progressive MS: an exploratory, randomized, controlled trial. Neurology. 2003;60(1):44–51.
99. Kalkers NF, Vrenken H, Uitdehaag BMJ, Polman CH, Barkhof F. Brain atrophy in multiple sclerosis: impact of lesions and of damage of whole brain tissue. Mult Scler. 2002;8(5):410–4.
100. Sastre-Garriga J, Ingle GT, Chard DT, et al. Grey and white matter volume changes in early primary progressive multiple sclerosis: a longitudinal study. Brain. 2005;128(Pt 6):1454–60.
101. Sepulcre J, Sastre-Garriga J, Cercignani M, et al. Regional gray matter atrophy in early primary progressive multiple sclerosis: a voxel-based morphometry study. Arch Neurol. 2006;63(8):1175–80.
102. Eshaghi A, Bodini B, Ridgway GR, et al. Temporal and spatial evolution of grey matter atrophy in primary progressive multiple sclerosis. Neuroimage. 2014;86(C):257–64.
103. Stevenson VL, Leary SM, Losseff NA, et al. Spinal cord atrophy and disability in MS: a longitudinal study. Neurology. 1998;51(1):234–8.
104. Agosta F, Absinta M, Sormani MP, et al. In vivo assessment of cervical cord damage in MS patients: a longitudinal diffusion tensor MRI study. Brain. 2007;130(Pt 8):2211–9.
105. Kearney H, Rocca M, Valsasina P, et al. Magnetic resonance imaging correlates of physical disability in relapse onset multiple sclerosis of long disease duration. Mult Scler (Houndmills, Basingstoke, England) 2014;20(1):72–80.
106. Daams M, Weiler F, Steenwijk MD, et al. Mean upper cervical cord area (MUCCA) measurement in long-standing multiple sclerosis: relation to brain findings and clinical disability. Mult Scler. 2014;20(14):1860–5.
107. Rocca MA, Horsfield MA, Sala S, et al. A multicenter assessment of cervical cord atrophy among MS clinical phenotypes. Neurology. 2011;76(24):2096–102.
108. Lukas C, Knol DL, Sombekke MH, et al. Cervical spinal cord volume loss is related to clinical disability progression in multiple sclerosis. J Neurol Neurosurg Psychiatry. 2015;86(4):410–8.
109. Brownlee WJ, Altmann DR, Alves Da Mota P, et al. Association of asymptomatic spinal cord lesions and atrophy with disability 5 years after a clinically isolated syndrome. Mult Scler. 2017;23(5):665–74.
110. Filippi M, Inglese M, Rovaris M, et al. Magnetization transfer imaging to monitor the evolution of MS: a 1-year follow-up study. Neurology. 2000;55(7):940–6.

111. Inglese M, van Waesberghe JHTM, Rovaris M, et al. The effect of interferon beta-1b on quantities derived from MT MRI in secondary progressive MS. Neurology. 2003;60(5):853–60.
112. Hayton T, Furby J, Smith KJ, et al. Longitudinal changes in magnetisation transfer ratio in secondary progressive multiple sclerosis: data from a randomised placebo controlled trial of lamotrigine. J Neurol. 2011;259(3):505–14.
113. Khaleeli Z, Sastre-Garriga J, Ciccarelli O, Miller DH, Thompson AJ. Magnetisation transfer ratio in the normal appearing white matter predicts progression of disability over 1 year in early primary progressive multiple sclerosis. J Neurol Neurosurg Psychiatry. 2007;78(10):1076–82.
114. Samann PG, Knop M, Golgor E, et al. Brain volume and diffusion markers as predictors of disability and short-term disease evolution in multiple sclerosis. Am J Neuroradiol. 2012;33(7):1356–62.
115. Harrison DM, Caffo BS, Shiee N, et al. Longitudinal changes in diffusion tensor-based quantitative MRI in multiple sclerosis. Neurology. 2011;76(2):179–86.
116. Rovaris M, Judica E, Gallo A, et al. Grey matter damage predicts the evolution of primary progressive multiple sclerosis at 5 years. Brain. 2006;129(Pt 10):2628–34.
117. Sajja BR, Narayana PA, Wolinsky JS, Ahn CW, PROMiSe Trial MRSI Group. Longitudinal magnetic resonance spectroscopic imaging of primary progressive multiple sclerosis patients treated with glatiramer acetate: multicenter study. Mult Scler. 2008;14(1):73–80.
118. Obert D, Helms G, Sättler MB, et al. Brain metabolite changes in patients with relapsing-remitting and secondary progressive multiple sclerosis: a two-year follow-up study. PLoS One. 2016;11(9):e0162583–15.
119. Choi I-Y, Lee P, Hughes AJ, Denney DR, Lynch SG. Longitudinal changes of cerebral glutathione (GSH) levels associated with the clinical course of disease progression in patients with secondary progressive multiple sclerosis. Mult Scler. 2016;7(7):1352458516669944.
120. Mostert JP, de Groot JC, Ramsaransing GSM, Koch MW, De Keyser J. Relationship between the extent of T2 lesions and the onset of secondary progression in multiple sclerosis. Eur J Neurol. 2007;14(11):1210–5.
121. Mostert JP, Koch MW, Steen C, et al. T2 lesions and rate of progression of disability in multiple sclerosis. Eur J Neurol. 2010;17(12):1471–5.
122. Confavreux C, Vukusic S. Natural history of multiple sclerosis: a unifying concept. Brain. 2006;129(Pt 3):606–16.
123. Khaleeli Z, Ciccarelli O, Mizskiel K, et al. Lesion enhancement diminishes with time in primary progressive multiple sclerosis. Mult Scler. 2010;16(3):317–24.
124. Khaleeli Z, Ciccarelli O, Manfredonia F, et al. Predicting progression in primary progressive multiple sclerosis: a 10-year multicenter study. Ann Neurol. 2008;63(6):790–3.
125. Weinshenker BG, Rice GP, Noseworthy JH, et al. The natural history of multiple sclerosis: a geographically based study. 4. Applications to planning and interpretation of clinical therapeutic trials. Brain. 1991;114(Pt 2):1057–67.
126. Altmann DR, Jasperse B, Barkhof F, et al. Sample sizes for brain atrophy outcomes in trials for secondary progressive multiple sclerosis. Neurology. 2009;72(7):595–601.
127. Chataway J. Biotin in progressive multiple sclerosis: a new lead? Multi Scler (Houndmills, Basingstoke, England). 2016;22(13):1640–1.
128. De Stefano N, Arnold DL. Towards a better understanding of pseudoatrophy in the brain of multiple sclerosis patients. Mult Scler. 2015;21(6):675–6.
129. Chard D. Brain atrophy measurements should be used to guide therapy monitoring in MS—Commentary. Mult Scler. 2016;22(12):1526–7.
130. De Stefano N, Stromillo ML, Giorgio A, et al. Establishing pathological cut-offs of brain atrophy rates in multiple sclerosis. J Neurol Neurosurg Psychiatry. 2016;87(1):93–9.
131. Frohman EM, Fujimoto JG, Frohman TC, et al. Optical coherence tomography: a window into the mechanisms of multiple sclerosis. Nature clinical practice. Neurology. 2008;4(12):664–75.
132. Gordon-Lipkin E, Calabresi PA. Optical coherence tomography: A quantitative tool to measure neurodegeneration and facilitate testing of novel treatments for tissue protection in multiple sclerosis. J Neuroimmunol. 2017;304(C):93–6.

133. Syc SB, Saidha S, Newsome SD, et al. Optical coherence tomography segmentation reveals ganglion cell layer pathology after optic neuritis. Brain. 2012;135(Pt 2):521–33.
134. Oberwahrenbrock T, Schippling S, Ringelstein M, et al. Retinal damage in multiple sclerosis disease subtypes measured by high-resolution optical coherence tomography. Mult Scler Int. 2012;2012(5035):1–10.
135. Siger M, Dziegielewski K, Jasek L, et al. Optical coherence tomography in multiple sclerosis: thickness of the retinal nerve fiber layer as a potential measure of axonal loss and brain atrophy. J Neurol. 2008;255(10):1555–60.
136. Trip SA, Schlottmann PG, Jones SJ, et al. Retinal nerve fiber layer axonal loss and visual dysfunction in optic neuritis. Ann Neurol. 2005;58(3):383–91.
137. Gelfand JM, Goodin DS, Boscardin WJ, et al. Retinal axonal loss begins early in the course of multiple sclerosis and is similar between progressive phenotypes. PLoS One. 2012;7(5):e36847.
138. Balk LJ, Tewarie P, Killestein J, et al. Disease course heterogeneity and OCT in multiple sclerosis. Mult Scler. 2014;20(9):1198–206.
139. Burkholder BM, Osborne B, Loguidice MJ, et al. Macular volume determined by optical coherence tomography as a measure of neuronal loss in multiple sclerosis. Arch Neurol. 2009;66(11):1366–72.
140. Saidha S, Al-Louzi O, Ratchford JN, et al. Optical coherence tomography reflects brain atrophy in multiple sclerosis: a four-year study. Ann Neurol. 2015;78(5):801–13.
141. Petracca M, Cordano C, Cellerino M, et al. Retinal degeneration in primary-progressive multiple sclerosis: a role for cortical lesions? Mult Scler. 2017;23(1):43–50.
142. Talman LS, Bisker ER, Sackel DJ, et al. Longitudinal study of vision and retinal nerve fiber layer thickness in multiple sclerosis. Ann Neurol. 2010;67(6):749–60.
143. Ratchford JN, Saidha S, Sotirchos ES, et al. Active MS is associated with accelerated retinal ganglion cell/inner plexiform layer thinning. Neurology. 2013;80(1):47–54.
144. Serbecic N, Aboul-Enein F, Beutelspacher SC, et al. High resolution spectral domain optical coherence tomography (SD-OCT) in multiple sclerosis: the first follow up study over two years. PLoS One. 2011;6(5):e19843–6.
145. Serbecic N, Aboul-Enein F, Beutelspacher SC, et al. High-resolution spectral domain-optical coherence tomography in multiple sclerosis, Part II—The Total Macular Volume. The First Follow-Up Study over 2 Years. Front Neurol. 2014;5:20.
146. Henderson APD, Trip SA, Schlottmann PG, et al. A preliminary longitudinal study of the retinal nerve fiber layer in progressive multiple sclerosis. J Neurol. 2010;257(7):1083–91.
147. Petzold A. Neuroprotection and visual function after optic neuritis. Curr Opin Neurol. 2017;30(1):67–73.
148. Martínez-Lapiscina EH, Arnow S, Wilson JA, et al. Retinal thickness measured with optical coherence tomography and risk of disability worsening in multiple sclerosis: a cohort study. Lancet Neurol. 2016;15(6):574–84.

Chapter 6
Biomarkers of Disease Progression

Axel Petzold

6.1 Introduction

Diagnostic criteria in multiple sclerosis (MS) continue to evolve [1]. Once a diagnosis is made a majority of patients will want to know about their long term prognosis [2]. The difficulty in providing an accurate long term prognosis relates to the unpredictability of the disease course [3]. Biomarkers for disease progression add valuable information in this context [4, 5].

More precisely when seen in clinic patients ask questions such as: "How bad is my disease?" or "What is my chance for another relapse?" [6]. There will be no completely accurate answer to these questions [2]. What can be said about disease progression will be based on an estimate of probabilities [7]. Biomarkers can be used to statistically model the probability of disease progression [8].

Disease progression due to axonal loss will be inoxerable [9]. In contrast to axonal loss, patients have a chance for recovery of function caused by demyelination and conduction block [10]. For this reason biomarkers which allow to assess axonal loss in MS are of particular interest for this chapter on disease progression [11, 12].

A. Petzold
Moorfields Eye Hospital, London, UK

Dutch Expertise Centre for Neuro–ophthalmology, VU Medical Center, Amsterdam,
The Netherlands & UCL Institute of Neurology, London, UK
e-mail: a.petzold@ucl.ac.uk

A. Wilkins (ed.), *Progressive Multiple Sclerosis*,
https://doi.org/10.1007/978-3-319-65921-3_6

6.2 Biomarker Definitions

The National Institutes of Health (NIH) workshop on biomarkers definitions are:

- Biomarker: "a characteristic that is objectively measured and evaluated as an indicator of normal biologic processes, pathogenic processes, or pharmacological responses to therapeutic intervention" [13]. Biomarkers may be sub-classified into:
  - Process biomarkers: biomarkers which allow monitoring of the dynamics and activity of pathological features.
  - Predictive biomarkers: biomarkers which can narrow the choices between treatment options [14].
  - Prognostic biomarkers: biomarkers which are associated with a clinical outcome, such as a time-to-event outcome [14].
- Surrogate endpoint: "defines a biomarker that is intended to serve as a substitute of a clinically meaningful endpoint and is expected to predict the effect of a therapeutic intervention or the evolution of disease [13]".
- Clinical endpoint: "defines a meaningful measure which captures how a patient feels, functions or survives [13]." Clinical endpoints can be broken down to:
  - Time-to-event outcome: The time until a predefined event occurs, e.g. the time to reaching a certain score on the Expanded Disability Status Scale score (EDSS) [15] ranging from 0 (normal) to 10 (death due to multiple sclerosis).
  - Intermediate endpoint: represents "a clinical endpoint that is not the ultimate outcome but is nonetheless of real clinical usefulness [13]" (e.g. a clinical scale [15, 16]).
  - Ultimate clinical outcome: represents "a clinical endpoint reflective of accumulation of irreversible morbidity and survival. [13]"

6.3 Biomarkers for Axonal Loss

Simplified, there are two types of biomarkers: those which are detectable during the acute phase of axonal loss [17]; and those which can document the loss of axons at a later stage [18]:

1. **Early** biomarkers of axonal loss:
   - Body fluid biomarkers released during axonal disintegration [11, 19]
   - *In vivo* apoptosis markers [20]
2. **Late** biomarkers of axonal loss:
   - Magnetic resonnance imaging (MRI) of the brain [21]
   - Optical coherence tomography (OCT) of the retina [22, 23]
   - Multimodal evoked potentials [24]

This chapter focuses on early biomarkers of axonal loss, which are body fluid biomarkers [25]. Historically, much of body fluid biomarker research in MS was conducted in the cerebrospinal fluid (CSF) [4]. This concept has substantially developed over the past years following discovery of the glympatic system [26].

6.4 The Cerebrospinal Fluid (CSF)

Normal CSF is clear and colourless and 70% of CSF water content originates from the choroid plexus [4]. The CSF represents an ultrafiltrate derived from the choroid plexus which has a filtration rate of about 40 mL/h [27]. Only about 30% of the CSF water comes from the meninges and the blood–nerve barrier which is located at level of the nerve roots. For biomarker research in MS it is important to realise that CSF water also comes from the interstial fluid (ISF) of the brain parenchyma [28]. Synonymous to ISF the literature used the term extracellular fluid (ECF) [28, 29]. Because plasma proteins diffuse through the blood-nerve barrier along the entire length of the spinal cord they are highest in the lumbar CSF.

About 80% of the CSF proteins originate from the plasma and only 20% come from the brain parenchyma. Overall, the CSF has a much lower protein concentration (350 g/L) compared to the serum (70,000 g/L). Nevertheless, biomarkers released by pathology of the brain parenchyma, such as formation of MS lesions or axonal loss will in most cases outweight the proportion of similar proteins transferred from the blood. This may change with a defective blood brain barrier which may allow for proteins to leak from the blood into the CSF.

6.4.1 The Blood Brain Barrier

The blood brain barrier (BBB) acts as a filter preventing the unselective diffusion of compounds into the human brain. To be precise, the anatomically defined BBB needs to be distinguished from the functionally defined blood–CSF barrier (BCB). The BCB is a sieve permitting small substances to diffuse from the blood into the CSF [30].

At time of writing the gold-standard for assessment of the BBB/BCB function is still based on the measurement of albumin in the CSF and serum [31]. With an intact BBB/BCB only a small amount of albumin can diffuse into the CSF (normal range ≈ 144–336 mg/L). In normal conditions, the CSF to serum albumin quotient is smaller than 0.0074. With breakdown of the BCB, serum albumin leaks into the ISF and CSF, the CSF albumin rises and the CSF to serum albumin quotient increases.

Sampling of the ISF is more challenging compared to the CSF and typically require microdialysis techniques [32]. Because it is not ethical to use this invasive technique in patients with MS progress in the field comes from neurointensive care units [29] and experimental studies [33]. There is a continuous fluid exchange between the CSF and ISF. Whilst conventional wisdom used to be that osmotic gradients were most relevant, more recent evidence points towards relevance of connective influx of the CSF [33].

6.4.2 The Glymphatic System

The brain glymphatic hypothesis states that hydrostatic pressure is relevant for trans-astrocytic water flow [33]. Pulsation of blood vessels drives water through AQP4 channels. The AQP4 channels are highly expressed at the astrocytic foot-processes which makes them a relevant autoimmune target in neuromyelitis optica [34]. The glymphatic system proposes that the CSF influx to the brain parenchyma promotes convective ICF flow, ultimately directed at the perivenous space. Because of similarities with the lymphatic system, and the special role taken by glial cells, the term 'glymphatic' was introduced [26]. The diurnal activity of the glymphatic system is considerable with highest activity during sleep. This has thought to be relevant for removal of compounds. The brain glymphatic system is particularly relevant for the clearance of proteins and protein breakdown products involved in neurodegenerative pathology.

The role of the glymphatic system in MS has not yet been studied in detail and its role for driving autoimmunity is unclear [35]. Given the access difficulties to the brain ICF *in vivo* in MS it will not be straightforward to address these questions. Because of developmental similarities between the brain and retina three different lines of research suggested presence of a retinal glymphatic system [36–38]. The existence of a retinal glymphatic system has not yet been shown experimentally. One advantage of investigating the presumed retinal glymphatic system in MS is that this can readily be done using non–invasive imaging techniques such as OCT [22, 23].

6.5 Early Biomarkers for Axonal Loss

In MS disintegration of the axonal membrane causes release of the cytoplasmatic content from injured axons the surrounding extracellular fluid (ECF, ISF) of the human brain [29]. The glymphatic system facilitates flux of these substances from the brain ECF/ISF into the blood stream from where they can be sampled and quantified. Sampling from blood, as opposed to CSF, has huge advantages for longitudinal studies in MS [39].

Of note, some biomarkers are only expressed by certain cell types. They are called cell–type–specific biomarkers. The measurement of cell–type specific biomarkers indirectly permits to estimate the degree of e.g. axonal loss.

6.6 Challenges for Biomarkers in MS

The challenges for biomarkers in MS are the pathological disease heterogeneity; the highly variable clinical course; and the subclinical disease course with acute relapse related damage on top of pre–existing damage. Probably this problem is greatest for any biomarker which is not specific for the neuro-axonal compartment. For example, the glial biomarkers S100B or glial fibrillary acidic protein (GFAP) will be increased following acute relapse related glial activation as well as after formation of a glial scar later in the disease course [41]. Even more difficult are biomarkers indicating systemic inflammation independent to whether or not there are acute MS lesions forming in the brain [42]. In contrast, a rise of biomarkers specific for the axonal compartment are likely to indicate acute damage to the one structure responsible for disability progression [43]. To add value, a biomarker should improve on the clinical prognostic accuracy.

At disease onset either the optic nerve, spinal cord or brainstem are affected in 85% of cases [44]. The risk for developing MS is higher with spinal cord involvement compared to isolated optic nerve pathology. About 85% of patients develop a relapsing remitting disease course [45]. Once patients reach an EDSS of 4 they disease course seems to progress inoxerably. A large proportion of these patients will lose their ability to walk independently (EDSS 6; within 20.1 years of disease onset and will be wheelchair–bound (EDSS 7) within 29.9 years of disease onset) [46]. The prognosis is much better in patients presenting with MS optic neuritis (MSON) [47]. Of note not all patients presenting with optic neuritis (ON) or transverse myelitis (TM) develop MS [6]. This implies that a biomarker result cannot be interpreted in isolation, but needs to be seen as an extension of the clinical assessment.

6.7 CSF Biomarkers in MS

There is no diagnostic biomarker for MS. Data from the available biomarkers are best interpreted in knowledge of a comprehensive CSF analysis.

6.7.1 *Routine CSF Analysis*

The reason for a standardised basic CSF analysis is that the specificity for any biomarker in the differential diagnosis of MS improves [4]. There are six core points to be considered:

1. Any biomarker should only be regarded as an extension of the clinical assessment
2. CSF cytology:
   - A high red blood cell count (5×10^9/L to 7×10^9/L) in the absence of bilirubin (assessed by spectrophotometry) suggests a traumatic tap. This may render other quantitative tests uninterpretable
   - A slightly raised white cell count ($>5 \times 10^6$/L) may be found in up to 34% of patients with MS
   - A high white cell count ($>50 \times 10^6$/L) is unusual in MS
3. CSF glucose: the CSF/serum ratio should be >0.4; low CSF glucose levels suggest an infectious process
4. CSF total protein: a very high CSF total protein content (>1 g/L) suggests an infectious or neoplastic process. High CSF total protein is occasionally seen in patients with chronic inflammatory demyelinating polyneuropathy (CIDP) who also have central demyelination
5. CSF/serum albumin quotient: allows assessment of the integrity of the blood–CSF barrier and is the basis for quantitative models on intrathecal immunoglobulins
6. CSF lactate: an increase in CSF lactate (>2.4 nmol/L) is unusual in MS and may suggest mitochondrial or infectious pathology

Good clinical selection and a basic CSF program help to minimise *pre-analytical* pitfalls leading to a false–positive or false–negative CSF biomarker results.

6.7.2 *Intrathecal IgG Synthesis—CSF Oligoclonal Bands*

Currently diagnosis of multiple sclerosis is based on dissemination in time and space. Before 2010 lack of MRI evidence for dissemination in space could be substituted by a paraclinical test, CSF oligoclonal bands (OCB). A debate followed discussing the value of cerebrospinal fluid (CSF) analysis [48–50]. These arguments have been refined over the subsequent 5 years [51, 52]. The authors have one point in common which is illustrated by a personal case.

6.7.2.1 Illustrative Clinical Case

In February 2011, a 41-year old, right–handed man experienced an episode of vertigo. His general practitioner noticed nystagmus and referred him to the Ear, Nose and Throat (ENT) specialist. The vertigo was thought to be central in origin and a

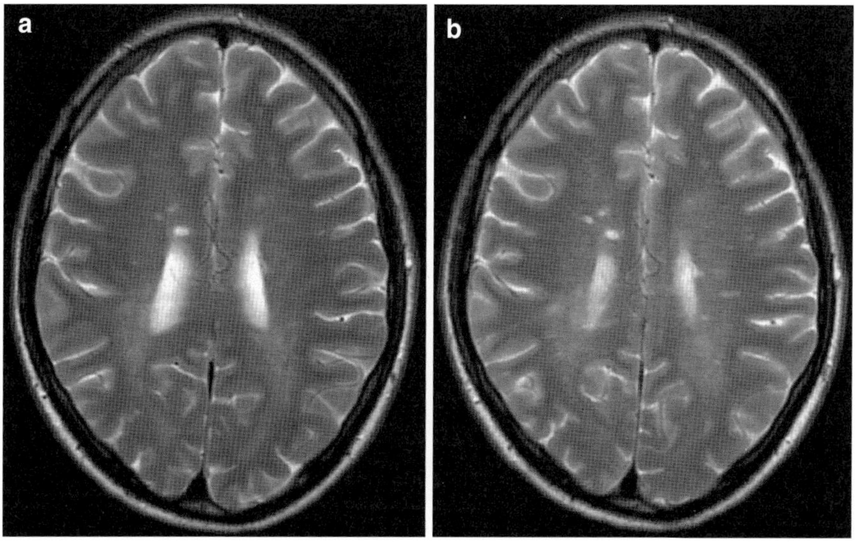

Fig. 6.1 MRI brain of a 41 year–old man demonstrating non–contrast enhancing T–2 lesions exclusively located in the paraventricular regions in (**a**) April 2011 and (**b**) July 2011

MRI was requested. This MRI demonstrated multiple paraventricular T2–lesions (Fig. 6.1a). By May 2011 the patient had made a full recovery.

In July 2011 he developed pain on eye–movements in his right eye. About 1 week later his vision started to deteriorate. He was referred to a Neurologist, who diagnosed optic neuritis. Visual evoked potentials (VEP) of the right eye were severely prolonged (P100, 125 ms). A repeat MRI did not show any new lesions (Fig. 6.1b). A subsequent lumbar puncture revealed intrathecally–synthesised oligoclonal bands (type 2 pattern, see below).

Taken together there were two attacks, one of which was clinically confirmed by a neurologist. Radiologically this patient did not fulfill DIS or DIT [53]. A diagnosis of MS could not be made in 2011 [53]. A year earlier, however the patient would been diagnosed with MS because evidence of intrathecally–produced IgG would have been a substitute for radiological DIS [54, 55].

6.7.2.2 CSF OCB—Analytical Aspects

One frequently cited criticism of CSF OCB has to do with reproducibility. Why does one laboratory get a different result compared to another laboratory? And which laboratory should one believe?

There is evidence that poor analytical quality can cause a loss of sensitivity (45–77%) much efforts had been made to optimise sample collection and processing [56]. Teunissen et al. have written an influential standardisation protocol for CSF analysis in MS [57]. In addition, specific recommendations for CSF OCB analysis have been developed [58].

Adhering to these guidelines an almost perfect inter–laboratory agreement (kappa >0.8) was found for 19 Spanish laboratories [59]. Likewise, data were excellent for 114 UK laboratories which participated in an external national quality assessment service (UK NEQAS) between 2008 to 2011. The analytical sensitivity ranged from 92 to 98% and the analytical specificity from 95 to 98%. Taken together these data suggest that lessons have been learned and a level of analytical accuracy has been reached which is acceptable.

6.7.2.3 The Source of CSF OCB

The immune system requires B–cells to produce IgG. Each of us has about 10^9 distinct B–cell clones. The B-cells reside in the meninges and parenchyma of the CNS [61, 62]. Only a small number of B–cell clones are present in the CNS [63]. Therefore any intrathecally–produced IgG can only ever be oligoclonal. This oligoclonal IgG is seen as a "band" on IEF, the preferred method [58]. Hence the name OCB.

Clonally–expanded B–cells from the CSF were shown to be the source of matching CSF IgG [64, 65].

The enormous diversity of IgG antibodies is achieved by IgG gene rearrangement (somatic hypermutation) during B–cell development (clonal expansion) [66]. This is done in a precise order. Firstly the heavy chain rearranges. Once a functional heavy chain results, the kappa chain rearranges. If kappa is unproductive (or cannot pair with the heavy chain) then lambda will rearrange.

This impressive antibody diversity is needed because of the potential threat any intruding molecule/organism poses to the human body. The immune system cannot risk leaving all the defense to one single clone of B–cells: the IgG may not be effective, e.g. because the target antigen may change, be masked or be shed. For these reasons any systemic infection triggers an oligoclonal response. Consequently a large number of B–cells are recruited and stimulated by cytokines. What is seen as polyclonal IgG in the serum is probably the result of this massive cytokine stimulation resulting in activity of B–cells. Each of these B–cell clones produces a slightly differently composed IgG molecule targeted at the potential antigen threat. Over time, particularly effective clones may be selected. This process is not fully understood and modification of B–cells in the germinal centers plays a role alongside somatic mutations and affinity maturation.

In the CNS only a small number of B–cell clones are present in the CNS. Hence the intrathecal B–cell immune response can only ever be oligoclonal. Further development of analytical techniques may reveal more about the different clones and their immunoglobulins.

From a biological point of view there appears to be a continuum from the systemic polycoclonal immune response to the oligoclonal, and occasionally monoclonal, immune response observed in the CNS. Any process triggering a B–cell response may lead to the presence of IgG in the CSF.

6.7.2.4 Five Keys to Understanding CSF OCB

Five simple keys to interprete OCBs results are:

- In normal CSF **all** IgG comes from the blood by passive diffusion
- In normal CSF and serum IgG is polyclonal
- Oligoclonal bands in blood give a mirror pattern in CSF
- Local synthesis is present when there are bands in the CSF that are absent from the serum
- Oligoclonal bands are (generally) a sign of pathology.

6.7.2.5 CSF OCB Are Not Specific for MS

Presence of CSF OCB has been described in MS and a range of other diseases [67–86]. The interpretation CSF OCB will depend on the clinical situation. Presence of CSF OCB can be taken as an indicator for a pathological relevant autoimmune process, an epiphenomenon or an inflammatory response. This interpretation will depend on the pattern of OCB seen on IEF.

6.7.2.6 Five OCB Patterns

The current recommendations are to use IEF for detection of OCB [58]. This is a qualitative technique. Therefore pattern recognition is crucial. It was suggested that the observed patterns be designated as "Type 1" to "Type 5" [58].

Figure 5 shows the five classical patterns and one more which can be relevant:

- **Type 1**: no bands in CSF and serum (S)
- **Type 2**: oligoclonal IgG bands in CSF, not in the serum, indicative of intrathecal IgG synthesis.
- **Type 3**: oligoclonal bands in the CSF (like Type 2) and additional identical oligoclonal bands in CSF and serum samples.
- **Type 4**: identical oligoclonal bands in CSF and serum indicating a systemic rather than an intrathecal immune reaction, with a leaky or normal or abnormal blood–CSF barrier and oligoclonal bands passively transferred into the CSF.
- **Type 5**: monoclonal bands in the CSF and serum sample seen in the presence of a paraprotein (monoclonal IgG component).

For didactic reasons *mnemonics* may come useful to remember the CSF OCB patterns.

- **Normal**: no bands in CSF and serum (type 1 [58])
- **Local**: oligoclonal bands in CSF but not in the serum, indicative of isolated intrathecal oligoclonal IgG synthesis (type 2 [58])

- **Mirror**: identical oligoclonal bands in CSF and serum, indicating a systemic rather than an intrathecal immune reaction where oligoclonal bands are passively transferred into the CSF (type 4 [58])
- **Mirror plus**: oligoclonal bands in the CSF and additional identical oligoclonal bands in CSF and serum samples, the space between bands is irregular (type 3 [58])
- **Mirror steps**: monoclonal bands in the CSF and serum sample seen in the presence of a paraprotein (monoclonal IgG component), spaced in symmetric steps (type 5 [58])
- **Artifact**: bands caused by pre–analytical or analytical problems.

6.7.2.7 Interpretation of OCB Patterns

Type 1 is easy: this is a negative test result. However, absence of evidence does not necessary provide evidence for absence. Figure 6.2 shows the IEF pattern of a patient with a clinical isolated syndrome (CIS) in 2004 and again 18 months later. Clearly a Type 2 pattern has developed and the patient then fullfilled the criteria for definite MS. If the clinical picture strongly suggests a diagnosis of MS, then a repeat lumbar puncture may be indicated in any patient with initially OCB–negative CSF.

Type 2 is also straight forward: specific bands are present in the CSF but not in the serum. This pattern is observed in patients with MS. It can be as discrete as shown in Fig. 6.2 or as strong as shown in Fig. 5. MS is probably the disease with the strongest stimulation of the B–cell clones within the CNS parenchyma. But, as mentioned above, OCBs are also seen in a number of other diseases, with the present list likely to be incomplete. An oligoclonal pattern in the CSF is pathological and requires further investigation.

The interpretation of Type 3 and 4 patterns is more complex [58]. In particular, Type 4 can be misinterpreted if the amount of IgG in the serum is too high, as this can blur the serum bands. This is one reason for adding equal amounts of IgG from

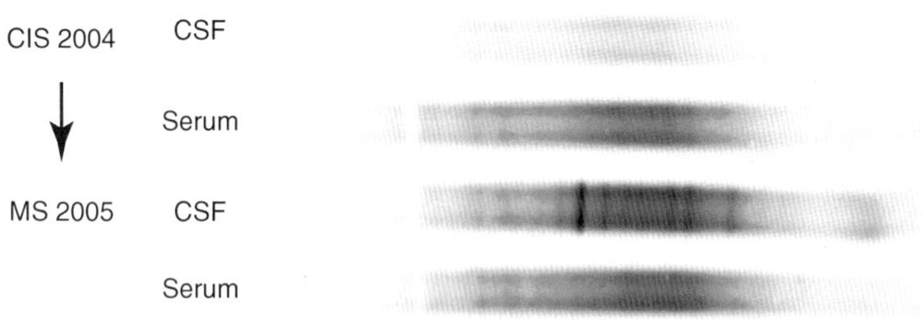

Fig. 6.2 The CSF in a patient presenting with CIS who showed no evidence of intrathecal IgG in 2004 but developed oligoclonal IgG bands in 2005

the CSF and the serum sample [58, 87]. Type 4 can be seen in conditions such as Guillain–Barré syndrome. Type 5 indicates the presence of a monoclonal gammopathy, but IEF resolves what would be a single band using other electrophoretic techniques, into multiple bands differing by 1 U of charge. This peculiarity is probably due to post–translational modifications such as glycosylation.

6.7.2.8 CSF Monoclonal Band

McCombe et al. found a CSF monoclonal band in 3/1490 of CSF samples [88]. The diagnoses were lymphoma or lymphomatoid granulomatosis within or adjacent to the nervous system in two patients and a chronic inflammatory demyelinating polyneuropathy in the third. Ben–Hur et al. (using the less sensitive agarose electrophoresis) described 20 patients with a CSF monoclonal band [89]. The diagnoses were clinically definite MS, probable MS, CIS, SLE, paraneoplastic syndrome, peripheral neuropathies, superficial siderosis and torsion dystonia.

Davies et al. performed a repeat lumbar puncture in 31 patients who had a monoclonal band in the CSF but not in the serum [90]. All patients who developed clinically definite MS also converted from an intrathecal monoclonal to a oligoclonal pattern.

6.7.2.9 Number CSF OCB Bands

It has been proposed that a higher number of bands may be of prognostic or diagnostic value. Bourahoui et al. concluded that the presence of ≥10 bands in the CSF was highly specific for MS [69].

In contrast, Koch et al. studied 143 patients (110 OCB positive, 33 OCB negative) and did not find any relationship between the presence and number (or absence) of CSF OCB bands and either disease progression or MS subgroups (RR, SP, PP disease) [91]. The percentage of OCB–negative.

MS patients (23%) in this study was higher compared to the studies shown in Table 3, with all groups using IEF followed by IgG specific immunofixation.

There are two potential problems:

- Absent OCBs in MS are rare. Are there any pre-analytical (diagnostic) or analytical (sensitivity) reasons for this?
- Counting the number of bands in the CSF may not be a true reflection of the number of B-cell clones producing the bands. Post–translational modification of IgG probably also includes changes in the disulfide bonds which changes the pI, resulting in a differential migration in the electric field. Therefore different IgG bands seen on the immunoblot may originate from the same clone. In order to address the biological relevance of OCBs, the number of clones producing the bands (reflecting the vigor of the immune response) may turn out to be more relevant than merely the number of bands present.

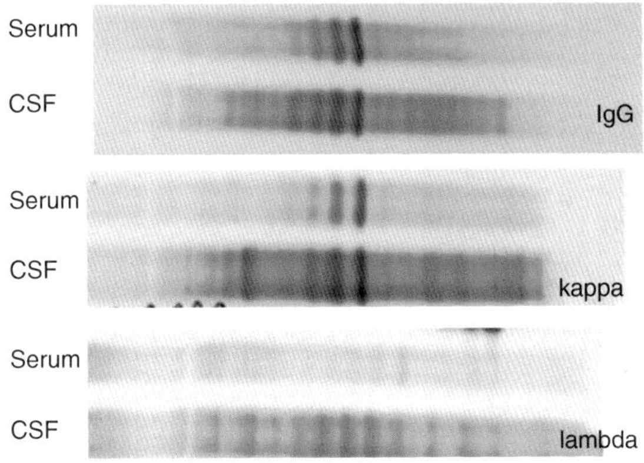

Fig. 6.3 A "ladder" is observed for total IgG. In this situation it is useful to stain for kappa and lambda light chains. (**a**) Total IgG, (**b**) free & bound kappa and (**c**) free & bound lambda

6.7.2.10 CSF Light Chains

As mentioned above, one B–cell clone can only express either kappa or lambda light chains. Because kappa is rearranged first, it is quantitatively the dominant light chain in the human body. Therefore the kappa light chain (free and bound) is found more frequently in the CSF than lambda.

In practise, immunoblotting for kappa/lambda light chains can be helpful in the following situations:

- When a ladder (Fig. 6.3) is seen with total IgG. This could be due to post-translational modifications of one single IgG molecule. Kappa/lambda staining decides whether this IgG is monoclonal. Monoclonal IgG only stains for one light chain.
- Where it is uncertain whether or not very faint bands are present. In one study [93] we found that the sensitivity for detecting OCBs in the CSF in clinically–definite MS patients increased from 89% to 98% using kappa/lamba staining (unpublished data). In view of this, it may be interesting to reanalyse the CSF of those MS patients reported to be OCB–negative, using kappa/lambda staining [91, 94, 95].
- Finally if there is "negative staining" (looking very white) at the beginning of the blot (towards the cathode). This may be due to IgM which is not picked up by the IgG staining and kappa/lambda can be of help.

6.7.2.11 CSF IgM OCB

Luisa Maria Villar has pioneered the investigation of CSF IgM bands in MS for the past decade [96]. The method has been validated [97]. As in any immune–response, IgM levels increase in the serum and CSF before IgG develops.

Sensitive and specific detection of CSF oligoclonal IgM bands is possible using IEF [96]. As with IgG, IgM is not specific for MS but is also found in other inflammatory CNS diseases [98]. CSF IgM was found to be of prognostic relevance in MS [99]. Importantly, CSF IgM OCB were found to be associated with axonal damage in MS [100]. In PPMS, IgM OCB were suggested to permit targetable inflammation [101]. Using OCT as an outcome measure it was possible to demonstrate an association between retinal nerve fibre atrophy and ganglion cell inner plexiform layer loss with presence of intrathecal lipid–specific CSF IgM OCBs [102].

6.7.2.12 CSF OCB and the Cause of MS

One intriguing hypothesis is that identification of the IgG antigens could reveal the cause of MS [103].

To illustrate this line of though an analogy will be used, which refers to high–affinity CSF IgG. In this example the CSF IgG OCBs will be mostly directed against viral antigens. A convenient laboratory technique for detecting such high–affinity viral antigen specific IgG is immunoblotting. This technique is readily available in a laboratory already using IEF for OCB detection [104]. An illustrative example of such a high–affinity IgG immunoblot is shown in Fig. 6.4.

Typically patients with subacute sclerosing panencephalitis (SSPE) have CSF IgG directed against the measles virus. An immunoblot against measles–specific antigens can help to identify them (see Fig. 6.5).

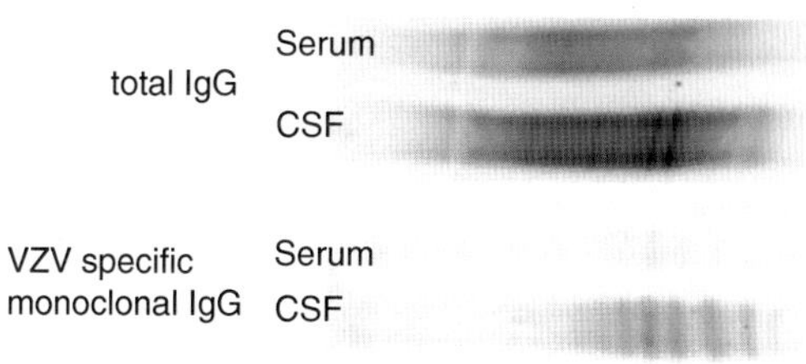

Fig. 6.4 The antigen specific immunoblot pulls out monoclonal IgG (the IgG is distributed in a ladder pattern) directed against VZV from the polyclonal background

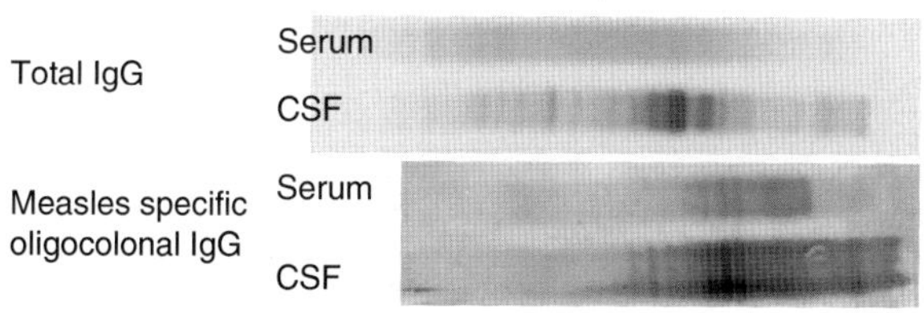

Fig. 6.5 Local synthesis of measles–specific oligoclonal IgG in Sub–acute Sclerosing Progressive Encephalomyelitis (SSPE)

The interpretation of antigen–specific bands needs to consider the following:

- If the total IgG and antigen–specific IgG patterns share >50% of bands, this probably indicates a causal relationship
- If there are multiple bands present against several viruses, this is probably an amnestic response
- Monoclonal antibodies may develop into oligoclonal antibodies
- The process is dynamic

To conclude with the analogy, CSF IgG is typically of high–affinity. However part of the problem in MS is that most of the CSF IgG in MS is of low affinity [105–107]. Unfortunately, attempts to identify the cause of MS using CSF OCB have not been successful. There is mounting evidence that much of the CSF OCB may represent an epiphenomenon of tissue damage.

6.7.2.13 CSF OCB in MS Target Debris

There is evidence that CSF OCBs are directed at self-proteins [108]. The CSF OCB may therefore contribute to waste clearance by targeting debris [109].

This interpretation may explain some of the points made above: firstly, the absence of CSF OCB at disease onset with limited tissue damage of short duration (see Fig. 6.2; with accumulation of tissue damage CSF OCB will develop); secondly, evolution of CSF monocolonal bands to CSF OCB in patients with MS over time; thirdly, the prognostic relevance of higher number of bands in patients with progressive tissue damage over a long period of time; fourthly, similarities of findings for IgG, IgM and light chains; fifthly, low diagnostic specificity of CSF OCB for MS if the differential diagnosis includes other inflammatory or autoimmune conditions with tissue damage; and sixthly, the low affinity of CSF OCB and the failure to discover a causative antigen.

6.8 Cell-Type Specific Protein Biomarkers in MS

The importance for biomarkers in neuro–axonal degeneration cannot be overestimated. For a patient, loss of function due to axonal loss is likely to be permanent [110]. Simplified, loss of function can be caused by demyelination and conduction block, both of which are reversible; and axonal loss which is irreversible. Disintegration of the axonal membrane leads to release of axonal proteins into the ECF and CSF as described above.

Biomarkers relevant for axonal degeneration in MS research have recently been reviewed [112–114]. Axonal biomarkers can distinguish between MS subtypes [115–118]. Of these, neurofilaments were most consistently found to be of prognostic relevance [115, 117–129]. There is evidence for axonal transport deficits in MS affecting Nf as a cargo of the motor protein KIF5A [130].

At present neurofilaments are probably one of the most promising axonal biomarkers in conditions with substantial axonal loss [116, 121, 127, 128, 131–141]. The concept has been validated in animal and cell-culture experiments [19, 142]. A number of analytical techniques have been developed to this purpose [39, 131, 143–148].

Firstly, immunohistochemistry was used to show the almost complete loss of axonal continuity, the presence of axonal end–bulbs and almost total loss of axons in the atrophied spinal cords from CREAE mice. Secondly, analysis of this spinal cord tissue homogenate using an ELISA technique showed that the proportion of tissue NfH^{SMI35} was significantly lower in CREAE animals compared to controls, and was consistent with axonal loss.

Another, important advantage is that the phosphorylated Nf heavy chain can also be quantified from the blood in patients with ON and MS [119, 125, 144].

6.9 The Challenge of Subclinical Disease Activity for Biomarkers in MS

An important question to answer is how biomarkers can be used in MS to distinguish a recent insult from biomarkers released by subclinical disease activity related to older MS lesions. It may be possible to address this difficult question by investigate post–translational modifications such as phosphorylation or glycosylation of cell–type–specific proteins.

In MS there is some evidence that the phosphorylation of NfH is changed in the MS brain [149]. This is consistent with the *in vivo* finding of increased CSF levels of NfH phosphorylation NfH in patients who reach the secondary progressive phase of their disease [117] and those who are more severely disabled, using the newly developed Global Multiple Sclerosis Severity Score (MSSS) [150]. Phosphorylation is only one of the many post–translational modifications biomarkers may undergo with disease.

6.9.1 Post-translational Modifications of Biomarkers

Many cell-type specific biomarkers are proteins. The biochemical properties of the amino acids used to design these proteins determines the structure. For example lysine is a small amino acid allowing a protein to bend. For this reason most coiled proteins such as collagen contain a high amount of lysine. Many of these proteins undergo physiological changes called *post-translational modification* (PTM). Again, the type of most PTMs are predetermined by the amino acid residues of the protein. For example the amino acids serine, threonine and tyrosine are particularly suitable for adding a phosphate atom (phosphorylation). As proteins age and get damaged and further PTMs such as oxidation occur. Most PTMs are targeted to "hot spots" in the protein. For example, oxidation and glycation are typically targeted on amino acid residues exposed at the protein surface, easily accessible to reactive molecules.

6.9.1.1 PTM: In General

Mechanisms of covalent protein modifications comprise co-translational, post-translational and spontaneous mechanisms. The mechanisms most relevant to CSF biomarker analysis have been summarised in Table 6.1, and fall principally into two categories:

- enzyme–mediated, these should only occur *in vivo* and can be scrutinized for disease–specific signatures,
- spontaneous, which will affect proteins *in vivo* and *in vitro* and are therefore difficult to study because of artefactual modifications.

Many of these PTMs are required to maintain normal cellular function. Under certain conditions they may, however, adversely affect protein and thus cell function, leading to disease. Additionally, non–physiological PTMs may alter the structure of a protein to such a degree that the acquired self–tolerance of the immune–system is breached and an autoimmune response results [151].

- **Glycosylation** Simplified, glycosylation occurs mainly on five amino acids: Asp → Asp-glycan, Ser → Ser-glycan, Thr → Thr-glycan, Hyl → Hyl-glycan, Hyp → Hypglycan. In humans N- and O–glycosylation have been described. C–glycosylation has not yet been described in humans, but is known to occur in bacteria. N-glycosylation occurs at the amino–group of Asn. Oglycosylation occurs at the hydroxy–group of Thr, Ser, hydroxylysine (Hyl) and hydroxyproline (Hyp). Protein glycosylation is central to a range of immune processes.

Table 6.1 Mechanisms of in vivo and in vitro post–translational modifications (PTM) relevant for CSF biomarker analysis

Mechanism	*In vitro*	*In vivo*
Glycosylation	No	Yes
Phosphorylation & dephosphorylation	No	Yes
Citrullination	No	Yes
N–terminal modifications	No	Yes
C–terminal modifications	No	Yes
Deamidation	Yes	Yes
Cross-linking	Yes	Yes
Oxidation	Yes	Yes
Nitrosylation	Yes	Yes
Glycation	Yes	Yes
Isomerisation	Yes	Yes
Racemisation	Yes	Yes
Proteolysis/clevage	Yes	Yes

Altered protein glycosylation may trigger an autoimmune–response [151]. Glycosylation may affect charge and susceptibility to proteolysis.

- **Phosphorylation & Dephosphorylation** Phosphorylation is essential for intracellular signaling. A range of kinases have been described, far exceeding the scope of this chapter (for selected reviews see references [152–164]). Phosphorylation affects manly three aminoacids: Thr → Thr(P), Ser → Ser(P) or Tyr → Tyr(P). It affects protein charge (more positive), molecular weight (heavier) and susceptibility to proteases (more stable with increased phosphorylation). Proteins can be immunogenic dependent on their phosphorylation status [151, 165]. There is data demonstrating that the affinity of Ser to phosphate is so high that it may occur *in vitro*. However, these experiments have been performed in solutions containing a non–physiologically high amount of phosphate. It is thought to be unlikely that spontaneous phosphorylation of proteins occurs to a significant degree in the CSF *in vitro*, because of the energy barrier.
- **Citrullination** Arg → Cit. Citrullination (synonymous: peptidylarginine deimination or just deimination) affects charge and susceptibility to proteolysis. The reaction is catalysed by peptidyl arginine deaminases in a Ca–dependent manner [166].
- **Deamidation** Asp, Gln → Glu and peptide bond hydrolysis, all of which affect protein charge and may also affect susceptibility to proteolysis. The reaction is catalysed by tissue transglutaminase (tTG) in a Ca–dependent manner. A range of autoantigens are substrates to tTG, the most popular being gliadin in coeliac disease [167].
- **Isomerisatoin** Asp → isoAsp, GLx → isoGly. Whilst susceptibility to proteolysis is always affected; the charge will only change if the modified residue is formed from Gln.
- **Racemisation** Axs → D-Asp (D-isoAsp), Glx → DGlu (D-isoGlu). Occasionally also other residues such as Ala, Ser, Thr, etc. may racemise. Again susceptibility to proteolysis is always affected, charge will only change if the modified residue is formed from Gln or Asn.
- **Glycation** Formation of advanced glycation end products (AGEs). The complex reactions leading to AGEs are caused by protein condensation, re–arrangement and fragmentation occurring in concentrated sugar solutions. Cross–links may occur (pentosidine, crossline, imidazolium, etc.), Lys → Amadori products, etc. Many AGEs are unstable and some are immunogenic [151]. Antibodies against AGE modified low density lipoprotein (LDL) have been demonstrated in patients with type I diabetes [168]. Protein charge and susceptibility to proteolysis can be changed.
- **Oxidation** The principal reactions are those of: Met → Met-sulphoxide, lysine → glycoxidation & lipoxidation products, Tyr → *ortho*-Tyr chloroTyr, nitroTyr, Pro & Arg → Glu & Glu–semialdehyde. Protein charge and susceptibility to proteolysis are changed. Enzymes involved in oxidative damage are nitric oxide synthethase (NOS), cyclo–oxygenase (COX), mono–amine oxidase B (MAO-B) [169]. The spectrum of oxidative stress related biomarkers in MS has

recently been reviewed in detail [42]. Spontaneous oxidation occurs with ionisading radiation, reduction of metal ions (Fe(II), Cu(I)) or chemical compounds. Oxidating compounds such as free radicals and are commonly known as reactive oxygen species (ROS).

- **Nitrosylation** S–nitrosylation (S–nitrosation) of the thiol side–chain of cystein with NO affects almost all proteins.
- **Cross-linking** Cross-linking and formation of bityrosin (S-S cross-links) happens with oxidation. There is also spontaneous formation of Cystine (–CH2-S-S-CH2–) disulfides, again particularly under oxidasing conditions. There are a number of further cross-links not summarised here.
- **N–terminal modifications** In humans the N–terminus is frequently Nacetyl "blocked" and common residues are: Ala, Ser, Met, Gly or Thr. Enzymatic removal of these residues is possible.
- **C-terminal modifications** Amidation of the C–terminus is common. Glycine is a frequent donor for the amide. Other mechanisms are methylation and isoprenylation for GPI anchors and ADP–dependent ribosylation of C–terminal Lys.
- **Proteolysis** The CSF is a body fluid rich in proteases, therefore proteins susceptible to proteolysis are quickly degraded. Generally phosphorylation of proteins protects to a certain degree from proteolysis. One example is the stability of the different neurofilament proteins, with NfL being less stable in the CSF than the phosphorylated form of NfH [131, 170–174]. This may be one of the reasons why the stoichemistry of phosphorylated NfH to NfL in the CSF was found to be 1:1.6 instead of the expected ratio of 1:3.

6.9.1.2 Analysis of PTMs

At present there is no simple method available detect all PTMs for any selected biomarker. In future, with the advent of highly sensitive mass–spectroscopy, this may change. There are a number of analytical pitfalls, but probably the most important one is related to sample collection and storage, both of which need to be standardised. One example is the cleavage of cystatin C [175, 176].

6.9.1.3 PTM: In Autoimmunity General

There is evidence that autoimmunity plays an important role in the pathophysiology of MS [177, 178].

Attempts have been made to characterise further the relationship between the cellular and humoral immune system and the antigens mentioned. Those studies provide evidence that PTMs may be of relevance in the development of autoimmunity.

6.9.1.4 PTM: In MS

Is MS a post–translational disease?

- Citrullination
  In MS citrullination is the most studied PTM from those listed in Table 6.1. MS leaves a signature using citrullination on MBP [151, 179–181] and GFAP [201]. Citrullination of MBP alters its conformation and interaction with other proteins and the myelin membrane [202, 203]. The change of charge (citrullination reduces the positive charge) of MBP results in loosening of the otherwise tight compaction of the major dense line between myelin and the axon. It has therefore been speculated that MS may be a post-translational disease where "molecular negativity" may expose MBP epitopes and cause an autoimmune response [204]. To think about MS as a post-translational disease is tempting and analogous to one approach taken for other autoimmune diseases [205–207]. However, much remains speculation and we still know too little about the aetiology of MS and are only just getting access to the analytical tools for detailed investigation of PTMs. Nevertheless, for the interested reader Harauz and Musse have summarised in their detailed review the known effects of citrullination on MBP and myelin stability (Table 1 in [166]). MBP citrullination is probably also of clinical relevance. Wood and Moscarello suggested in the 1980s that there was a relationship between the severity of MS, the degree of myelin degeneration and the characteristics of MBP. Using cation-exchange chromatography it was shown that the citrullination of MBP was about 6.7 to eightfold higher in severe disease, including one case of the Marburg variant, when compared to patients with milder forms of MS [180, 209]. In other words, in normal humans about 20% of MBP is citrullinated, in chronic MS about 45% and in the case report on the Marburg variant about 80% [180, 209]. Peptidylarginine deiminases (PAD or PADI, EC 3.5.3.15) are the enzymes responsible for the conversion of peptide-linked arginine to citrulline in vivo in a Ca-dependent manner. Some of the PAD isoforms were shown to be in increased in MS brain tissue by some [210–213], but not by other investigators [214]. Increased protein citrullination makes EAE worse [166, 215–217].
- Phosphorylation
  Tau An increase of tau phosphorylation in the brain tissue of rat with EAE has been shown [218, 219]. Figure 6.6 shows that for equal amounts of total tau (antibody tau-5) there is a relatively larger proportion of phosphorylated tau (antibodies AT8, AT100, AT-180 and 12E8) in brain tissue from rats with EAE when compared to controls. CSF studies on tau phosphoforms in MS are still lacking. The technology for these studies is available and tau phosphoforms have been studied intensively in the CSF of patients with Alzheimer's disease. It would be interesting to test whether an increase of tau phosphorylation is found in the CSF from patient with MS and whether this relates to disease severity/subtype. One study measured total tau and p-tau levels in the CSF of patients with MS [220], but we do not know about the ratio of p-tau/tau as an estimate for

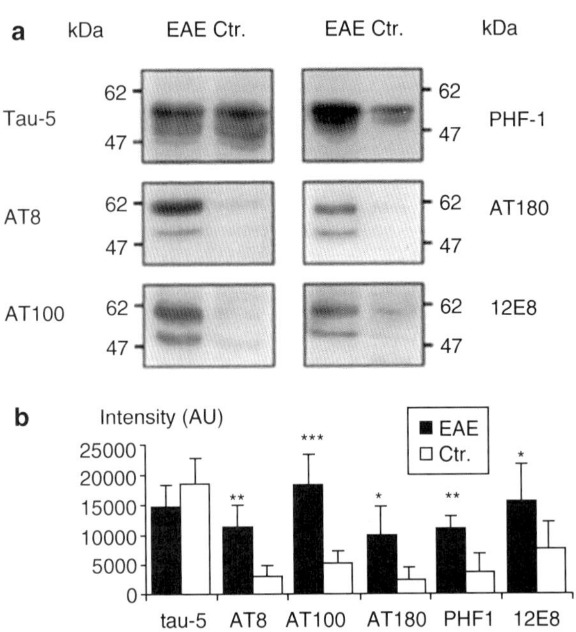

Fig. 6.6 Hyperphosphorylation of tau in rats with EAE. (**a**) Protein lysates prepared from EAE brainstems and controls containing equal amounts of proteins were subjected to Western blot analysis with phosphorylation–dependent antibodies PHF-1 (pS396/pS404), AT-8 (pS202/pT205), AT-100 (pT212/pS214), AT-180 (pT231/pS235), and 12E8 (pS262) in addition to the pan-tau antibody tau-5. (**b**) Quantitative analysis of tau expression and phosphorylation of tau epitopes in EAE and control brains. Values are mean ± S.D., n = 5 for each value. Three independent experiments showed similar results (*$p < 0.05$; **$p < 0.01$; ***$p < 0.001$). Copied from reference [219]

tau phosphorylation. Such a ratio would extend on previous work showing an increase of total tau in the CSF of patients with MS [118, 220–223], a finding not replicated by others [224, 225].

Neurofilaments An increase of NfH phosphorylation has been described in the CSF of patients with secondary progressive MS when compared to those with relapsing remitting disease [117]. Neurofilament phosphorylation was increased about eightfold in patients with optic neuritis compared to other neurological controls [226]. Recently a new clinical score for the severity of MS, the MS severity score (MSSS) has been developed [227]. A re-analysis of the samples from our initial study [117] showed that patients with more severe disease had an eightfold higher degree of NfH phosphorylation [150].

- Glycosylation

  Kaj Blennow's group recently described a new ELISA which allows for the measurement of glycosolyated forms of clusterin in the CSF [228]. Figure 17 demonstrates that enzymatic deglycosylation of clusterin enhances the antibody affinity. There is no data on clusterin glycoforms in the CSF of patients with MS.

Acknowledgements The author's work described in this chapter is supported by the Dutch MS Research Foundation, the University College London Comprehensive Bio-medical Research Centre and the Moorfields Biomedical Research Centre.

References

1. Filippi M, Rocca MA, Ciccarelli O, De Stefano N, Evangelou N, Kappos L, Rovira A, Sastre-Garriga J, Tintorè M, Frederiksen JL, Gasperini C, Palace J, Reich DS, Banwell B, Montalban X, Barkhof F, MAGNIMS Study Group. MRI criteria for the diagnosis of multiple sclerosis: MAGNIMS consensus guidelines. Lancet Neurol. 2016;15(3):292–303.
2. Dennison L, McCloy Smith E, Bradbury K, Galea I. How do people with multiple sclerosis experience prognostic uncertainty and prognosis communication? A qualitative study. PLoS One. 2016;11:e0158982.
3. Larochelle C, Uphaus T, Prat A, Zipp F. Secondary progression in multiple sclerosis: neuronal exhaustion or distinct pathology? Trends Neurosci. 2016;39:325–39.
4. Stangel M, Fredrikson S, Meinl E, Petzold A, Stüve O, and Tumani H. The utility of cerebrospinal fluid analysis in patients with multiple sclerosis. Nat Rev Neurol. 2013;9:267–76.
5. Kuhle J. Comment: "if you can't measure it, you can't improve it" (lord kelvin). Neurology. 2016;87:1335.
6. Petzold A. Isolated, relapsing and progressive demyelinating diseases of the central nervous system. J Neurol. 2008;255(Suppl 6):69–76.
7. Mandel M, Mercier F, Eckert B, Chin P, Betensky RA. Estimating time to disease progression comparing transition models and survival methods—an analysis of multiple sclerosis data. Biometrics. 2013;69:225–34.
8. Petzold A, Bowser R, Calabresi P, Zetterberg H, Uitdehaag BM. Biomarker time out. Mult Scler. 2014;20(12):1560–3.
9. Petzold A. Neurodegeneration and multiple sclerosis. In: Neurodegenerative diseases. London: Springer; 2014. p. 227–45.
10. Friese MA, Schattling B, and Fugger L. Mechanisms of neurodegeneration and axonal dysfunction in multiple sclerosis. Nat Rev Neurol. 2014;10(4):225–38.
11. Petzold A. Neurofilament phosphoforms: surrogate markers for axonal injury, degeneration and loss. J Neurol Sci. 2005;233:183–98.
12. Fitzner B, Hecker M, and Zettl UK. Molecular biomarkers in cerebrospinal fluid of multiple sclerosis patients. Autoimmun Rev. 2015;14(10):903–13.
13. Martin R, Bielekova B, Hohlfeld R, Utz U. Biomarkers in multiple sclerosis. Dis Markers. 2006;22:183–5.
14. McShane LM, Altman DG, Sauerbrei W, Taube SE, Gion M, Clark GM. REporting recommendations for tumor MARKer prognostic studies (REMARK). Breast Cancer Res Treat. 2006;100:229–235.
15. Kurtzke JF. Rating neurological impairment in multiple sclerosis: an expanded disability status scale (EDSS). Neurology. 1983;33:1444–52.
16. Uitdehaag BM, Ader HJ, Roosma TJ, de Groot V, Kalkers NF, Polman CH. Multiple sclerosis functional composite: impact of reference population and interpretation of changes. Mult Scler. 2002;8(5):366–71.
17. Kuhle J, Petzold A. What makes a prognostic biomarker in cns diseases: strategies for targeted biomarker discovery? Part 1: Acute and monophasic diseases. Expert Opin Med Diagn. 2011;5:333–46.
18. Kuhle J, Petzold A. What makes a prognostic biomarker in cns diseases: strategies for targeted biomarker discovery? Part 2: Chronic progressive and relapsing diseases. Expert Opin Med Diagn. 2011;5:393–410.

19. Bacioglu M, Maia LF, Preische O, Schelle J, Apel A, Kaeser SA, Schweighauser M, Eninger T, Lambert M, Pilotto A, Shimshek DR, Neumann U, Kahle PJ, Staufenbiel M, Neumann M, Maetzler W, Kuhle J, Jucker M. Neurofilament light chain in blood and csf as marker of disease progression in mouse models and in neurodegenerative diseases. Neuron. 2016;91:494–6.
20. Macrez R, Stys PK, Vivien D, Lipton SA, Docagne F. Mechanisms of glutamate toxicity in multiple sclerosis: biomarker and therapeutic opportunities. Lancet Neurol. 2016;15(10):1089–102.
21. Hagens M, van Berckel B, Barkhof F. Novel mri and pet markers of neuroinflammation in multiple sclerosis. Curr Opin Neurol. 2016;29(3):229–36.
22. Petzold A, de Boer JF, Schippling S, Vermersch P, Kardon R, Green A, Calabresi PA, and Polman C. Optical coherence tomography in multiple sclerosis: a systematic review and meta-analysis. Lancet Neurol. 2010; Expert Opin Med Diagn. 2011;9(9):921–32.
23. Martinez-Lapiscina EH, Arnow S, Wilson JA, Saidha S, Preiningerova JL, Oberwahrenbrock T, Brandt AU, Pablo LE, Guerrieri S, Gonzalez I, Outteryck O, Mueller AK, Albrecht P, Chan W, Lukas S, Balk LJ, Fraser C, Frederiksen JL, Resto J, Frohman T, Cordano C, Zubizarreta I, Andorra M, Sanchez-Dalmau B, Saiz A, Bermel R, Klistorner A, Petzold A, Schippling S, Costello F, Aktas O, Vermersch P, Oreja-Guevara C, Comi G, Leocani L, Garcia-Martin E, Paul F, Havrdova E, Frohman E, Balcer LJ, Green AJ, Calabresi PA, Villoslada P; IMSVISUAL consortium. Retinal thickness measured with optical coherence tomography and risk of disability worsening in multiple sclerosis: a cohort study. Send toLancet Neurol. 2016:15(6):574–84.
24. Giffroy X, Maes N, Albert A, Maquet P, Crielaard J-M, Dive D. Do evoked potentials contribute to the functional follow-up and clinical prognosis of multiple sclerosis? Acta Neurol Belg. 2017;117(1):53–59.
25. Petzold A and Plant GT. Diagnosis and classification of autoimmune optic neuropathy. Autoimmun Rev. 2014;13:539–45.
26. Jessen NA, Munk ASF, Lundgaard I, Nedergaard M. The glymphatic system: a beginnerâs guide. Neurochem Res. 2015;40(12):2583–99.
27. Nilsson C, Stahlberg F, Thomsen C, Henriksen O, Herning M, Owman C. Circadian variation in human cerebrospinal fluid production measured by magnetic resonance imaging. Am J Physiol. 1992;262:R20–4.
28. Ratner V, Gao Y, Lee H, Nedergaard M, Benveniste H, Tannenbaum AR. Cerebrospinal fluid and interstitial fluid motion via the glymphatic pathway modelled by optimal mass transport. bioRxiv. 2016:043281.
29. Petzold A, Tisdall MM, Girbes AR, Martinian L, Thom M, Kitchen N, and Smith M. In vivo monitoring of neuronal loss in traumatic brain injury: a microdialysis study. Brain. 2011; 134(Pt 2):464–83.
30. Saunders NR, Habgood MD, Møllgård K, Dziegielewska KM. The biological significance of brain barrier mechanisms: help or hindrance in drug delivery to the central nervous system? F1000 Res. 2016;5
31. LeVine SM. Albumin and multiple sclerosis. BMC Neurol. 2016;16(1):1.
32. Young B, Kalanuria A, Kumar M, Burke K, Balu R, Amendolia O, McNulty K, Marion BA, Beckmann B, Ciocco L, et al. Cerebral microdialysis. Crit Care Nurs Clin N Am. 2016;28(1):109–24.
33. Iliff JJ, Wang M, Liao Y, Plogg BA, Peng W, Gundersen GA, Benveniste H, Edward Vates G, Deane R, Goldman SA, et al. A paravascular pathway facilitates CSF flow through the brain parenchyma and the clearance of interstitial solutes, including amyloid. Sci Transl Med. 2012;4(147):147ra111.
34. Hinson SR, Lennon VA, and Pittock SJ. Autoimmune aqp4 channelopathies and neuromyelitis optica spectrum disorders. Handb Clin Neurol. 2016;133:377–403.
35. Hemmer B, Kerschensteiner M, and Korn T. Role of the innate and adaptive immune responses in the course of multiple sclerosis. Lancet Neurol. 2015;14(4):406–19.
36. Petzold A. Retinal glymphatic system: an explanation for transient retinal layer volume changes? Brain. 2016;139:2816–26.

37. Wostyn P, De Groot V, Van Dam D, Audenaert K, Killer HE, De Deyn PP. Age-related macular degeneration, glaucoma and alzheimerâs disease: amyloidogenic diseases with the same glymphatic background? Cell Mol Life Sci. 2016;73(22):4299–301.
38. Spaide RF. Retinal vascular cystoid macular edema: review and new theory. Retina. 2016;36(10):1823–42.
39. Gaiottino J, Norgren N, Dobson R, Topping J, Nissim A, Malaspina A, Bestwick JP, Monsch AU, Regeniter A, Lindberg RL, Kappos L, Leppert D, Petzold A, Giovannoni G, and Kuhle J. Increased neurofilament light chain blood levels in neurodegenerative neurological diseases. PLoS One. 2013;8(9):e75091.
40. Petzold A. Biomarker for early diagnosis of Alzheimer's disease (chapter). The CSF analysis in dementia, 1st ed. New York: NOVA Science Publishers, Inc. pp 123–156.
41. Petzold A. Glial fibrillary acidic protein is a body fluid biomarker for glial pathology in human disease. Brain Res. 2015;1600:17–31.
42. Ibitoye R, Kemp K, Rice C, Hares K, Scolding N, Wilkins A. Oxidative stress-related biomarkers in multiple sclerosis: a review. Biomark Med. 2016;10(8):889–902.
43. Wilkins A, Scolding N. Protecting axons in multiple sclerosis. Mult Scler. 2008;14(8):1013–25.
44. Miller D, Barkhof F, Montalban X, Thompson A, Filippi M. Clinically isolated syndromes suggestive of multiple sclerosis, part I: natural history, pathogenesis, diagnosis, and prognosis. Lancet Neurol. 2005;4(5):281–8.
45. Lublin FD, Reingold SC. Defining the clinical course of multiple sclerosis: results of an international survey National Multiple Sclerosis Society (USA) Advisory Committee on Clinical Trials of New Agents in Multiple Sclerosis. Neurology. 1996;46:907–11.
46. Confavreux C, Vukusic S, and Adeleine P. Early clinical predictors and progression of irreversible disability in multiple sclerosis: an amnesic process. Brain. 2003;126:770–82.
47. Petzold A, Wong S, Plant GT. Autoimmunity in visual loss. Handb Clin Neurol. 2016;133:353–76.
48. Galea I, Freedman MS, and Thompson EJ. Cerebrospinal fluid analysis in the 2010 revised mcdonald's multiple sclerosis diagnostic criteria. Ann Neurol. 2011;70(1):183; author reply 183–183; author reply 184.
49. Tumani H, Deisenhammer F, Giovannoni G, Gold R, Hartung H-P, Hemmer B, Hohlfeld R, Otto M, Stangel M, Wildemann B, Zettl UK. Revised mcdonald criteria: the persisting importance of cerebrospinal fluid analysis. Ann Neurol. 2011;70(3):520; author reply 521.
50. Chris H Polman and for the international panel on diagnosis of multiple sclerosis. Ann Neurol. 2011.
51. Schwenkenbecher P, Sarikidi A, Wurster U, Bronzlik P, Süns K-W, Raab P, Stangel M, Pul R, Skripuletz T. Mcdonald criteria 2010 and 2005 compared: persistence of high oligoclonal band prevalence despite almost doubled diagnostic sensitivity. Int J Mol Sci. 2016;17(9):1592.
52. Huss AM, Halbgebauer S, Öckl P, Trebst C, Spreer A, Borisow N, Harrer A, Brecht I, Balint B, Stich O, et al. Importance of cerebrospinal fluid analysis in the era of McDonald 2010 criteria: a German–Austrian retrospective multicenter study in patients with a clinically isolated syndrome. J Neurol. 2016;263(12):2499–504.
53. Polman CH, Reingold SC, Banwell B, Clanet M, Cohen JA, Filippi M, Fujihara K, Havrdova E, Hutchinson M, Kappos L, Lublin FD, Montalban X, O'Connor P, Sandberg-Wollheim M, Thompson AJ, Waubant E, Weinshenker B, and Wolinsky JS. Diagnostic criteria for multiple sclerosis: 2010 revisions to the mcdonald criteria. Ann Neurol. 2011;69(2):292–302.
54. Polman CH, Reingold SC, Edan G, Filippi M, Hartung HP, Kappos L, Lublin FD, Metz LM, McFarland HF, O'Connor PW, Sandberg-Wollheim M, Thompson AJ, Weinshenker BG, Wolinsky JS. Diagnostic criteria for multiple sclerosis: 2005 revisions to the "McDonald Criteria". Ann Neurol. 2005;58:840–6.
55. McDonald WI, Compston A, Edan G, et al. Recommended diagnostic criteria for multiple sclerosis: guidelines from the International Panel on the diagnosis of multiple sclerosis. Ann Neurol. 2001;50:121–7.
56. Keren DF. Optimizing detection of oligoclonal bands in cerebrospinal fluid by use of isoelectric focusing with IgG immunoblotting. Am J Clin Pathol. 2003;120:649–51.

57. Teunissen CE, Petzold A, Bennett JL, Berven FS, Brundin L, Comabella M, Franciotta D, Frederiksen JL, Fleming JO, Furlan R, Hintzen RQ, Hughes SG, Johnson MH, Krasulova E, Kuhle J, Magnone MC, Rajda C, Rejdak K, Schmidt HK, van Pesch V, Waubant E, Wolf C, Giovannoni G, Hemmer B, Tumani H, and Deisenhammer F. A consensus protocol for the standardization of cerebrospinal fluid collection and biobanking. Neurology. 2009;73(22):1914–22.
58. Freedman MS, Thompson EJ, Deisenhammer F, Giovannoni G, Grimsley G, Keir G, Ohman S, Racke MK, Sharief M, Sindic CJ, Sellebjerg F, and Tourtellotte WW. Recommended standard of cerebrospinal fluid analysis in the diagnosis of multiple sclerosis: a consensus statement. Arch Neurol. 2005;62:865–870.
59. Abraira V, Alvarez-Cermeño JC, Arroyo R, Cámara C, Casanova B, Cubillo S, de Andrés C, Espejo C, Fernández O, et al. Utility of oligoclonal IgG band detection for ms diagnosis in daily clinical practice. J Immunol Methods. 2011;371(1–2):170–73.
60. Petzold A. Intrathecal oligoclonal igg synthesis in multiple sclerosis. J Neuroimmunol. 2013;262(1–2):1–10.
61. Lovato L, Willis SN, Rodig SJ, Caron T, Almendinger SE, Howell OW, Reynolds R, O'Connor KC, and Hafler DA. Related b cell clones populate the meninges and parenchyma of patients with multiple sclerosis. Brain. 2011;134(Pt 2):534–541.
62. Harp C, Lee J, Lambracht-Washington D, Cameron E, Olsen G, Frohman E, Racke M, and Monson N. Cerebrospinal fluid b cells from multiple sclerosis patients are subject to normal germinal center selection. J Neuroimmunol. 2007;183(1–2):189–99.
63. Racke MK. The role of b cells in multiple sclerosis: rationale for b-cell-targeted therapies. Drugs. 2010;21(Suppl 1):S9–18.
64. Obermeier B, Mentele R, Malotka J, Kellermann J, Kümpfel T, Wekerle H, Lottspeich F, Hohlfeld R, Dornmair K. Matching of oligoclonal immunoglobulin transcriptomes and proteomes of cerebrospinal fluid in multiple sclerosis. Nat Med. 2008;14(6):688–93.
65. Monson NL, Brezinschek H-P, Brezinschek RI, Mobley A, Vaughan GK, Frohman EM, Racke MK, and Lipsky PE. Receptor revision and atypical mutational characteristics in clonally expanded b cells from the cerebrospinal fluid of recently diagnosed multiple sclerosis patients. J Neuroimmunol. 2005;158(1–2):170–181.
66. Qin Y, Duquette P, Zhang Y, Talbot P, Poole R, Antel J. Clonal expansion and somatic hypermutation of V(H) genes of B cells from cerebrospinal fluid in multiple sclerosis. J Clin Invest. 1998;102:1045–50.
67. Arneth B and Birklein F. High sensitivity of free lambda and free kappa light chains for detection of intrathecal immunoglobulin synthesis in cerebrospinal fluid. Acta Neurol Scand. 2009;119(1):39–44.
68. Bednárová J, Stourac P, and Adam P. Relevance of immunological variables in neuroborreliosis and multiple sclerosis. Acta Neurol Scand. 2005;112(2):97–102.
69. Bourahoui A, De Seze J, Guttierez R, Onraed B, Hennache B, Ferriby D, Stojkovic T, and Vermersch P. CSF isoelectrofocusing in a large cohort of ms and other neurological diseases. Eur J Neurol. 2004;11(8):525–529.
70. Caudie C, Birouk AM, Bancel J, Claudy D, Gignoux L, Vukusic S, Confavreux C. Cytoimmunological profile of cerebrospinal fluid in diagnosis of multiple sclerosis. Pathol Biol (Paris). 2005;53(2):68–74.
71. Falip M, Tintoré M, Jardí R, Duran I, Link H, and Montalbán X. [Clinical usefulness of oligoclonal bands]. Rev Neurol. 2001;32(12):1120–4.
72. Fortini AS, Sanders EL, Weinshenker BG, Katzmann JA. Cerebrospinal fluid oligoclonal bands in the diagnosis of multiple sclerosis. Isoelectric focusing with IgG immunoblotting compared with high-resolution agarose gel electrophoresis and cerebrospinal fluid IgG index. Am J Clin Pathol. 2003;120(5):672–5.
73. Franciotta D, Zardini E, Bergamaschi R, Grimaldi LM, Andreoni L, and Cosi V. Analysis of chlamydia pneumoniae-specific oligoclonal bands in multiple sclerosis and other neurologic diseases. Acta Neurol Scand. 2005;112(4):238–41.
74. Franciotta D, Di Stefano AL, Jarius S, Zardini E, Tavazzi E, Ballerini C, Marchioni E, Bergamaschi R, Ceroni M. Cerebrospinal baff and epsteinbarr virus-specific oligoclonal bands in multiple sclerosis and other inflammatory demyelinating neurological diseases. J Neuroimmunol. 2011;230(1–2):160–3.

75. Gama PD, Machado Ldos R, Livramento JA, Gomes HR, Adoni T, Lino AM, Marchiori PE, Morales Rde R, Lana-Peixoto MA, Callegaro D. Study of oligoclonal bands restricted to the cerebrospinal fluid in multiple sclerosis patients in the city of São Paulo. Arq Neuropsiquiatr. 2009;67(4):1017–22.
76. Heard RN, Teutsch SM, Bennetts BH, Lee SD, Deane EM, and Stewart GJ. Lack of restriction of t cell receptor beta variable gene usage in cerebrospinal fluid lymphocytes in acute optic neuritis. J Neurol Neurosurg Psychiatry. 1999;67(5):585–90.
77. Li B, Dong H, Zhang J, Song X, and Guo L. Cerebrospinal fluid IgG profiles and oligoclonal bands in Chinese patients with multiple sclerosis. Acta Neurol Scand. 2007;115(5):319–24.
78. Mygland A, Trydal T, Vinje BU, and Vedeler C. Isoelectric focusing is superior to immunofixation electrophoresis in diagnosing CNS inflammation. Acta Neurol Scand. 2007;115(2):122–25.
79. Piazza F, DiFrancesco JC, Fusco ML, Corti D, Pirovano L, Frigeni B, Mattavelli L, Andreoni S, Frigo M, Ferrarese C, Tredici G, and Cavaletti G. Cerebrospinal fluid levels of BAFF and APRIL in untreated multiple sclerosis. J Neuroimmunol. 2010;220(1–2):104–7.
80. Presslauer Stefan, Milosavljevic Dejan, Brücke T, Bayer P, Hübl W. Elevated levels of kappa free light chains in CSF support the diagnosis of multiple sclerosis. J Neurol. 2008;255(10):1508–14.
81. Sá MJ, Sequeira L, Rio ME, and Thompson EJ. [Oligoclonal IgG bands in the cerebrospinal fluid of portuguese patients with multiple sclerosis: negative results indicate benign disease]. Arq Neuropsiquiatr. 2005;63(2B):375–9.
82. Sellebjerg F and Christiansen M. Qualitative assessment of intrathecal IgG synthesis by isoelectric focusing and immunodetection: interlaboratory reproducibility and interobserver agreement. Scand J Clin Lab Invest. 1996;56(2):135–43.
83. Villar LM, Masjuan J, Sádaba MC, González-Porqué P, Plaza J, Bootello A, and Alvarez-Cermeño JC. Early differential diagnosis of multiple sclerosis using a new oligoclonal band test. Arch Neurol. 2005;62(4):574–7.
84. Vogt MH, Teunissen CE, Iacobaeus E, Heijnen DA, Breij EC, Olsson T, Brundin L, Killestein J, Dijkstra CD. Cerebrospinal fluid anti-myelin antibodies are related to magnetic resonance measures of disease activity in multiple sclerosis. J Neurol Neurosurg Psychiatry. 2009;80(10):1110–5.
85. Xiao BG, Zhang GX, Ma CG, and Link H. The cerebrospinal fluid from patients with multiple sclerosis promotes neuronal and oligodendrocyte damage by delayed production of nitric oxide in vitro. J Neurol Sci. 1996;142(1–2):114–20.
86. Yao SY, Stratton CW, Mitchell WM, and Sriram S. CSF oligoclonal bands in MS include antibodies against chlamydophila antigens. Neurology. 2001;56(9):1168–76.
87. Link H and Huang YM. Oligoclonal bands in multiple sclerosis cerebrospinal fluid: an update on methodology and clinical usefulness. J Neuroimmunol. 2006;180:17–28.
88. McCombe PA, Brown NN, Barr AE, Parkin L. Monoclonal immunoglobulin bands in the cerebrospinal fluid. Aust N Z J Med. 1991;21:227–9.
89. Ben-Hur T, Abramsky O, River Y. The clinical significance of a single abnormal immunoglobulin band in cerebrospinal fluid electrophoresis. J Neurol Sci. 1996;136:159–61.
90. Davies G, Keir G, Thompson EJ, Giovannoni G. The clinical significance of an intrathecal monoclonal immunoglobulin band: a follow-up study. Neurology. 2003;60:1163–6.
91. Koch M, Heersema D, Mostert J, Teelken A, and J. De Keyser. Cerebrospinal fluid oligoclonal bands and progression of disability in multiple sclerosis. Eur J Neurol. 2007;14:797–800.
92. Walsh G, Jefferis R. Post-translational modifications in the context of therapeutic proteins. Nat Biotechnol. 2006;24:1241–52.
93. Petzold A, Eikelenboom MJ, Gveric D, Keir G, Chapman M, Lazeron RH, et al. Markers for different glial cell responses in multiple sclerosis: clinical and pathological correlations. Brain. 2002;125:1462–73.
94. Zeman AZ, Kidd D, McLean BN, Kelly MA, Francis DA, Miller DH, Kendall BE, Rudge P, Thompson EJ, and McDonald WI. A study of oligoclonal band negative multiple sclerosis. J Neurol Neurosurg Psychiatry. 1996;60:27–30.
95. Amato MP, Ponziani G. A prospective study on the prognosis of multiple sclerosis. Neurol Sci. 2000;21(4 Suppl 2):S831–8.

96. Villar LM, Gonzalez-Porque P, Masjuan J, Alvarez-Cermeno JC, Bootello A, Keir G. A sensitive and reproducible method for the detection of oligoclonal IgM bands. J Immunol Methods. 2001;258:151–5.
97. Espiño M, Abraira V, Arroyo R, Bau L, Cámara C, Campos-Ruiz L, Casanova B, Espejo C, Fernández O, García-Merino A, García-Sánchez MI, Gómez M, Gosis A, Izquierdo G, Meca J, Montalban X, Morandeira F, Olascoaga J, Prada A, Quintana E, Ramió-Torrentà L, Rodríguez-Antigüedad A, Salgado G, Santiago JL, Sarasola E, Simó-Castelló M, Alvarez-Cermeño JC, Villar LM. Assessment of the reproducibility of oligoclonal IgM band detection for its application in daily clinical practice. Clin Chim Acta. 2015;438:67–9. doi:10.1016/j.cca.2014.08.004.
98. Villar LM, Masjuan J, P González-Porqué, Plaza J, Sádaba MC, Roldán E, Bootello A, and Alvarez-Cermeño JC. Intrathecal IgM synthesis in neurologic diseases: relationship with disability in MS. Neurology. 2002;58(5):824–6.
99. Villar LM, Masjuan J, Gonzalez-Porque P, Plaza J, Sadaba MC, Roldan E, Bootello A, Alvarez-Cermeno JC. Intrathecal IgM synthesis is a prognostic factor in multiple sclerosis. Ann Neurol. 2003;53:222–6.
100. Villar LM, Costa-Frossard L, Alenda R, García-Caldentey J, Espiño M, Muriel A, Álvarez-Cermeño JC. Cerebrospinal fluid immunological biomarkers associated with axonal damage in multiple sclerosis. Eur J Neurol. 2015;22(8):1169–75. doi:10.1111/ene.12579.
101. Villar LM, Casanova B, Ouamara N, Comabella M, Jalili F, Leppert D, de Andrés C, Izquierdo G, Arroyo R, Avşar T, Lapin SV, Johnson T, Montalbán X, Fernández O, Álvarez-Lafuente R, Masterman D, García-Sánchez MI, Coret F, Siva A, Evdoshenko E, Álvarez-Cermeño JC, Bar-Or A. Immunoglobulin M oligoclonal bands: biomarker of targetable inflammation in primary progressive multiple sclerosis. Ann Neurol. 2014;76(2):231–40. doi:10.1002/ana.24190.
102. Álvarez-Cermeño JC, Muñoz-Negrete FJ, Costa-Frossard L, Sainz de la Maza S, Villar LM, Rebolleda G. Intrathecal lipid-specific oligoclonal IgM synthesis associates with retinal axonal loss in multiple sclerosis. J Neurol Sci. 2016;360:41–4. doi:10.1016/j.jns.2015.11.030.
103. Franciotta D, Salvetti M, Lolli F, Serafini B, Aloisi F. B cells and multiple sclerosis. Lancet Neurol. 2008;7:852–8.
104. Morris P, Davies NW, and Keir G. A screening assay to detect antigenspecific antibodies within cerebrospinal fluid. J Immunol Methods. 2006;311:81–86.
105. Luxton RW, Thompson EJ. Affinity distributions of antigen-specific IgG in patients with multiple sclerosis and in patients with viral encephalitis. J Immunol Methods. 1990;131:277–82.
106. Sindic CJ, Van Antwerpen MP, Goffette S. The intrathecal humoral immune response: laboratory analysis and clinical relevance. Clin Chem Lab Med. 2001;39:333–40.
107. O'Connor KC, Chitnis T, Griffin DE, Piyasirisilp S, Bar-Or A, Khoury S, Wucherpfennig KW, Hafler DA. Myelin basic proteinreactive autoantibodies in the serum and cerebrospinal fluid of multiple sclerosis patients are characterized by low-affinity interactions. J Neuroimmunol. 2003;136:140–8.
108. SM Brändle, Obermeier B, Senel M, Bruder J, Mentele R, Khademi M, Olsson T, Tumani H, Kristoferitsch W, Lottspeich F, Wekerle H, Hohlfeld R, and Dornmair K. Distinct oligoclonal band antibodies in multiple sclerosis recognize ubiquitous self-proteins. Proc Natl Acad Sci U S A. 2016;113(28):7864–9.
109. Winger RC, Zamvil SS. Antibodies in multiple sclerosis oligoclonal bands target debris. Proc Natl Acad Sci U S A. 2016;113(28):7696–8.
110. Trapp BD, Peterson JP, et al. Axonal transection in the lesions of multiple sclerosis. N Engl J Med. 1998;338:278–85.
111. Stubbs EB Jr, Lawlor MW, et al. Anti-neurofilament antibodies in neuropathy with monoclonal gammopathy of undetermined significance produce experimental motor nerve conduction block. Acta Neuropathol. 2003;105:109–16.
112. Gastaldi M, Zardini E, Franciotta D. An update on the use of cerebrospinal fluid analysis as a diagnostic tool in multiple sclerosis. Expert Rev Mol Diagn. 2017;17:31–46.
113. Correale J, Gaitán MI, Ysrraelit MC, Fiol MP. Progressive multiple sclerosis: from pathogenic mechanisms to treatment. Brain. 2017;140(3):537–46.

114. Comabella M, Sastre-Garriga J, Montalban X. Precision medicine in multiple sclerosis: biomarkers for diagnosis, prognosis, and treatment response. Curr Opin Neurol. 2016;29:254–62.
115. Malmeström C, Haghighi S, Rosengren L, Andersen O, Lycke J. Neurofilament light protein and glial fibrillary acidic protein as biological markers in MS. Neurology. 2003;61(12):1720–5.
116. Semra YK, Seidi OA, Sharief MK. Heightened intrathecal release of axonal cytoskeletal proteins in multiple sclerosis is associated with progressive disease and clinical disability. J Neuroimmunol. 2002;122:132–9.
117. Petzold A, Eikelenboom MJ, Keir G, et al. Axonal damage accumulates in the progressive phase of multiple sclerosis: a 3–year follow–up study. J Neurol Neurosurg Psychiatry. 2005;76:206–11.
118. Brettschneider J, Petzold A, Junker A, Tumani H. Axonal damage markers in cerebrospinal fluid of patients with clinically isolated syndrome improve predicting conversion to definite MS. Mult Scler. 2006;12:143–8.
119. Petzold A, Rejdak K, Plant GT. Axonal degeneration and inflammation in acute optic neuritis. J Neurol Neurosurg Psychiatry. 2004;75:1178–80.
120. Teunissen CE, Iacobaeus E, Khademi M, Brundin L, Norgren N, Koel-Simmelink MJ, Schepens M, Bouwman F, Twaalfhoven HA, Blom HJ, Jakobs C, Dijkstra CD. Combination of CSF n-acetylaspartate and neurofilaments in multiple sclerosis. Neurology. 2009;72(15):1322–9.
121. Kuhle J, Leppert D, Petzold A, Regeniter A, Schindler C, Mehling M, Anthony DC, Kappos L, and Lindberg RL. Neurofilament heavy chain in CSF correlates with relapses and disability in multiple sclerosis. Neurology. 2011;76(14):1206–13.
122. Lycke J, Andersen O, Rosengren L. Neurofilament in cerebrospinal fluid: a potential marker of activity in multiple sclerosis. Eur J Neurol. 1996;3:100.
123. Lycke JN, Karlsson JE, Andersen O, Rosengren LE. Neurofilament protein in cerebrospinal fluid: a potential marker of activity in multiple sclerosis. J Neurol Neurosurg Psychiatry. 1998;64:402–4.
124. Gunnarsson M, Malmeström C, Axelsson M, Sundström P, Dahle C, Vrethem M, Olsson T, Piehl F, Norgren N, Rosengren L, Svenningsson A, Lycke J. Axonal damage in relapsing multiple sclerosis is markedly reduced by natalizumab. Ann Neurol. 2011;69(1):83–89.
125. Petzold A, Mondria T, Kuhle J, Rocca MA, Cornelissen J, Te Boekhorst P, Lowenberg B, Giovannoni G, Filippi M, Kappos L, and Hintzen R. Evidence for acute neurotoxicity after chemotherapy. Ann Neurol. 2010;68(6):806–15.
126. Petzold A. The prognostic value of csf neurofilaments in multiple sclerosis at 15-year follow-up. J Neurol Neurosurg Psychiatry. 2015;88:1388–90.
127. Arrambide G, Espejo C, Eixarch H, Villar LM, Alvarez-Cermeño JC, Picón C, Kuhle J, Disanto G, Kappos L, Sastre-Garriga J, Pareto D, Simon E, Comabella M, Río J, Nos C, Tur C, Castilló J, Vidal-Jordana A, Galán I, Arévalo MJ, Auger C, Rovira A, Montalban X, Tintore M. Neurofilament light chain level is a weak risk factor for the development of MS. Neurology. 2016;87(11):1076–84. doi:10.1212/WNL.0000000000003085.
128. Kuhle J, Barro C, Disanto G, Mathias A, Soneson C, Bonnier G, Yaldizli Ã, Regeniter A, Derfuss T, Canales M, Schluep M, Du Pasquier R, Krueger G, Granziera C. Serum neurofilament light chain in early relapsing remitting MS is increased and correlates with CSF levels and with MRI measures of disease severity. Mult Scler. 2016;22:1550–9.
129. Petzold A, Steenwijk MD, Eikelenboom JM, Wattjes MP, Uitdehaag BM. Elevated CSF neurofilament proteins predict brain atrophy: a 15-year follow-up study. Mult Scler. 2016;22:1154–62.
130. Hares K, Redondo J, Kemp K, Rice C, Scolding N, Wilkins A. Axonal motor protein kif5a and associated cargo deficits in multiple sclerosis lesional and normal-appearing white matter. Neuropathol Appl Neurobiol. 2017;43(3):227–41.
131. Petzold A, Keir G, Green AJE, Giovannoni G, Thompson EJ. A specific ELISA for measuring neurofilament heavy chain phosphoforms. J Immunol Methods. 2003;278:179–90.
132. Rosengren LE, Karlsson JE, Karlsson JO, Persson LI, Wikkelso C. Patients with amyotrophic lateral sclerosis and other neurodegenerative diseases have increased levels of neurofilament protein in CSF. J Neurochem. 1996;67:2013–8.

133. N Norgren, L Rosengren, and T Stigbrand. Elevated neurofilament levels in neurological diseases. Brain Res. 2003;987(1):25–31.
134. Modvig S, Degn M, Sander B, Horwitz H, Wanscher B, Sellebjerg F, and Frederiksen JL. Cerebrospinal fluid neurofilament light chain levels predict visual outcome after optic neuritis. Mult Scler. 2016;22(5):590–8.
135. Disanto G, Adiutori R, Dobson R, Martinelli V, Costa GD, Runia T, Evdoshenko E, Thouvenot E, Trojano M, Norgren N, Teunissen C, Kappos L, Giovannoni G, Kuhle J, International Clinically Isolated Syndrome Study Group. Serum neurofilament light chain levels are increased in patients with a clinically isolated syndrome. J Neurol Neurosurg Psychiatry. 2016;87:126–9.
136. Disanto G, Adiutori R, Dobson R, Martinelli V, G. Dalla Costa, Runia T, Evdoshenko E, Thouvenot E, Trojano M, Norgren N, Teunissen C, Kappos L, Giovannoni G, and Kuhle J. Serum neurofilament light chain levels are increased in patients with a clinically isolated syndrome. J Neurol Neurosurg Psychiatry. 2016;87(2):126–9.
137. Kuhle J, Disanto G, Lorscheider J, Stites T, Chen Y, Dahlke F, Francis G, Shrinivasan A, Radue E-W, Giovannoni G, and Kappos L. Fingolimod and CSF neurofilament light chain levels in relapsing-remitting multiple sclerosis. Neurology. 2015;84(16):1639–1643.
138. Tortorella C, Direnzo V, Taurisano P, Romano R, Ruggieri M, Zoccolella S, Mastrapasqua M, Popolizio T, Blasi G, Bertolino A, and Trojano M. Cerebrospinal fluid neurofilament tracks fmri correlates of attention at the first attack of multiple sclerosis. Mult Scler. 2015;21(4):396–401.
139. Amor S, van der Star BJ, Bosca I, Raffel J, Gnanapavan S, Watchorn J, Kuhle J, Giovannoni G, Baker D, Malaspina A, and Puentes F. Neurofilament light antibodies in serum reflect response to natalizumab treatment in multiple sclerosis. Mult Scler. 2014;20(10):1355–62.
140. Gresle MM, Liu Y, Dagley LF, Haartsen J, Pearson F, Purcell AW, Laverick L, Petzold A, Lucas RM, Van der Walt A, Prime H, Morris DR, Taylor BV, Shaw G, and Butzkueven H. Serum phosphorylated neurofilament-heavy chain levels in multiple sclerosis patients. J Neurol Neurosurg Psychiatry. 2014;85(11):1209–13.
141. Kuhle J, Malmeström C, Axelsson M, Plattner K, Yaldizli O, Derfuss T, Giovannoni G, Kappos L, Lycke J. Neurofilament light and heavy subunits compared as therapeutic biomarkers in multiple sclerosis. Acta Neurol Scand. 2013;128(6):e33–6.
142. Petzold A, Baker D, Pryce G, et al. Quantification of neurodegeneration by measurement of brain–specific proteins. J Neuroimmunol. 2003;138:45–8.
143. Hares K, Kemp K, Gray E, Scolding N, and Wilkins A. Neurofilament dot blot assays: novel means of assessing axon viability in culture. J Neurosci Methods. 2011;198(2):195–203.
144. G Shaw, C Yang, R Ellis, K Anderson, et al. Hyperphosphorylated neurofilament NF-H is a serum biomarker for axonal injury. Biochem Biophys Res Commun. 2005;336:1268–77.
145. J Kuhle, A Regeniter, D Leppert, M Mehling, L Kappos, RLP Lindberg, and A Petzold. A highly sensitive electrochemiluminescence immunoassay for the neurofilament heavy chain protein. J Neuroimmunol. 2010;220:114–9.
146. Abdo WF, van de Warrenburg BP, Munneke M, van Geel WJ, Bloem BR Kremer HP, and Verbeek MM. CSF analysis differentiates multiple-system atrophy from idiopathic late-onset cerebellar ataxia. Neurology. 2006;67:474–9.
147. Kuhle J, Barro C, Andreasson U, Derfuss T, Lindberg R, Sandelius Ã, Liman V, Norgren N, Blennow K, Zetterberg H. Comparison of three analytical platforms for quantification of the neurofilament light chain in blood samples: elisa, electrochemiluminescence immunoassay and simoa. Clin Chem Lab Med. 2016;54:1655–61.
148. Limberg M, Disanto G, Barro C, Kuhle J. Neurofilament light chain determination from peripheral blood samples. Methods Mol Biol. 2016;1304:93–8.
149. Petzold A, Gveric D, Groves M, Schmierer K, Grant D, Chapman M, Keir G, Cuzner L, and Thompson EJ. Phosphorylation and compactness of neurofilaments in multiple sclerosis: indicators of axonal pathology. Exp Neurol. 2008;213:326–35.
150. Petzold A, Eikelenboom MJ, Keir G, et al. The new Global Multiple Sclerosis Severity Score (MSSS) correlates with axonal but not glial biomarkers. Mult Scler. 2006;12:325–8.

151. Cloos PA and Christgau S. Post-translational modifications of proteins: implications for aging, antigen recognition, and autoimmunity. Biogerontology. 2004;5(3):139–58.
152. Delom F and Chevet E. Phosphoprotein analysis: from proteins to proteomes. Proteome Sci. 2006;4:15.
153. Yao X, Kwan HY, and Huang Y. Regulation of TRP channels by phosphorylation. Neurosignals. 2005;14:273–80.
154. Ventura JJ, Nebreda AR. Protein kinases and phosphatases as therapeutic targets in cancer. Clin Transl Oncol. 2006;8:153–60.
155. Forrest AR, Taylor DF, Fink JL, Gongora MM, Flegg C, Teasdale RD, Suzuki H, Kanamori M, Kai C, Hayashizaki Y, and Grimmond SM. PhosphoregDB: the tissue and sub-cellular distribution of mammalian protein kinases and phosphatases. BMC Bioinformatics. 2006;7:82.
156. Wang JQ, Arora A, Yang L, Parelkar NK, Zhang G, Liu X, Choe ES, and Mao L. Phosphorylation of AMPA receptors: mechanisms and synaptic plasticity. Mol Neurobiol. 2005;32:237–49.
157. Rye CSand Baell JB. Phosphate isosteres in medicinal chemistry. Curr Med Chem. 2005;12:3127–41.
158. Lieser SA, Aubol BE, Wong L, Jennings PA, Adams JA. Coupling phosphoryl transfer and substrate interactions in protein kinases. Biochim Biophys Acta. 1754;191–109:2005.
159. Shen K, Hines AC, Schwarzer D, Pickin KA, and Cole PA. Protein kinase structure and function analysis with chemical tools. Biochim Biophys Acta. 2005;1754:65–78.
160. Roskoski R Jr. Src kinase regulation by phosphorylation and dephosphorylation. Biochem Biophys Res Commun. 2005;331:1–14.
161. Lua BL and Low BC. Cortactin phosphorylation as a switch for actin cytoskeletal network and cell dynamics control. FEBS Lett. 2005;579:577–85.
162. Horbinski C, Chu CT. Kinase signaling cascades in the mitochondrion: a matter of life or death. Free Radic Biol Med. 2005;38:2–11.
163. Chen F, David D, Ferrari A, and Gotz J. Posttranslational modifications of tau–role in human tauopathies and modeling in transgenic animals. Curr Drug Targets. 2004;5:503–15.
164. Krupa A, Preethi G, and Srinivasan N. Structural modes of stabilization of permissive phosphorylation sites in protein kinases: distinct strategies in Ser/Thr and Tyr kinases. J Mol Biol. 2004;339:1025–39.
165. Carden MJ, Schlaepfer WW, and Lee VM. The structure, biochemical properties, and immunogenicity of neurofilament peripheral regions are determined by phosphorylation state. J Biol Chem. 1985;260:9805–17.
166. Harauz G, Musse AA. A tale of two citrullines—structural and functional aspects of myelin basic protein deimination in health and disease. Neurochem Res. 2007;32(2):137–58.
167. Piacentini M, Colizzi V. Tissue transglutaminase: apoptosis versus autoimmunity. Immunol Today. 1999;20:130–4.
168. Virella G, Thorpe SR, Alderson NL, Stephan EM, Atchley D, Wagner F, and MF Lopes-Virella. Autoimmune response to advanced glycosylation end-products of human LDL. J Lipid Res. 2003;44:487–93.
169. Witherick J, Wilkins A, Scolding N, Kemp K. Mechanisms of oxidative damage in multiple sclerosis and a cell therapy approach to treatment. Autoimmune Dis. 2010;2011:164608.
170. Schlaepfer WW, Lee C, Lee VMY, Zimmerman UJP. An immunoblot study of neurofilament degradation in situ and during calcium–activated proteolysis. J Neurochem. 1985;44:502–9.
171. Wang S, Lees GJ, Rosengren LE, Karlsson JE, Hamberger A, Haglid KG. Proteolysis of filament proteins in glial and neuronal cells after in vivo stimulation of hippocampal NMDA receptors. Neurochem Res. 1992;17:1005–9.
172. Van Geel WJA, Rosengren LE, and Verbeek MM. An enzyme immunoassay to quantify neurofilament light chain in cerebrospinal fluid. J Immunol Methods. 2005;296:179–85.
173. Goldstein ME, Sternberger NH, Sternberger LA. Phosphorylation protects neurofilaments against proteolysis. J Neuroimmunol. 1987;14:149–60.

174. Pant HC. Dephosphorylation of neurofilament proteins enhances their susceptibility to degradation by calpain. Biochem J. 1988;256:665–8.
175. Irani DN, Anderson C, Gundry R, Cotter R, Moore S, Kerr DA, McArthur JC, Sacktor N, Pardo CA, Jones M, Calabresi PA, and Nath A. Cleavage of cystatin C in the cerebrospinal fluid of patients with multiple sclerosis. Ann Neurol. 2006;59:237–247.
176. Carrette O, Burkhard PR, Hughes S, Hochstrasser DF, Sanchez JC. Truncated cystatin C in cerebrospiral fluid: technical [corrected] artefact or biological process? Proteomics. 2005;5:3060–5.
177. Steinman L. Multiple approaches to multiple sclerosis. Nat Med. 2000;6:15–6.
178. Steinman L. Multiple sclerosis: a coordinated immunological attack against myelin in the central nervous system. Cell. 1996;85:299–302.
179. Zamvil SS, Mitchell DJ, Moore AC, Kitamura K, Steinman L, and Rothbard JB. T-cell epitope of the autoantigen myelin basic protein that induces encephalomyelitis. Nature. 1986;324:258–60.
180. Moscarello MA, Wood DD, Ackerley C, Boulias C. Myelin in multiple sclerosis is developmentally immature. J Clin Invest. 1994;94:146–54.
181. Pritzker LB, Joshi S, Harauz G, Moscarello MA. Deimination of myelin basic protein. 2. Effect of methylation of MBP on its deimination by peptidylarginine deiminase. Biochemistry. 2000;39:5382–8.
182. Fujii N, Ishibashi Y, Satoh K, Fujino M, Harada K. Simultaneous racemization and isomerization at specific aspartic acid residues in alpha B-crystallin from the aged human lens. Biochim Biophys Acta. 1994;1204:157–63.
183. van Stipdonk MJ, Willems AA, Amor S, Persoon-Deen C, Travers PJ, Boog CJ, van Noort JM. T cells discriminate between differentially phosphorylated forms of alphaB-crystallin, a major central nervous system myelin antigen. Int Immunol. 1998;10:943–50.
184. Voorter CE, de Haard-Hoekman WA, van den Oetelaar PJ, Bloemendal H, de Jong WW. Spontaneous peptide bond cleavage in aging alpha-crystallin through a succinimide intermediate. J Biol Chem. 1988;263:19020–3.
185. Corthay A, Backlund J, Broddefalk J, Michaelsson E, Goldschmidt TJ, Kihlberg J, and Holmdahl R. Epitope glycosylation plays a critical role for T cell recognition of type II collagen in collagen-induced arthritis. Eur J Immunol. 1998;28:2580–2590.
186. Masson-Bessiere C, Sebbag M, Girbal-Neuhauser E, Nogueira L, Vincent C, Senshu T, and Serre G. The major synovial targets of the rheumatoid arthritis-specific antifilaggrin autoantibodies are deiminated forms of the alpha- and beta-chains of fibrin. J Immunol. 2001;166:4177–4184.
187. Girbal-Neuhauser E, Durieux JJ, Arnaud M, Dalbon P, Sebbag M, Vincent C, Simon M, Senshu T, Masson-Bessiere C, Jolivet-Reynaud C, Jolivet M, and Serre G. The epitopes targeted by the rheumatoid arthritis-associated antifilaggrin autoantibodies are posttranslationally generated on various sites of (pro)filaggrin by deimination of arginine residues. J Immunol. 1999;162:585–594.
188. Asaga H, Yamada M, Senshu T. Selective deimination of vimentin in calcium ionophore-induced apoptosis of mouse peritoneal macrophages. Biochem Biophys Res Commun. 1998;243:641–6.
189. Inagaki M, Takahara H, Nishi Y, Sugawara K, and Sato C. Ca^{2+}-dependent deimination-induced disassembly of intermediate filaments involves specific modification of the amino-terminal head domain. J Biol Chem. 1989;264:18119–27.
190. Newkirk MM, Goldbach-Mansky R, Lee J, Hoxworth J, McCoy A, Yarboro C, Klippel J, El-Gabalawy HS. Advanced glycation endproduct (AGE)-damaged IgG and IgM autoantibodies to IgG-AGE in patients with early synovitis. Arthritis Res Ther. 2003;5:R82–90.
191. Brange J, Langkjaer L, Havelund S, and Volund A. Chemical stability of insulin. 1. Hydrolytic degradation during storage of pharmaceutical preparations. Pharm Res. 1992;9:715–26.
192. Trigwell SM, Radford PM, Page SR, Loweth AC, James RF, Morgan NG, Todd I. Islet glutamic acid decarboxylase modified by reactive oxygen species is recognized by antibodies from patients with type 1 diabetes mellitus. Clin Exp Immunol. 2001;126:242–9.

193. Young AL, Carter WG, Doyle HA, Mamula MJ, Aswad DW. Structural integrity of histone H2B in vivo requires the activity of protein L-isoaspartate O-methyltransferase, a putative protein repair enzyme. J Biol Chem. 2001;276:37161–5.
194. Kim JH, Nam KH, Kwon OS, Kim IG, Bustin M, Choy HE, Park SC. Histone cross-linking by transglutaminase. Biochem Biophys Res Commun. 2002;293:1453–7.
195. Mamula MJ, Gee RJ, Elliott JI, Sette A, Southwood S, Jones PJ, Blier PR. Isoaspartyl post-translational modification triggers autoimmune responses to self-proteins. J Biol Chem. 1999;274:22321–7.
196. Monneaux F, Lozano JM, Patarroyo ME, Briand JP, and Muller S. T cell recognition and therapeutic effect of a phosphorylated synthetic peptide of the 70K snRNP protein administered in MR/lpr mice. Eur J Immunol. 2003;33:287–96.
197. Cao L, Sun D, Whitaker JN. Citrullinated myelin basic protein induces experimental autoimmune encephalomyelitis in Lewis rats through a diverse T cell repertoire. J Neuroimmunol. 1998;88:21–9.
198. Hill JA, Southwood S, Sette A, Jevnikar AM, Bell DA, and Cairns E. Cutting edge: the conversion of arginine to citrulline allows for a high-affinity peptide interaction with the rheumatoid arthritis-associated HLA-DRB1*0401 MHC class II molecule. J Immunol. 2003;171:538–41.
199. Sollid LM. Molecular basis of celiac disease. Annu Rev Immunol. 2000;18:53–81.
200. Wuttge DM, Bruzelius M, Stemme S. T-cell recognition of lipid peroxidation products breaks tolerance to self proteins. Immunology. 1999;98:273.
201. Nicholas AP, Sambandam T, Echols JD, and Tourtellotte WW. Increased citrullinated glial fibrillary acidic protein in secondary progressive multiple sclerosis. J Comp Neurol. 2004;473(1):128–36.
202. Harauz G, Ishiyama N, Hill CM, Bates IR, Libich DS, and Fares C. Myelin basic protein-diverse conformational states of an intrinsically unstructured protein and its roles in myelin assembly and multiple sclerosis. Micron. 2004;35:503–42.
203. Boggs JM. Myelin basic protein: a multifunctional protein. Cell Mol Life Sci. 2006;63(17):1945–61.
204. Musse AA, Boggs JM, Harauz G. Deimination of membrane-bound myelin basic protein in multiple sclerosis exposes an immunodominant epitope. Proc Natl Acad Sci U S A. 2006;103:4422–7.
205. Doyle HA and Mamula MJ. Post-translational protein modifications in antigen recognition and autoimmunity. Trends Immunol. 2001;22(8):443–9.
206. Doyle HA, Mamula MJ. Posttranslational protein modifications: new flavors in the menu of autoantigens. Curr Opin Rheumatol. 2002;14:244–9.
207. Doyle HA and Mamula MJ. Posttranslational modifications of selfantigens. Ann N Y Acad Sci. 2005;1050:1–9.
208. Husted C. Structural insight into the role of myelin basic protein in multiple sclerosis. Proc Natl Acad Sci U S A. 2006;103:4339–4340.
209. Wood DD, Bilbao JM, O'Connors P, and Moscarello MA. Acute multiple sclerosis (Marburg type) is associated with developmentally immature myelin basic protein. Ann Neurol. 1996;40:18–24.
210. Lamensa JW and Moscarello MA. Deimination of human myelin basic protein by a peptidylarginine deiminase from bovine brain. J Neurochem. 1993;61:987–96.
211. Pritzker LB, Nguyen TA, Moscarello MA. The developmental expression and activity of peptidylarginine deiminase in the mouse. Neurosci Lett. 1999;266:161–4.
212. Moscarello MA, Pritzker L, Mastronardi FG, and Wood DD. Peptidylarginine deiminase: a candidate factor in demyelinating disease. J Neurochem. 2002;81:335–43.
213. Mastronardi FGand Moscarello MA. Molecules affecting myelin stability: a novel hypothesis regarding the pathogenesis of multiple sclerosis. J Neurosci Res. 2005;80:301–8.
214. De Keyser J, Schaaf M, Teelken A. Peptidylarginine deiminase activity in postmortem white matter of patients with multiple sclerosis. Neurosci Lett. 1999;260:74–6.

215. de Seze J, Dubucquoi S, Lefranc D, Virecoulon F, Nuez I, Dutoit V, Vermersch P, Prin L. IgG reactivity against citrullinated myelin basic protein in multiple sclerosis. J Neuroimmunol. 2001;117:149–55.
216. Raijmakers R, Vogelzangs J, Raats J, Panzenbeck M, Corby M, Jiang H, Thibodeau M, Haynes N, Van Venrooij WJ, Pruijn GJ, and Werneburg B. Experimental autoimmune encephalomyelitis induction in peptidylarginine deiminase 2 knockout mice. J Comp Neurol. 2006;498:217–26.
217. Bizzozero OA, DeJesus G, Callahan K, and Pastuszyn A. Elevated protein carbonylation in the brain white matter and gray matter of patients with multiple sclerosis. J Neurosci Res. 2005;81:687–695.
218. Anderson JM, Hampton DW, Patani R, Pryce G, Crowther RA, Reynolds R, Franklin RJM, Giovannoni G, Compston DAS, Baker D, Spillantini MG, and Chandran S. Abnormally phosphorylated tau is associated with neuronal and axonal loss in experimental autoimmune encephalomyelitis and multiple sclerosis. Brain. 2008;131(Pt 7):1736–48.
219. Schneider A, Wright Araujo G, Trajkovic K, et al. Hyperphosphorylation and aggregation of tau in experimental autoimmune encephalomyelitis. J Biol Chem. 2004;279(53):55833–9.
220. Bartosik-Psujek H and Stelmasiak Z. The CSF levels of total-tau and phosphotau in patients with relapsing-remitting multiple sclerosis. J Neural Transm. 2006;113(3):339–345.
221. Brettschneider J, Maier M, Arda S, Claus A, Sussmuth SD, Kassubek J, and Tumani H. Tau protein level in cerebrospinal fluid is increased in patients with early multiple sclerosis. Mult Scler. 2005;11(3):261–265.
222. Bartosik-Psujek H, Archelos JJ. Tau protein and 14-3-3 are elevated in the cerebrospinal fluid of patients with multiple sclerosis and correlate with intrathecal synthesis of IgG. J Neurol. 2004;251:414–20.
223. Kapaki E, Paraskevas GP, Michalopoulou M, and Kilidireas K. Increased cerebrospinal fluid tau protein in multiple sclerosis. Eur Neurol. 2000;43:228–32.
224. Guimaraes I, Cardoso MI, Sa MJ. Tau protein seems not to be a useful routine clinical marker of axonal damage in multiple sclerosis. Mult Scler. 2006;12:354–6.
225. Jimenez-Jimenez FJ, Zurdo JM, Hernanz A, Medina-Acebron S, de Bustos F, Barcenilla B, Sayed Y, Ayuso-Peralta L. Tau protein concentrations in cerebrospinal fluid of patients with multiple sclerosis. Acta Neurol Scand. 2002;106:351–4.
226. Lim ET, Grant D, Pashenkov M, Keir G, Thompson EJ, Söderström M, Giovannoni G. Cerebrospinal fluid levels of brain specific proteins in optic neuritis. Mult Scler. 2004;10(3):261–265.
227. Roxburgh RH, Seaman SR, Masterman T, Hensiek AE, Sawcer SJ, Vukusic S, et al. Multiple sclerosis severity score. Using disability and disease duration to rate disease severity. Neurology. 2005;64:1144–51.
228. Nilselid AM, Davidsson P, Nagga K, Andreasen N, Fredman P, and Blennow K. Clusterin in cerebrospinal fluid: analysis of carbohydrates and quantification of native and glycosylated forms. Neurochem Int. 2006;48:718–28.

Chapter 7
Symptomatic Treatment for Progressive Multiple Sclerosis

Steven M. Bailey and Claire M. Rice

7.1 Introduction

The symptoms of progressive MS are thought to be driven by neuronal loss within the CNS and the widespread distribution of the disease can manifest in a wide variety of symptoms. Typically, however, a stereotyped pattern emerges in progressive disease—an upper motor neuron syndrome with the character of a high spinal cord lesion and superimposed ataxia and cognitive impairment. This results in symptoms such as impaired mobility, spasticity, tremor and incoordination, bladder and bowel dysfunction and cognitive difficulties. In addition, fatigue, mood disturbance and paroxysmal symptoms such as trigeminal neuralgia may be troublesome. In the absence of a curative intervention for progressive disease, reducing the burden of symptoms will lead to improvement in quality of life for patients and carers, as well as reducing the significant socioeconomic impact of a chronic, disabling condition. Indeed, such a combined approach which prioritises the identification of disease modifying and improved symptom-relieving therapies is supported by the International Collaborative on Progressive MS Alliance [1].

Neurorehabilitation programmes require that the patient is assessed by a proficient multidisciplinary team who, taking the perspective of the patient into account, draw up a goal-orientated programme which is regularly evaluated [2]. These basic principles are directly applicable to the management of symptoms in progressive disease, notwithstanding the knowledge that full recovery is not possible. Indeed, this is explicitly acknowledged by the World Health Organization's definition of rehabilitation [3], and is further emphasised by the focus placed upon 'activities' and 'participation' (as opposed to 'disability' and 'handicap') in the International Classification of Functioning, Disability and Health [4, 5].

S.M. Bailey • C.M. Rice (✉)
Clinical Neurosciences, University of Bristol,
Learning and Research Building, Southmead Hospital, Bristol, UK
e-mail: c.m.rice@bris.ac.uk

A. Wilkins (ed.), *Progressive Multiple Sclerosis*,
https://doi.org/10.1007/978-3-319-65921-3_7

Within this context, the specific needs of the patient with progressive MS have been highlighted in a number of government documents both in the United Kingdom (UK) [6] and elsewhere [7, 8]. Attention has been drawn to the relatively weak standard of evidence underpinning the value of neurorehabilitation in progressive MS [2, 9], but progress undoubtedly has been made in the development of more sensitive evaluation tools (particularly those which incorporate the patient's perspective [10]) and the establishment of robust clinical trials [2, 11].

A Cochrane review of neurorehabilitation interventions for patients with MS suggested that there was "moderate evidence" to support an improvement in activity levels, participation and bladder function up to 12 months following an inpatient or outpatient rehabilitation intervention [12]. Evidence was stronger for a short-term effect on activity levels and participation at 6 weeks post-intervention, but this was true only for inpatient rehabilitation, not for outpatient or home-based rehabilitation programmes [12]. More recently, improved physical fitness has been shown to correlate with improved cognition in MS [13] and robotics may have potential to facilitate high-intensity training in those with disability [14]. Overall however, further research is needed to determine appropriate outcome measures, optimal intensity, frequency, cost, and effectiveness of rehabilitation therapy over a longer time periods [12].

7.2 Spasticity

Spasticity is a component of the upper motor neuron syndrome and has been traditionally defined as an inappropriate, velocity-dependent, increase in muscle tonic stretch reflexes [15]. However, this definition excluded spasms and clonus and fails to acknowledge the contribution to spasticity of abnormal activity in afferent and supraspinal pathways, as well as changes in the visco-elastic properties of musculoskeletal tissues. An updated definition has therefore been proposed: 'disordered sensorimotor control, resulting from an upper motor neuron lesion, presenting as intermittent or sustained involuntary activation of muscles' [16].

Spasticity is a particularly common symptom in patients with MS. Although estimates of the proportion of patients affected vary [17, 18], some report that up to 90% are affected at some point [19]. Approximately one-third of patients with MS report an impact of spasticity on activities of daily living [17]. It may contribute to disability, causing pain, spasms, contractures and deformity, and some evidence points to improvement in function with treatment [20]. However, spasticity may also contribute to preserved lower limb function in otherwise weak limbs [21, 22]. Although spasticity is associated with worse health status, its relationship with overall quality of life has not been established [23]. It follows, therefore, that treatment should only be undertaken if it is negatively impacting upon function or otherwise causing distress. In addition, aggravating factors such as pain, urinary and bowel dysfunction, poor posture or infection should be addressed first, and careful attention should be paid during the titration of pharmacological agents in those who remain mobile. Treatment options will vary depending on whether the spasticity is generalised or more localised to a group of muscles, and will also differ depending on the goal—appropriate interventions for the patient in whom the aim is improvement or preservation of ambulation will be very different from those for an immobile patient, where improvement of sitting posture, hygiene and comfort have been prioritised.

7.2.1 Physical Therapy for Spasticity

Physical interventions for spasticity secondary to a chronic, progressive condition such as progressive MS should ideally be incorporated into the patient's daily regimen. The goals and nature of the therapy will, of course, vary depending on the patient's condition, but examples range from exercises to improve muscle strength and cardiovascular fitness, to the use of positioning aids to improve seating and/or prevent the adoption of abnormal postures secondary to spasms or spasticity. Although immediate benefit from passive stretching in conditions causing spasticity is reported, there is very little evidence to support the persistence of such effects [24–30]. The evidence supporting active movement [31] and standing [32, 33] is somewhat stronger. Exercise has been demonstrated to have beneficial effects in a number of studies, and a meta-analysis concluded that there was strong evidence in favour of exercise for improving muscle power, exercise tolerance and mobility as well as a significant effect on mood enhancement [34]. There is little evidence available currently to guide decisions regarding the optimum frequency and duration of such interventions, which are likely to depend upon the individual and their particular circumstances [34–36]. The mechanisms underlying the effects of exercise are likely to be multifactorial [37–39] and require further investigation. Intriguingly, however, these effects have recently been reported to be susceptible to 'priming' by transcranial magnetic stimulation [40], which may itself reduce spasticity secondary to MS [41–43], perhaps by facilitating synaptic plasticity [44–46].

Orthotic devices may complement physical therapy, but their use and evaluation require specialist expertise if complications are to be avoided, particularly in a patient group that may have sensory impairments. Soft splinting, which may be used in combination with botulinum toxin injection, can be particularly helpful for some patients [35].

Functional electrical stimulation (FES) has been demonstrated to be of benefit to patients with MS in a number of studies [47, 48]. Interestingly, the benefits of long-term use persist even when the FES is switched off, an effect which has been postulated to be due to increased activation of motor cortex and corticospinal connections [49].

7.2.2 *Oral Medications for the Treatment of Spasticity*

The more commonly prescribed treatments for spasticity are summarised in Table 7.1. A Cochrane review of anti-spasticity agents for MS published in 2003 found that there was insufficient evidence to compare the effectiveness of treatments [50]. This is, at least in part, due to the well-recognised limitations of the Ashworth scale, which has been the most commonly used assessment tool [51]. UK guidelines published by NICE in 2014, taking clinical efficacy and health economic factors into account, advise baclofen or gabapentin as first-line monotherapy for MS-related spasticity, with consideration of combination therapy when these are ineffective individually or poorly tolerated on dose escalation [6]; tizanidine or

Table 7.1 Pharmacological therapies for spasticity which can be administered orally as tablets or oromucosal spray

Drug	Proposed mechanism of action	Frequent or serious side effects
Baclofen	GABA analogue which binds to $GABA_B$ receptors with consequent inhibition of spinal reflexes	Sedation, weakness, hallucinations, mood and sleep disturbance, myalgia, respiratory and cardiovascular depression
Tizanidine	Activation of α2-adrenergic receptors increasing pre-synaptic inhibition of motor neurons	Sedation, hypotension, hepatotoxicity (necessitating monitoring of liver function)
Benzodiazepines	Increase GABA release from $GABA_A$ neurons	Somnolence and sedation, dependence
Dantrolene	Ryanodine receptor-mediated reduction of calcium release from sarcoplasmic reticulum	Sedation, weakness, gastrointestinal upset and hepatotoxicity (necessitating monitoring of liver function)
Gabapentin	GABA analogue but also binds to α2-δ subunit protein of voltage-gated calcium channels with consequent reduction in release of excitatory neurotransmitters	Drowsiness, sedation, gastrointestinal upset, dizziness
Pregabalin	Increased GABA activity and reduction in excitatory neurotransmission via voltage-gated calcium channels	Somnolence, gastrointestinal upset, mood disturbance
Levetiracetam	Acts on $GABA_A$ and glycine receptors	Drowsiness, dizziness, gastrointestinal upset, mood disturbance
Carbamazepine	Sodium channel blocker	Dizziness, sedation, gastrointestinal upset, hyponatraemia, blood dyscrasiae
Phenytoin	Sodium channel blocker	Sedation, dizziness, rash, blood dyscrasiae, paraesthesiae, gingival hypertrophy, hirsutism, hepatotoxicity
Cannabis based medicinal extract	Pre-synaptic CB1 receptors with inhibition of calcium influx at axon terminals and activation of somatic and dendritic potassium channels	Gastrointestinal upset, cognitive impairment, sedation, mood disturbance, alteration in appetite

dantrolene are recommended as second-line therapies, and benzodiazepines (such as diazepam and clonazepam) as third-line therapies and for the treatment of nocturnal spasms [6]. Nabiximols oromucosal spray (tradename Sativex®) is licensed but not approved for prescription on the NHS in England, Wales and Scotland (discussed later). A systematic review and consensus paper published in 2016 made broadly similar recommendations, except that tizanidine was promoted to first-line, diazepam was promoted to second-line, and Sativex® was endorsed as add-on therapy in patients with poor response and/or tolerance to other treatments [52]. The review authors noted the variable methodological quality of studies on which current practice is based, and identified the need for large, well-designed trials in order to confirm the effectiveness of antispasticity agents and produce evidence-based treatment algorithms [52].

Oral baclofen is probably the most widely used drug for the treatment of spasticity, although the evidence basis supporting it is weak; benefit, which has generally been assessed in terms of reduction of hypertonia and spasms, was demonstrated in only three of eight placebo-controlled trials reviewed as part of the Cochrane analysis [50]. Doses of up to 60 mg daily are usually required for control of symptomatic spasticity, with a maximum daily dose of 100 mg [53]. Baclofen is an analogue of gamma-aminobutyric acid (GABA) and binds to $GABA_B$ receptors, inhibiting the excitatory activity of spinal reflexes. It is associated with a significant number of potential adverse effects—sedation and weakness may occur in up to 45% of patients [54], but hallucinations, mood and sleep disturbances, myalgia, and respiratory and cardiovascular depression have all been reported. The drug therefore necessitates careful titration and withdrawal.

Like baclofen, tizanidine has not consistently demonstrated benefit in randomised placebo-controlled trials (RCTs) [55–57], although in a meta-analysis it was found to have similar efficacy to baclofen and diazepam but improved tolerability [58]. The average effective dose is 12–24 mg daily, with a starting dose of 2 mg and a maximum dose of 36 mg daily in three to four divided doses [59]. Its mechanism of action has not been fully elucidated [60], but it is thought to act at α2-adrenergic receptor sites to increase pre-synaptic inhibition of motor neurons. Some patients complain of sedation, and hypotension may also be a limiting factor. In view of the possibility of liver toxicity, monitoring of liver function tests is advised for at least 4 months following commencement of treatment and thereafter in anyone complaining of symptoms compatible with liver dysfunction.

The use of benzodiazepines which act upon $GABA_A$ receptors is frequently complicated by somnolence and sedation, but in selected cases these may be helpful drugs, particularly for the treatment of difficult nocturnal spasticity. Diazepam has been compared with other benzodiazepines and, although efficacy appears comparable, it is probably the least well tolerated drug.

Dantrolene is believed to act at the ryanodine receptor, reducing calcium release from the sarcoplasmic reticulum [61]. The usual starting dose is 25 mg daily, increasing gradually to a maximum of 100 mg four times a day [62]. As with other agents in widespread clinical use, the evidence basis for functional benefit is not strong, although benefit has been shown on other measures [63]. Given that dantrolene is thought to work peripherally, it may be a useful additional treatment for those already on centrally-acting drugs, although monitoring of liver function tests is mandatory due to the potential for hepatotoxicity. Other reported side-effects include sedation, weakness and gastro-intestinal upset.

Gabapentin has been shown to be efficacious in the treatment of spasticity in a number of double-blind, placebo-controlled crossover studies [64, 65] and a small RCT [66]. It is normally prescribed at a starting dose of 300 mg daily, increasing gradually to a maximum of 3600 mg [67]. It may have advantages as a symptomatic treatment for spasticity, given that it may also treat other co-existent symptoms such as neuropathic pain and oscillopsia. The related drug, pregabalin, also binds with high affinity to the α2-δ subunit protein of voltage-gated calcium channels [68], reducing the release of excitatory neurotransmitters. Its effect upon spasticity has been examined only in a very limited sense; a modest benefit was observed in a single, small open-label study, in which only some of the patients had spasticity secondary to MS [69].

Levetiracetam is an anticonvulsant agent that is thought to act upon $GABA_A$ and glycine receptors [70]. A small, retrospective study has raised the possibility of benefit for intermittent spasms rather than tonic spasticity in patients with MS [70], an effect also reported in small numbers of patients with spasticity due to conditions other than MS [71, 72].

Tolperisone is a piperidine derivative that is thought to be a centrally-acting muscle relaxant. It has undergone only limited evaluation in patients with MS [73], although the outcome of a double-blind, randomised controlled trial in stroke patients did have a favourable outcome in terms of tolerability and reduction of measurable spasticity [74]. The possibility that other sodium channel blockers, including the related eperisone [75, 76], may be of benefit in the treatment of spasticity is beginning to be evaluated, whilst the use of others such as carbamazepine and phenytoin should be reserved for those patients who require simultaneous treatment for neuropathic pain.

Cannabis sativa or marijuana has been used both recreationally and medicinally for centuries [77]. Of the 60 cannabinoids found in natural *Cannabis*, tetrahydrocannabinol (THC) and cannabidol (CBD) are the two most abundant [78], and THC is the main psychoactive component [79]. There are at least two classes of cannabinoid receptors; CB1 receptors are widely distributed throughout the CNS, particularly in the basal ganglia, cerebellum and hippocampus [80–82], but CB2 receptors are mostly expressed in the immune system, with some restricted expression in the brainstem and cerebellum [83, 84]. CB1 receptors are located pre-synaptically, and their activation inhibits calcium influx at axon terminals and activates somatic and dendritic potassium channels. Together, these effects lead to reduced neuronal excitability [85, 86], and this, combined with the changes noted in CB1 receptors following the induction of spasticity, has led some to postulate that endogenous cannabinoids may play a role in the tonic control of spasticity [87–90].

A significant minority of patients with MS use *Cannabis* on a regular basis for relief of symptoms including anxiety, sleep disturbance, pain and spasticity caused by the disease [91, 92]. Early studies (mainly using THC) were complicated by concerns regarding tolerability [93]. Later studies have looked at whole plant extracts containing both THC and CBD (only THC is psychoactive), and the safety data generated by these relatively short studies indicate that the risk of serious adverse effects is low. With the exception of one longer follow-up study using THC [94], treatment with cannabinoids has not been associated with statistically significant objective benefit, although this is at odds with consistently reported subjective benefit [95–98]. It has been suggested that this may reflect the deficiencies of the rating scales employed to measure spasticity objectively [50, 97], and alternatives are being developed [99].

The recent licensing of *Cannabis* based medicinal extract (CBME, Sativex® oromucosal spray) in the UK for treatment of moderate to severe MS-related spasticity unresponsive to other medications, together with the relatively new appreciation that cannabinoids may promote remyelination and have anti-inflammatory and/or neuroprotective effects [100], has reignited interest in the potential of *Cannabis*-based treatments in MS, although the potential for adverse effects on cognition cannot be overlooked [101].

Syed et al. have extensively reviewed the trial data, real-world observational data and health economic considerations that pertain to prescribing Sativex® for refractory, moderate to severe spasticity in patients with MS [102]. Trial evidence largely derives from four multi-centre, double-blind, randomised, placebo-controlled, phase III studies, which studied treatment over a period of 6–14 weeks [103–106]. The pivotal and largest of these trials [106], which was the only one to use the approved treatment regimen, used an 'enriched study design' to select 'responders' during a 4-week single-blind trial of add-on therapy with Sativex®. 47.6% of patients were deemed to be 'responders' and were then randomised to either Sativex® or placebo as add-on therapy for 12 weeks; this may have introduced a patient selection bias, but also reflects real-world practice. Seventy-four percent of patients receiving Sativex® had a clinically meaningful reduction in spasticity, compared with 51% receiving placebo ($p < 0.001$). Real-world observational data from risk management registries in the UK, Germany and Switzerland (which require voluntary retrospective reporting), and a prospective study undertaken in Spain [107], also support the drug's efficacy for this indication and show similar response rates to the key clinical trial, and also suggest that it is safe and relatively well tolerated, with no evidence of addiction, misuse or abuse [108]. The largest study of Sativex use in daily practice comes from an Italian registry of 1615 patients, which again demonstrated safety and efficacy of the drug [109]. However, there are concerns about its cost-effectiveness compared to standard anti-spasticity treatment, and as such, it cannot be prescribed on the NHS in England and Wales [6, 110], nor in Scotland where marketing authorisation has not been applied for. In contrast, it was found to be cost-effective in Germany and dominant in Spain [102, 111].

A large multi-centre trial that set out to determine whether THC can slow the course of progressive MS—the Cannabinoid Use in Progressive Inflammatory brain Disease (CUPID) trial—has recently concluded with disappointing results. There was no significant reduction of disability progression or of any of the secondary outcomes, which included spasticity [112]. This result may in part relate to poor medication compliance and the fact that patients were more disabled than in previous studies, possibly reducing the ability to detect treatment effects. Further research is warranted into the potential symptomatic and neuroprotective benefits of cannabinoids.

Naltrexone is an oral semi-synthetic opiate antagonist, originally licensed for the treatment of heroin and alcohol addiction [113]. However, at off-label doses below or equal to 5 mg/day, naltrexone is said to stimulate prolonged release of endogenous opioids such as β-endorphin [114]. This is perhaps even more noteworthy considering the growing body of literature documenting interactions between the opioid and cannabinoid systems [115]. The safety, tolerability and efficacy of low-dose naltrexone in primary progressive MS has been studied in a 6 month, open-label, uncontrolled pilot trial. Five out of forty patients dropped out of the study, and there were two serious adverse events that were probably unrelated to the treatment. However, the drug was found to be relatively safe and well-tolerated, and in an intention-to-treat analysis of secondary end-points, there was a reduction in spasticity as assessed by the Modified Ashworth Scale (improved in 47.4% of participants, stable in 42.1%, worsened in 10.5%). There was no effect of treatment on pain, fatigue, depression or quality of life. Mean β-endorphin levels in peripheral blood mononuclear cells were also shown to progressively and significantly increase throughout the 6-month trial period and at 1 month after discontinuation of low-dose naltrexone. Low-dose naltrexone cannot be recommended for use in clinical practice until further research can verify the reported reduction in spasticity, particularly as a 17-week double-blind, randomised, placebo-controlled, cross-over design clinical trial was unable to demonstrate any change in quality of life outcomes in 96 patients with relapsing-remitting or secondary progressive MS treated with low-dose naltrexone.

7.2.3 *Other Pharmacological Therapies for Spasticity*

Inhibition of acetylcholine release at the neuromuscular junction by injection of botulinum toxin A [116] is the most commonly used focal pharmacological therapy for spasticity. The resultant reduction in muscle overactivity allows for stretching and lengthening and attempts to restore the balance between antagonist muscle groups disturbed as part of the upper motor neuron syndrome [117]. Although the blockade is permanent, nerve sprouting and re-innervation means that repeat injections are usually required after 3–6 months. Patients with MS who have focal increases in spasticity in the lower limbs causing adductor spasticity, hip flexor spasticity, hip extensor spasticity, spastic talipes equinus and striatal toe, for example, may derive particular benefit [118]. The upper limbs are less frequently targeted in MS, but severe adductor spasm of the shoulder is a recognised indication [118]. Some limited studies have demonstrated efficacy of botulinum toxin A, at least in terms of tone reduction and aiding passive functions leading to ease of nursing care (reviewed in Habek et al. [119]), but emphasis is placed on the need to combine such therapy with physiotherapy if benefits are to be optimised [120]. Botulinum toxin injections are expensive treatments, given the cost of the drugs, need for repeated administration, and specialist training required to perform the treatment. Analyses of its cost-effectiveness in spasticity due to MS and other conditions are on-going [121, 122].

Chemical neurolysis with phenol or alcohol is a potential alternative therapy for nerves with motor predominance, with the potential for post-injection sensory dysaesthesia limiting its use elsewhere. Although often considered permanent, the effects may wear off after several months due to partial nerve regeneration and sprouting. Nonetheless, careful assessment and consideration must be undertaken prior to performing these more destructive procedures, which may also cause tissue fibrosis, potentially rendering any subsequent surgical intervention more difficult. A transient motor block may be performed prior to injection to give a clearer indication of potential benefit [123], and such treatments are usually reserved for patients with spasticity affecting a relatively wide region that has been resistant to other treatments [124].

Intrathecal therapy may be also useful in patients who have not responded to oral therapies and who have severe, predominantly lower limb spasticity. The high concentration of GABAergic receptors in the spinal cord allows lower doses of medication to be effective, whilst reducing the likelihood of side effects. Intrathecal baclofen reduces both spasticity and spasms in patients with MS, as well as having beneficial effects on pain and sleep [125–127]. Long-term treatment appears to be effective and well tolerated [128, 129], although there are reports of increased seizure frequency [130] and impaired response to treatment developing with time [131]. Intrathecal phenol is an alternative intervention, but, although it has been used in the treatment of spasticity for many years [132, 133], the consequences of bowel and bladder incontinence, limb weakness and painful dysaesthesiae preclude its current use in all but a minority of carefully selected (and consented) patients [134].

7.2.4 Surgical Procedures for Spasticity

Many surgical procedures have been attempted to reduce spasticity. Most, including ventral rhizotomy, longitudinal myelotomy and distal cordectomy, have been complicated by severe side effects [135]. Posterior rhizotomy has been employed for the treatment of spasticity since the beginning of the twentieth century [136], following on from the observation that decerebrate rigidity could be abolished in animals by sectioning the dorsal roots [137]. Early surgical procedures were complicated by severe sensory disturbances, and the procedure was subsequently modified so that a proportion of the dorsal roots were spared in an effort to reduce the sensory disturbances—the so-called selective dorsal rhizotomy [138]. Although it is not commonly performed in patients with MS, it may be useful in a small proportion of patients [139]. Similarly, peripheral neurotomy can be undertaken in an effort to restore the normal balance between agonists and antagonists in focal spasticity [140, 141] but is rarely undertaken. Other surgical interventions are directed at correcting the consequences of spasticity and include tendon lengthening, tendon transfers and tendotomy, as well as osteotomy and arthrodesis.

7.3 Pain

The prevalence of pain in patients with MS has been examined frequently, but methodological problems have resulted in a wide variation between reported estimates (29–90%) for prevalence of pain of any description [142, 143]. However, it is undoubtedly a common problem faced by patients with MS and some have suggested that it may be the MS symptom most frequently treated pharmacologically [144]. Types of pain directly attributable to MS include persistent central neuropathic pain, painful tonic spasms, and paroxysmal sensory disturbances including trigeminal neuralgia and Lhermitte's phenomenon. With the notable exception of the paroxysmal phenomena, pain is rarely the presenting symptom of MS (1–2% for central dysaesthetic pain [145, 146]), and most studies have demonstrated an association with disability and disease duration [146–151], although the negative impact of pain early in disease course has also been highlighted [152].

Other pains frequently experienced by those with MS, but which will not be dealt extensively with here, include headache and low back pain [148, 149, 153]. Directly attributing these to MS is difficult, given that they occur widely in the otherwise normal population, and low back pain in particular may arise secondary to musculoskeletal problems. It is worth noting, however, that mechanisms have been proposed for how headache might arise due to MS pathophysiology [154–157], and that headache may increase, perhaps temporarily, with disease-modifying treatment [148, 158].

7.3.1 Central Dysaesthetic Pain

Stimuli that are either noxious or have the potential to damage tissues activate primary nociceptive afferents. These signals are subsequently processed in the nociceptive system, giving rise to the sensation of pain. This is physiological and can be contrasted with central neuropathic pain, in which activity is generated within the nociceptive system without stimulation of the primary afferents, and which has been defined as "pain arising as a direct consequence of a lesion or disease affecting the somatosensory system" [159].

The lifetime prevalence of central dysaesthetic pain in those with MS has been estimated to be between 12–28% [146–149, 160], but it should be noted that this type of pain is difficult to assess and is frequently reported in control populations [153]. The character of the pain is similar to that described by patients with neuropathic pain secondary to other conditions, but it tends not to respect dermatomal borders and is associated with sensory loss [146]. Many patients with MS and central dysaesthetic pain have thalamic lesions and spinal cord disease [146], but the pathophysiology is not clearly understood.

There are few high-quality trials to provide an evidence basis for the treatment of central dysaesthetic pain in MS, and treatment guidelines have tended to extrapolate from data gathered from clinical trials of agents for the treatment of peripheral neuropathic pain [158, 161–163]. The most recent UK guideline on the management of MS in primary and secondary care [164] defers to recommendations made in the NICE guideline on the pharmacological management of neuropathic pain in adults in non-specialist settings [165]. In this guideline, they did not differentiate between central dysaesthetic pain in MS and neuropathic pain in other diseases, although separate recommendations were made for trigeminal neuralgia [165]. Recommended first-line treatment is with amitriptyline, duloxetine, gabapentin or pregabalin, trialling one agent at a time [165]. Although combination therapy is common and may help to minimise adverse effects, there is a lack of trial evidence comparing the efficacy, tolerability and cost-effectiveness of different drug combinations [165]. In specialist settings, other tricyclic antidepressants, anticonvulsant agents (*e.g.* carbamazepine, levetiracetam) and selective noradrenaline reuptake inhibitors (*e.g.* venlafaxine) may also be of use, as well as lidocaine patches or topical capsaicin cream for patients who do not tolerate or wish to avoid oral medication.

Patients have frequently reported benefit in the treatment of neuropathic pain with cannabinoids, although none is presently licensed for this indication in the UK. Their potential as pharmacological modulators of neuropathic pain has been explored in a variety of contexts [166]. While there is some evidence for an analgesic effect of various cannabinoid compounds, their safety and long-term effects on cognition still need to be evaluated in MS patients [167]. A systematic review and meta-analysis published by the American Academy of Neurology in 2015 [168] concluded, based on two class I studies, that oral cannabis extracts containing a combination of THC (delta-9 tetrahydrocannabinol) and CBD (cannabidiol) were effective at reducing central pain in MS, and those containing only THC were "probably effective". The same review concluded, based on one class I study, that nabiximols (tradename Sativex®) oromucosal spray was "probably effective". Nabilone, a synthetic cannabinoid that mimics THC, has been studied as an adjunctive treatment to gabapentin (≥1800 mg/day) in MS patients with refractory pain in a small double-blind, randomised, placebo-controlled trial that recruited 15 patients [169]. The nabilone group showed a statistically significant improvement in the rate of decline of visual analogue pain intensity scores compared to the placebo group, however it is possible that there could have been unmasking because of the psychoactive nature and adverse effects of nabilone. There is a suggestion that opioids may be more effective in MS than is the case with other central causes of persistent pain [170, 171], although not all patients may respond [172]. While these drugs can undoubtedly have a role in pain control in MS [158], their side effect profile limits their usefulness.

A variety of non-pharmacological treatments have been purported to be helpful in the treatment of central neuropathic pain, but have generally not been rigorously tested. Various forms of non-invasive neurostimulation therapy are widely available, often as preliminary or add-on therapy, and include high-frequency transcutaneous electrical nerve stimulation (TENS) [173], electro-acupuncture, and repetitive transcranial magnetic stimulation (r-TMS). More invasive options, including spinal cord stimulation (SCS) [174], epidural motor cortex stimulation (MCS) [175, 176] and deep brain stimulation (DBS) [176, 177], are generally reserved for those with chronic pain that has proved resistant to other interventions. This also applies to intrathecal infusion of baclofen and/or morphine [178] or anaesthetic agents such as bupivacaine [179].

7.3.2 *Painful Tonic Spasms*

Painful tonic spasms are paroxysmal episodes of limb posturing, lasting seconds or minutes, which can occur many times a day for weeks to months before spontaneous remission. They may be associated with pain or other sensory symptoms, and although they may spread to adjacent body parts, they are typically unilateral. An important differential diagnosis is tonic seizures, which are most frequently bilateral, commonly with preserved consciousness, and may be preceded by an aura [180]. Tonic spasms are believed to arise from ephaptic activation of demyelinated motor axons of the pyramidal tract, particularly in relation to lesions of the posterior limb of the internal capsule or the cerebral peduncle, where radial spread of an ectopic impulse is facilitated by close proximity of the motor axons [181]. While tonic spasms are more common in those with progressive disease [148, 149], they may occasionally occur in the setting of acute relapse [180]. Anti-epileptic drugs have been reported to be of benefit, including tiagabine [182], levetiracetam [183] and gabapentin [184]. The use of botulinum toxin for painful tonic spasms remains controversial [185, 186]. The possibility that lidocaine, a sodium channel blocker, may have a positive effect on the treatment of painful tonic spasms was raised following the results of a small, open trial [187]. Mexiletine, which is a derivative of lidocaine that can be administered orally, had a lesser effect.

7.3.3 *Trigeminal Neuralgia*

The pain of trigeminal neuralgia is paroxysmal and frequently triggered by environmental stimuli. It occurs in the distribution of the trigeminal nerve, sensation in which is preserved. Although indistinguishable in terms of character from those who do not have MS, trigeminal neuralgia occurs much more commonly in the MS patient population (approximately 2–6%) [145, 148, 149, 188] and is also far more likely to be bilateral (estimated at 18% [189]). The dorsal root entry zone of the trigeminal nerve is the most common site of vascular compression in those with trigeminal neuralgia unrelated to MS, and is a transition zone between peripheral, Schwann cell-derived myelin and central myelin from oligodendrocytes. A study examining operative specimens from a small number of MS patients undergoing partial trigeminal rhizotomy revealed not only demyelination and gliosis but also remyelination and axons lying directly next to each other [190], which may predispose to both spontaneous firing and ephaptic transmission [191]. The relative contribution of vascular compression (a common cause in trigeminal neuralgia unrelated to MS) as opposed to an MS plaque affecting the primary afferents of the trigeminal nerve remains unclear [192].

Carbamazepine is recognised to be first-line treatment for trigeminal neuralgia [165, 193], but may exacerbate other symptoms due to MS [194, 195]. The potential of other pharmacological agents has therefore been explored, if only in small, uncontrolled studies, and some benefit has been demonstrated with lamotrigine [196–198], gabapentin [198–200], topiramate [201, 202] and misoprostol [203, 204].

The relative role of vascular compression of the trigeminal nerve at the root entry zone in the pathogenesis of trigeminal neuralgia in patients with MS assumes increased importance now that microvascular decompression (MVD) is well-established as a successful treatment for trigeminal neuralgia occurring outside the context of MS [205]. Traditionally, patients with MS have tended not to be offered MVD, given that the results of MVD in MS patients have not been as good as in the otherwise normal population and that vascular compression of the trigeminal nerve is a frequent incidental finding [206, 207]. More recently, however, it has been appreciated that patients with trigeminal neuralgia and MS can benefit from MVD, and a diagnosis of MS should not necessarily preclude the intervention being considered [208–212] (Fig. 7.1). Debate continues, and a clear consensus has not been reached as to whether a posterior fossa craniectomy and decompression with consequent risk of mortality (0.2–0.4%) or ipsilateral hearing loss (2–4%) [213] is preferable to the proven safety and efficacy of percutaneous neuroablative procedures at the level of the Gasserian ganglion [214–216] or gamma-knife radiosurgery [189, 217], albeit with an acquired sensory deficit and need for repeat procedures [218].

Other paroxysmal discomfort may arise in patients with MS due to Lhermitte's phenomenon or glossopharyngeal neuralgia. The former rarely requires treatment but, like glossopharyngeal neuralgia, it may respond to carbamazepine [219, 220]. Alternative sodium channel blockers have also been reported to be helpful [187].

Optic neuritis is classically associated with pain on eye movement. The pain may not require treatment but, if particularly distressing, could be treated with non-steroidal anti-inflammatory drugs or may respond to corticosteroids [221].

7.4 Urogenital System

7.4.1 Bladder Dysfunction

Bladder symptoms are a common problem for patients with MS with one study reporting that 70% rate them to be of 'moderate' or 'high' impact [222]. There are numerous CNS regions involved in the control of micturition including the periaqueductal grey matter, pontine micturition centre, medial frontal cortex, hypothalamus and sacral micturition centre [223]. However, in patients with MS the majority

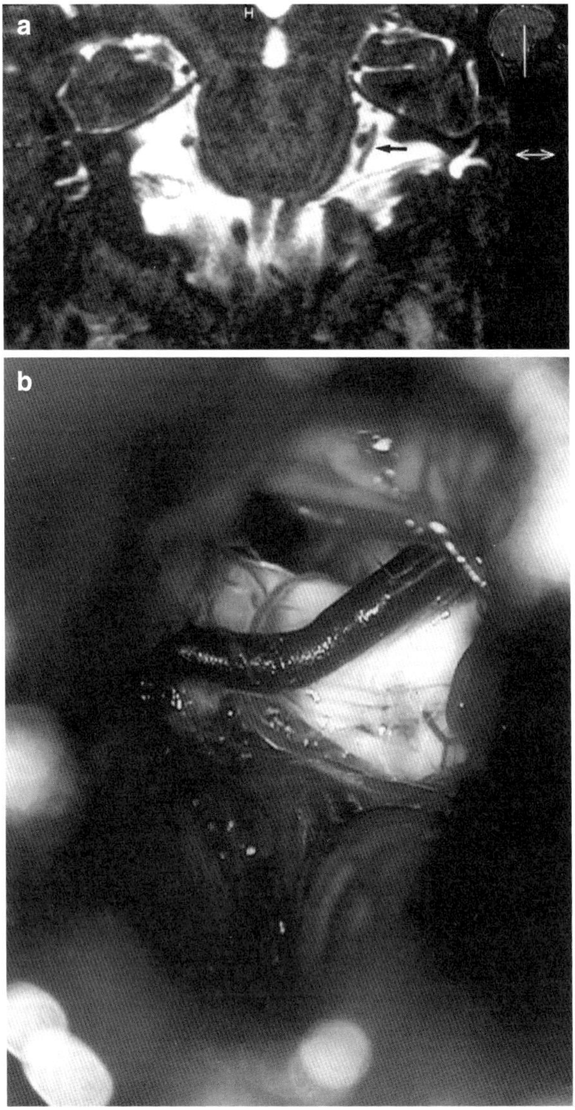

Fig. 7.1 Although microvascular decompression of the trigeminal nerve may still be undertaken with good effect in patients with MS and trigeminal neuralgia, overall the operation is not as successful in those with MS as in those who do not have the disease. (**a**) Shows a T2-weighted MRI with a prominent vessel in contact with the lateral aspect of the right trigeminal root. (**b**) Is an operative photograph of the right trigeminal root compressed laterally by a trigeminal vein. Reproduced with permission from Athanasiou et al., British Journal of Neurosurgery, 2005 [208]

of urinary symptoms are thought to be due to impaired signalling between the pons and sacral spinal cord [224]. The pathophysiology varies between patients with detrusor over-activity causing urgency, frequency and urge incontinence; detrusor inefficiency leading to frequency and incomplete emptying; and detrusor sphincter dyssynergia causing hesitancy, incomplete emptying and interrupted stream. There may also be superimposed problems due to common conditions unrelated to MS such as stress incontinence in women and prostatic hypertrophy in men.

Consensus guidelines have been published in the UK for management of bladder symptoms in MS [225] and these stress the importance of careful regular review by appropriately trained professionals, exclusion of a urinary tract infection and checking a post-micturition residual bladder volume with abdominal ultrasound. In contrast to other published guidelines [226], the UK group do not recommend routine urodynamics, reserving these for more complicated cases such as those with refractory symptoms, upper urinary tract disease, superimposed urinary problems such as stress incontinence in women or anyone in whom a surgical or an intra-vesical procedure is contemplated.

It is important to reinforce to patients that general measures such as good hydration, reducing caffeine intake, avoiding constipation and pelvic floor exercises (for both stress incontinence and detrusor overactivity as pelvic floor activity inhibits the detrusor) may be helpful and individualised bladder rehabilitation programmes have been proven to be of demonstrable benefit [227].

For those with persistent post-void residual volumes of greater than 100 mL, clean intermittent self-catheterisation (ISC) is recommended [225]. Other measures which can be considered include α-adrenergic antagonists [228] and suprapubic vibration [229] although in practice many feel that the benefit of both is minimal unless there is concomitant obstruction secondary to prostatic disease when the combination of α-blockers and 5α-reductase inhibitors can be beneficial [230]. If an indwelling catheter becomes a necessity, a suprapubic catheter is preferable to avoid urethral damage and careful consideration should be given to which type of catheter is most appropriate for the individual [163, 231]. Botulinum toxin injection can be helpful if urethral leakage (catheter by-passing) is problematic [232].

Anti-muscarinic medications are available for the treatment of detrusor overactivity and can reduce symptoms of frequency, urgency and incontinence [233]. A small number of studies have examined this in the specific context of MS [234–236], but not all available agents have been so examined. Consideration can be given to combination therapy if single agents are not effective, although the trial which explored this included only two patients with MS [237]. Anti-muscarinics are not recommended without concurrent ISC in those who have impaired voiding as they may further impair bladder emptying. For the same reason, anyone who fails treatment with anti-muscarinics should have repeat abdominal ultrasound to assess the post-void micturition volume. Other possible side effects include worsening cognitive impairment, a risk which may be minimised by using those anti-muscarinics which either do not cross the blood-brain barrier (trospium chloride) or which selectively block receptors not involved in cognition (darifenacin—M3 receptor blocker) [238, 239]. An additional option which may be suitable for some patients includes intravesical drug delivery [240, 241].

Considerable attention has been focused recently on the use of botulinum toxin A injections into the detrusor for the treatment of detrusor overactivity [242]. OnabotulinumtoxinA (typically a dose of 100–300 U) is the toxin most commonly used by urologists [243]. A positive effect was observed in a randomised, double-blind placebo-controlled trial which has recently been published [244], and a long-term follow-up study of those having repeat injections (approximately once per year) has reported an improved quality of life, albeit with reliance on ISC [245]. A randomised, double-blind, placebo-controlled trial has also reported that botulinum toxin A injections (at a dose of either 200 or 300 units) can improve quality of life measures in patients with neurogenic detrusor over-activity not adequately managed with anticholinergic therapy [246].

Desmopressin may be considered for some patients with urinary frequency, including nocturia [247], although the side effect profile, which includes fluid retention and hyponatraemia, precludes use in many patients, particularly those over 65 years of age [248]. Diuretics taken in the afternoon may also reduce nocturia, particularly if there is dependent oedema [225, 249].

Participants in the ‘Cannabinoids in Multiple Sclerosis Study’ completed incontinence diaries and the results of this sub-study demonstrated a benefit for cannabinoids over placebo in the treatment of urge incontinence [250]. This followed on from the benefit observed with cannabis extracts upon urinary urgency, incontinence, frequency and nocturia in an open-label study [251]. More recently, however, a randomised, placebo-controlled trial of nabiximols (Sativex®) as add-on therapy failed to reach statistical significance for the primary endpoint of reduction of number of daily incontinence episodes, although the authors concluded that some benefit in terms of symptoms attributable to bladder overactivity was observed [252]. It therefore remains to be determined how useful cannabinoids will be in the treatment of urinary dysfunction attributable to MS [253].

Intravesical treatment with either capsaicin [254] or an analogue thereof [255] has also been explored for the symptoms of neurogenic bladder dysfunction, in trials which included a number of patients with MS, and shown some promise.

The evidence for sacral nerve neuromodulation as a treatment for urinary dysfunction in patients with MS is limited to small retrospective studies [243]. An observational, retrospective, case-control study has reported on the effect of sacral nerve neuromodulation (SNM) in patients with MS, and documented a reduction in the post-void residual volume and increase in number of patients who could void spontaneously [256]. Magnetic resonance imaging is contraindicated following implantation, however, which is a significant disadvantage in this patient group [243]. Further investigation is required before this treatment can be recommended. This also applies to electro-acupuncture [257], percutaneous posterior tibial nerve stimulation [258] and stimulation of the dorsal penile/clitoral nerve [259].

Urinary diversion remains an option for a minority of patients who remain intolerant of a urinary catheter despite best medical management, although the risks are not inconsiderable [260]. This procedure may also be required for the small number of patients who have intractable urge incontinence, although bladder augmentation surgery may be an alternative intervention [225]..

7.4.2 Sexual Dysfunction

Sexual dysfunction is recognised as being a common problem for patients with MS, with the incidence being estimated at approximately 70% in both males [261, 262] and females [263], although detection rates are low [264]. It is thought to arise primarily due to spinal cord disease [261, 265]. Men report impotence, ejaculatory and orgasmic dysfunction, and reduced libido. Women may also experience reduced libido and orgasmic dysfunction, along with reduced lubrication and an increase in spasticity with sexual activity. In both sexes, sexual dysfunction tends to increase with disease severity [266]. Sexual problems may be exacerbated by coexistent fatigue, spasticity, and depression, as well as concerns about incontinence [267, 268]. The complex nature of sexual dysfunction in MS necessitates a sensitive and often multidisciplinary team approach [269].

Pharmacological interventions, particularly for erectile dysfunction, are available and are beginning to be assessed in the context of MS. Two double-blind, randomised, placebo-controlled trials have investigated the short-term efficacy and safety of sildenafil, a phosphodiesterase-5 inhibitor, as a treatment for erectile dysfunction in MS [270, 271], with both trials reporting a positive outcome. The possibility of un-blinding due to side effects has been raised [11], while a Cochrane review noted a high risk of attrition bias [272]. Intriguingly, sildenafil has been reported to be protective in mouse models of demyelination (both experimental autoimmune encephalomyelitis [273, 274] and cuprizone-induced demyelination [275, 276]), through a combination of immunoregulatory and neuroprotective effects and by enhancing remyelination. Other phosphodiesterase-5 inhibitors have not been extensively investigated in MS, although tadalafil has been reported to be both safe and efficacious in an open label study [277]. Apomorphine administered sub-lingually has not been tested in patients with MS and might be expected to be less efficacious than in patients with erectile dysfunction due to a cause other than MS, due to its mechanism of action being *via* the spinal cord [278]. Although agents available for intra-cavernosal or intraurethral application and vacuum devices are effectual in neurogenic impotence, their requirement for manual dexterity and other side effects may reduce their potential benefit for some patients with MS [278]. There has been a suggestion that patients with MS who have ejaculation failure may benefit from midodrine (an alpha-1-adrenergic receptor agonist), but the relevant trial included only a very small number of patients with MS and further studies are required [279].

Some female patients may benefit from either topical or systemic oestrogen replacement therapy or co-treatment with methyltestosterone and oestrogen. However, as for any other patient, the relative risks and benefits of hormonal treatment must be considered. A double-blind, placebo-controlled trial of sildenafil for female sexual dysfunction in participants with MS showed benefit only in lubrication and not in quality of life, and other treatments have not yet been formally examined [280].

7.5 Bowel Dysfunction

Bowel symptoms may be particularly distressing for patients with MS and occur frequently—studies report prevalence rates of 35–54% for constipation and 29–51% for faecal incontinence [281–284]. Unsurprisingly, bowel problems are associated with impaired quality of life [285], yet despite the scale of the problem, there is relatively little published data on which to base treatment recommendations. Constipation may be due to slow colonic transit and/or abnormal rectal function; while faecal incontinence can result from impaired sensation of rectal fullness, poor contraction of the pelvic musculature, reduced rectal compliance and weakness of the anal sphincter [278, 286]. In addition, there may be effects of medications or concomitant disease. To optimise treatment recommendations, careful assessment of the nature of bowel symptoms is therefore required [287].

Following careful medication review, general measures which are often recommended include increasing fluid and dietary fibre, as well as increasing physical exercise. However, increasing fluid intake may be poorly adhered to by patients with urinary symptoms and, whilst it may be helpful in those with mild symptoms, increased dietary fibre has been shown to have adverse effects in chronic constipation [288].

Behavioural techniques have been shown to have some benefit in some patients with MS, particularly those with less severe disease, and involve increased awareness of rectal fullness, techniques for anal sphincter relaxation and recto-anal co-ordination, as well as habit training [289]. A recent pilot study of abdominal massage also suggested a positive effect [290].

A range of pharmacological agents are available but have not been tested in MS specifically. Stimulant laxatives can be very helpful, although osmotic laxatives are less likely to cause liquid stool and may therefore be advantageous if there is co-existent incontinence. Sodium docusate has both a stimulant and stool softener effect which may be useful. Timing of defecation may be regulated using rectal stimulants, although direct comparison of agents has been examined only in patients with spinal injury [291].

In some patients, mechanical evacuation will be required using digital evacuation [292] or trans-anal colonic irrigation [293]. Surgical procedures including formation of a stoma will be required in a minority of patients refractory to other interventions [287, 294]. Depending on the site of stoma formation, laxatives or irrigation may still be required due to impaired gut motility. It should also be recognised that while colostomy is frequently considered a last resort and is not without considerable risk, it has been demonstrated to improve quality of life in those with spinal cord injury [295].

Treatment interventions for faecal incontinence remain sub-optimal. Following medication review and the exclusion of diarrhoea secondary to other causes including faecal overloading, anti-motility agents such as codeine and loperamide may be tried. Anal plugs can be helpful for those with impaired anorectal sensation.

7.6 Ataxia and Tremor

Ataxia ultimately affects up to 80% of patients with MS [296], and can occur due to cerebellar disease or impaired proprioception related to problems with sensory afferent input. Postural and intention tremors are also common and have been reported to involve the head, neck, vocal cords, trunk and limbs, while rest and rubral tremors are relatively rare [297, 298]. MS tremor is thought to arise predominantly as a consequence of cerebellar or thalamic disease [299]. An increase in long-latency stretch reflexes has also been implicated in the case of intention tremor [300], which may explain the effect of peripheral cooling in dampening intention tremor [301, 302].

A wide variety of conservative treatment measures have been proposed and evaluated to some extent. These include limb cooling, exposure to electromagnetic fields [303], weighted bracelets [304], orthoses [305], physiotherapy [306], Pilates exercises [307], specialised software [308], robot training [309], and mechanical focal vibration [310]. Whilst they may provide assistance to some patients, the need for improved treatments remains. A systematic review concluded that there is weak evidence to suggest that physiotherapy improves balance in MS patients with mild to moderate disability, although the effect is relatively small, and evidence is lacking for severely disabled patients [311].

There is no strong evidence basis on which to guide pharmacological treatment. A 2007 Cochrane review of treatments for ataxia in MS concluded that no recommendations could be made [312], and little has changed in the interim. Benefit has been reported for the treatment of tremor with a wide range of drugs in small open-label studies or case reports, including primidone [313], glutethimide [314], intrathecal baclofen [315], topiramate [316], and isoniazid [317–320]. Negative outcomes were seen in controlled trials performed with propranolol [321], isoniazid [321], ethanol [321], levetiracetam [322] and dolasetron [323], but the number of patients involved was generally very low. Some degree of improvement was observed in other controlled trials with isoniazid [324, 325], as well as with carbamazepine [326] and ondansetron [327]. Cannabinoids appear to have no beneficial effect on tremor due to MS, given the outcome of a number of well-conducted, randomised, controlled trials of cannabis extracts [103, 328, 329] or THC [328].

Surgical options that may be considered for drug-resistant tremor secondary to MS include deep brain stimulation (DBS) and stereotactic thalamotomy. DBS has the advantage of being a reversible treatment with a better risk profile, although it is slightly less efficacious than thalamotomy [330]. Bilateral DBS is also considered safer than bilateral thalamotomy in patients requiring treatment of bilateral tremor [331]. The mainly retrospective, observational studies published to date have generally targeted thalamic structures with promising results (reviewed by Koch et al. [299] and Yap et al. [332]). DBS has historically targeted the thalamic nucleus ventralis intermedius, although more recently the ventralis oralis posterior (Vop) and zona incerta (ZI) have gained favour for distal and proximal tremors, respectively [331]. These studies will undoubtedly be refined as microelectrode placement and gamma-knife surgery are evaluated, but concerns regarding the risks of the procedure, including seizures [333] and adverse effects on cognition [334], will need to be addressed. Clearly, careful patient selection and consent will be required but, encouragingly, consensus statements are already emerging [335].

7.7 Walking Speed: Fampridine SR

A symptomatic treatment that could meaningfully improve a patient's walking speed would be highly desirable to patients with MS. Indeed, in one large survey of patients with MS, gait function was rated the most valuable bodily function [336]. Fampridine sustained-release (fampridine SR), a formulation of 4-aminopyridine, is thought to improve action potential conduction in demyelinated nerve fibres by blocking potassium channels, and in this way, it was hoped that it might be able to ameliorate some of the symptoms of MS.

Fampridine SR has been shown to improve walking speed in some patients with MS in two double-blind, randomised, placebo-controlled trials [337, 338]. The original trial, which also reported an improvement in lower limb strength, only reported an improvement in walking speed in the *post-hoc* analysis [337]. In the larger, more definitive trial, which recruited 239 patients, fampridine SR was shown to meaningfully improve walking speed in up to a third of patients, who were termed 'responders' [338]. Specifically, the proportion of 'timed walk responders' was 42.9% in the treatment arm compared to 9.3% in the control arm, and the approximately 25% reduction in the timed walk was sustained at 9 weeks. Open-label extensions to the original two double-blind, randomised, placebo-controlled trials have reported that these findings persisted over the up to 5 years of follow-up, although the mean improvement in walking speed declined with time [339].

In addition, three prospective, uncontrolled studies of fampridine SR in patients with MS have been published, reporting improvements from baseline in walking speed [337, 340, 341], manual dexterity [340, 342], cognition [341], self-reported fatigue [341, 342], mood [341, 342], and quality of life [340, 342]. Such results should be interpreted with caution, as they derive from class III evidence, but they present avenues for further research.

The drug is marketed as Fampyra in Europe and Ampyra in the US. It was approved by the United States FDA in January 2010 to improve walking in patients with MS, and it was granted conditional marketing authorisation by the European Medicines Agency in July 2011, which requires the manufacturer to carry out further research into clinical efficacy and long-term safety. Currently it cannot be prescribed on the NHS in England and Wales, because it was not deemed by NICE to be a cost-effective treatment for reduced mobility [6], and more recently it was rejected by the Scottish Medicines Consortium for similar reasons.

7.8 Psychiatric Manifestations of MS

Neuropsychiatric symptoms are rarely the presenting symptoms of MS but overall are common and can negatively impact upon quality of life for both patients and their care-givers [343].

7.8.1 Depression

Depression not only occurs more frequently in patients with MS than in the general population, but also more commonly than in other chronic disease [344]. It is the most frequent psychiatric manifestation of MS, occurring with a prevalence of 40–60% [345, 346], and has adverse effects not only on quality of life but also on cognition [347–349]. It remains under-diagnosed in the MS population [350].

The effect of behavioural treatments, such as cognitive behavioural therapy, mindfulness and other group interventions, is beginning to be evaluated for depression in MS, with some encouraging results [329, 351–354]. A recent Cochrane review of the pharmacological treatment highlighted the need for further dedicated studies of anti-depressants in MS [355], whilst another systematic review and meta-analysis of anti-depressants in neurological diseases concluded that there was evidence for their efficacy, although not for improvement of quality of life or cognition [356]. A more recent systematic review and meta-analysis of pharmacological and psychological interventions for depression and anxiety in MS identified 13 randomised controlled trials. It was concluded that both antidepressants and psychological interventions (primarily CBT) were generally effective in reducing depressive symptoms, although no effect was found on fatigue or quality of life [327]. The positive effect reported for antidepressants contrasts with the negative outcome in the Cochrane meta-analysis, despite analysing the same three trials of antidepressant therapy (using paroxetine, sertraline and desipramine). This inconsistency may relate to the fact that the Cochrane reviewers analysed categorical outcomes, while the more recent review analysed continuous outcomes.

7.8.2 Psychosis

The prevalence of psychosis and bipolar disorder in patients with MS has been reported to be two to three times that in the general population [357], although not all studies, particularly older ones, corroborate this ([358]; reviewed by Kosmidis et al. [359]). Clearly, psychosis may also be induced by medications taken by those with MS, such as corticosteroids [360, 361] and, more rarely, beta-interferons [362, 363]. One study has reported that psychosis is associated with increased MRI lesion load in MS [364]. It has not been definitively established whether psychosis in MS generally occurs as a separate condition or as a manifestation of demyelinating disease, but features such as a relative lack of family history and the demonstration of temporal lobe disease, associated with psychosis in other contexts, suggests that there may be a direct causal link [359]. Little evidence exists to guide treatment, but success has been reported with clozapine [365, 366], as well as newer atypical antipsychotics such as risperidone [367] and ziprasidone [368].

7.8.3 Bipolar Disorder

The prevalence of bipolar disorder has been estimated as being twice that expected in the MS patient population [369]. No evidence basis exists for treatment but, anecdotally, conventional mood stabilisers, antipsychotics and benzodiazepines can be recommended [370].

7.8.4 Pathological Laughing and Crying

Outbursts of uncontrollable laughing and/or crying, which are either disproportionate to or incongruent with the precipitating emotional stimulus and underlying feelings, may be referred to as pathological laughing and crying, emotional incontinence, or pseudobulbar affect. These symptoms have been recognised in 10% of patients with MS and are more often exhibited by those with more severe disease [371]. In MS, there is some evidence that treatment with dextromethorphan and quinidine can be helpful [372, 373], although there is probably more clinical experience, if not evidence, for the use of amitriptyline [374] and selective serotonin reuptake inhibitors [375, 376].

7.9 Cognition

Estimates of the prevalence of cognitive impairment associated with MS range from 40–70% [377]. Although cognitive impairment can undoubtedly occur at any stage and in any subtype of disease [378, 379], it increases with disease duration [380], is most severe in those with greatest disability [379, 381] and has an adverse effect on quality of life [382]. Speed of information processing, memory and executive function are the domains of function most likely to be affected, whilst language tends to be relatively preserved [377].

Following exclusion of concurrent systemic infection and review of medication to eliminate drugs contributing to excessive sedation, formal neuropsychometry is advised to determine the relative contribution of other deficits such as depression and fatigue to cognitive dysfunction. This clearly has implications for determining not only an accurate diagnosis but also treatment options, although the interplay between these symptoms is not straightforward.

At present, there is not a strong evidence basis for the use of cognitive rehabilitation in MS, with no class I trials in this area. A Cochrane review from 2006 concluded that there was some evidence that cognitive rehabilitation could improve cognitive outcomes, but the range of outcome measures employed made definitive conclusions impossible [354]. A systematic review published in 2015 analysed 33 studies and came to a similar conclusion [383]: although the studies generally showed some improvement in cognitive performance, there were conflicting findings in the published literature about the effectiveness of various forms of cognitive rehabilitation.

Trials of disease modifying therapies have not tended to include primary outcome measures that include tests of cognitive function, possibly because longitudinal studies with relatively short follow-up periods typically show little change [384, 385]. Nonetheless, the suggestion has been raised that treatment with interferon beta-1a and interferon beta-1b might confer some benefit, although this has not been definitively addressed [386–390]. Analysis of pooled data from two landmark natalizumab trials, AFFIRM and SENTINEL, has shown that natalizumab treatment reduced the risk of confirmed progression of cognitive deficits by 43% compared with placebo ($P = 0.013$) [391]. In addition, several class III studies have indicated that natalizumab treatment in relapsing-remitting MS is associated with a reduction in the rate of decline, or even an improvement and stabilisation, of aspects of cognitive function [392–398].

The rationale behind the use of anticholinesterases in MS arises due to the possibility that diffuse cholinergic connections from the nucleus basalis of Meynert could be disrupted due to the presence of deep white matter lesions and the fact that cholinergic deficits contribute to cognitive impairments in a disease model of MS [399]. Although some trials pointed towards a possible benefit with donepezil, a larger more recent trial provided class I evidence for lack of effect [400]. Similarly, benefit was not observed following treatment with rivastigmine [401]. A trial of memantine, a non-competitive inhibitor of N-methyl-D-aspartic acid (NMDA) receptors, for cognitive impairment in MS was limited by the emergence of reversible dose-related deterioration in neurological disability [402]. A study using a lower dose of memantine was reasonably well tolerated, but benefit was not observed [403]. A number of other agents have also been associated with negative outcomes in clinical trials for cognitive impairment in MS including amantadine [404], pemoline [404] and gingko biloba [405]. Although a trial of L-amphetamine sulfate showed benefit in some tests of learning and memory, improvement was not seen in the primary outcome measures and the duration of the trial was very short, so further investigation is required before L-amphetamine sulfate can be recommended [406].

7.10 Fatigue

Fatigue is one of the most commonly reported and disabling symptoms in people with MS. It has been estimated to occur throughout the course of the illness in approximately 75% of patients, with significant impact upon quality of life and employment [407–410], although not upon the potential for benefit from rehabilitation [411]. Individuals with MS-related fatigue commonly describe it as "tiredness or the need to rest", usually occurring in the late afternoon or evening, potentially exacerbated by exertion and warm environments, and sometimes associated with worsening of other MS symptoms [412]. It has been defined as a "subjective lack of physical and/or mental energy that is perceived by the individual or caregiver to interfere with usual and desired activities" [413], but a single, accepted and objective definition of MS-related fatigue is lacking [414].

The pathophysiology of MS-related fatigue remains poorly understood but is probably multi-factorial, consisting of primary and secondary mechanisms [415]:

Primary mechanisms may include high circulating levels of inflammatory cytokines [416–418], endocrine changes [419–421], axonal loss [422, 423], and abnormal patterns of cerebral activation [424–427]. There are contradictory reports regarding the role of lesion load and location and the degree of grey and white matter atrophy [414, 428, 429]. Controversially, there are recent reports of an association between fatigue and slightly higher endogenous body temperature in patients with relapsing-remitting MS, which will require further evaluation [430, 431].

Secondary mechanisms may include co-existent medical conditions, such as anaemia, thyroid disorders, anxiety and depression [409], and sleep disorders [432–434], as well as medication side-effects [435]. Multiple factors can contribute to fatigue, including pain, mood, sleep, coping ability, and degree of psychosocial support [408]. Indeed, a subjective loss of control over one's environment is an independent predictor for fatigue [436].

7.10.1 General Approach to Treating Fatigue

Once treatable co-morbidities have been excluded, lifestyle measures which should be addressed include sleep hygiene, optimisation of exercise regimens, and dietary review. Careful attention should be paid to identifying and treating depression and anxiety, which are prevalent throughout the MS disease course and tend to associate with fatigue [437, 438]. Fatigue should be managed by a multidisciplinary team consisting of neurologists, MS nurses, occupational therapists and physiotherapists [439], although chronic fatigue may prove refractory even to this approach [440].

7.10.2 Pharmacological Treatment of Fatigue

Patients on disease-modifying drugs report less fatigue [441, 442], and there is growing evidence that the highly-effective disease-modifying treatments improve fatigue in parallel with their stronger immunomodulatory effects [443]. A cross-sectional case-controlled study suggested that the effect was greater with natalizumab than with interferon-beta or glatiramer acetate [444]. Longitudinal follow-up studies of patients commenced on natalizumab have also highlighted a reduction in fatigue [445–447]. Equivalent evidence is not yet available for alemtuzumab [448].

Specific pharmacological interventions for the treatment of fatigue may be considered, although there is little supportive evidence for their use. This reflects both the lack of highly efficacious medications and the difficulties encountered in accurately measuring fatigue. On the basis of positive outcomes in a number of randomised controlled trials, some guidelines have suggested that a trial of amantadine might be helpful [163, 449]. However, the effect size reported is small and the validity of the outcome measures has been questioned [450–452].

Small randomised controlled trials of modafinil (a central stimulant used in narcolepsy) for MS-related fatigue have had mixed results, and there are also concerns about the drug's safety following a European Medicines Agency directive in 2010 [439]. Two trials showed generally no effect of modafinil on fatigue [453] [454], one trial showed benefit at 200 mg daily but not 400 mg daily [455], while another trial reported improvements in fatigue, focused attention and dexterity, and enhanced motor cortex excitability with modafinil [456]. The primary outcome measure was not met in a more recent, and much larger, double-blind, randomised, placebo-controlled trial [457]. As a result, some national guidelines do not recommend modafinil for treating fatigue in MS [6]. Interestingly, however, a retrospective analysis suggested that modafinil may show more promise in MS patients who experience fatigue in association with daytime sleepiness [458].

The effect of the CNS stimulant, pemoline, on MS-related fatigue has been examined in double-blind, randomised cross-over [459] and parallel-arm [460] studies, but a lack of effect was observed. Furthermore, liver toxicity has been reported and it has not been widely used.

Aminopyridines have been associated with improvements in fatigue in some [341, 342, 461, 462] but not all [337] trials, and safety concerns still remain [463], notwithstanding the recent licensing of fampridine sustained-release (dalfampridine) in the United States and Europe for the symptomatic treatment of walking difficulty due to MS [464].

The effects of carnitine on MS-related fatigue have been examined in a number of studies, but only one completed study met the criteria for inclusion in a Cochrane review [465]. On the basis of this randomised, double-blind, active-comparator (no placebo), cross-over trial comparing carnitine with amantadine, there was insufficient evidence to support a recommendation [466]. Another randomized, placebo-controlled, cross-over trial, comparing amantadine, carnitine and modafinil with placebo has reported a positive result for amantadine but not for carnitine or modafinil [467].

The use of many complementary therapies has not been rigorously examined, although a single-centre, randomised, placebo-controlled trial of ginseng was not associated with benefit [468].

7.10.3 Non-pharmacological Interventions for Fatigue

Behavioural and patient education approaches using cognitive behavioural therapy (CBT) [469], energy conservation techniques [470], or a combination of the two [471], have reported positive patient outcomes with respect to MS-related fatigue. A systematic review of CBT for MS-related fatigue was published in 2016 [472]. This identified 994 randomised controlled trials where CBT was the intervention and fatigue was the primary outcome measure. Four studies were included in the meta-analysis, which revealed a moderately positive short-term effect of CBT on fatigue, but this fell after cessation of treatment [472].

Exercise therapy has also attracted interest as a treatment for MS-related fatigue. Although patients with MS were once advised to avoid physical activity, evidence has mounted that exercise is not only safe but may confer health benefits [473]. A Cochrane review published in 2015, which examined 45 randomised controlled trials of exercise therapy versus a no-exercise control intervention, concluded that exercise therapy is safe for patients with MS and may reduce self-reported fatigue, without increasing relapse frequency [474]. However, the reviewers have cautioned against clinical implementation of exercise therapy specifically for the treatment of fatigue, citing a lack of evidence for clinically meaningful impact, as well as unanswered questions about tolerability and efficacy for MS patients with severe fatigue [475].

A set of three nearly-identical, single-blind randomised controlled trials is currently underway, comparing aerobic training, CBT and energy conservation management against the same control intervention. This promises to allow a useful comparison between different approaches, which until now has been hindered by the use of different definitions and rating scales for fatigue between studies [476].

Cooling has been reported to make many MS patients feel transiently better [477]. To date, most studies of cooling therapy in patients with MS have been limited by uncontrolled designs, unblinded evaluations, reliance on subjective outcome measures, and small sample sizes [478]. A temporary benefit in terms of physical performance and levels of fatigue has been reported with cooling garments or pre-cooling by immersion prior to exercise, compared to sham cooling [479, 480]. In a double-blind, randomised, sham-controlled study of acute and chronic cooling in MS patients, the control group unintentionally received low-dose cooling [478]. The investigators were unable to demonstrate significant differences in outcome measures between the groups that received high-dose and low-dose cooling. A significant improvement from baseline, however, was reported in the MS Functional Composite score and the Timed 25 Foot Walk following an hour of high-dose cooling. There was also a significant improvement from baseline in visual acuity/contrast sensitivity after both high- and low-dose cooling. Patients reported a greater reduction in fatigue after daily sessions of cooling for 4 weeks compared to observation without sham therapy, but the patients were unblinded and the outcome measures were entirely subjective and susceptible to a strong placebo effect [478]. As such, further research into the effects of chronic cooling with blinded comparisons and a combination of subjective and objective outcome measures would be justified.

Repeated exposure to a magnetic field for the treatment of MS-related fatigue has been studied in two randomised controlled trials [481, 482]. There was a marked placebo effect in both trials owing to the nature of the intervention. Only one of the trials reported a positive treatment effect [481], although the trials employed very different treatment protocols.

7.11 Sleep Disorders

Sleep disorders occur with increased prevalence in MS patients [434, 483, 484], and yet they frequently go unrecognised in this population [485] and may represent a treatable cause of daytime fatigue [486]. Examples of sleep disorders in MS include insomnia, circadian rhythm disorders, drug-induced sleep disorders, nocturnal movement disorders, respiratory disorders during sleep, narcolepsy and REM sleep disorder. The precise relationship between such conditions and MS-related fatigue remains to be determined [433], although current evidence suggests that sleep disorders account for approximately quarter of the variance of fatigue in MS, more than either depression (7–10%) or disease severity (9%) [487–489]. Treatment recommendations for MS patients are no different to those of the general population, given the current lack of disease-specific data.

7.12 Neuro-Ophthalmological Symptoms

Optic neuritis is a common ophthalmological problem in those with MS and is frequently the presenting clinical manifestation. Spontaneous improvement in visual acuity is anticipated, and treatment with corticosteroids can be considered to accelerate this. Although any part of the visual pathway may be affected in MS, symptomatic retrochiasmal field defects are relatively unusual. Uveitis is approximately ten times more common in those with MS than in the normal population, yet the presence of ocular inflammation requires screening for other conditions including syphilis, sarcoidosis, Lyme disease, tuberculosis, Behçet's and rheumatological disease [490, 491]. Eye movement disorders are a common problem for MS patients, and this is unsurprising given the predilection for lesions to occur in the brainstem and cerebellum. Symptomatic treatments for oscillopsia include optical dampening using spectacles and contact lenses [492]; NICE guidelines in the UK also recommend considering off-license use of gabapentin (first-line) or memantine (second-line) [6]. Treatment for pendular nystagmus is frequently unsatisfactory, but there is some evidence to support a trial of memantine or gabapentin [493]. A recent cross-over trial included three patients with MS and showed little benefit of one drug over the other [494], and concerns have been raised regarding the association of memantine with worsening neurological symptoms in patients with MS, therefore use of this drug will necessitate careful patient selection and dose titration [402]. Downbeat nystagmus may be suppressed by either 3,4-diaminopyridine [495] or fampridine [496], although fampridine may have a greater effect at equivalent doses [497]. Clonazepam may be an alternative for the treatment of downbeat nystagmus, baclofen for periodic alternating nystagmus and carbamazepine or acetazolamide for paroxysmal nystagmus [498]. Reports have emerged regarding the use of retrobulbar botulinium toxin A for the treatment of oscillopsia, but there is currently insufficient evidence to recommend it [499, 500]. Surgical intervention is undertaken only rarely but may be appropriate for a few, carefully selected patients [501].

7.13 Dysphagia

Swallowing problems are common in patients with MS and should be specifically asked about, as they may not always be reported by the patient [502]. Although frequently associated with brainstem and cerebellar dysfunction, there are a variety of reasons why this symptom should develop, and careful assessment should be made to establish the nature of the problem, which typically involves the oral and pharyngeal phases of swallow. This generally necessitates the involvement of a speech therapist. In addition to careful clinical assessment, video fluoroscopy will often be required [503] and electrophysiological studies may have a role in some patients [504]. Mild dysphagia may be managed simply by providing the patient and their carers with appropriate advice regarding attention to swallow, posture and food consistency. With increasing severity, exercises to employ breath-holding, diaphragmatic breathing and voluntary cough can be useful. Intermittent exacerbations may require temporary use of a nasogastric tube, although more persistent requirement for enteral feeding is best met by placement of a percutaneous gastrostomy (PEG). It should be noted, however, that siting a PEG to supply adequate caloric intake does not obviate the need to continue oral care, and on-going speech and language therapy may still be required to try to preserve residual function [503]. Pharmacological therapies are not routinely available to treat dysphagia in MS. However, interest is increasing in the development of botulinum toxin A injection of cricopharyngeus to treat over-activity of the upper oesophageal sphincter (either as a treatment in its own right or to identify those who might benefit from surgical myotomy [505]) and in the use of vagal nerve stimulation [506].

7.14 Speech and Communication

Communication may be impaired in patients with MS, due to problems with speech production and articulation, as well as higher level cognitive impairment [507]. The proportion of patients affected has been reported to vary between 23–51% [508–511], and the classical speech pattern is dysarthric (mixed spastic and ataxic), hypernasal speech. The evidence basis for intervention is weak, and guidelines which encourage the early involvement of speech and language therapists have generally been established on the basis of consensus agreement between experts [163, 164]. No pharmacological interventions are available, but technological advances continue to increase the range of options available regarding communication aids [512].

Paroxysmal dysarthria resulting from brainstem dysfunction infrequently manifests as sudden onset, transient impairment of speech initiation and control, which can occur very frequently throughout the day [513, 514]. As with other paroxysmal symptoms, treatment with carbamazepine [513] or lamotrigine [515] may be helpful. Success with levetiracetam has also been reported [516]. Acetazolamide can be considered as an alternative, although it is frequently poorly tolerated [517].

7.15 Autonomic System Dysregulation

Disturbances of the autonomic nervous system may contribute greatly to urogenital and gastrointestinal symptoms as well sleep disturbances, and the symptomatic treatment of these problems has been discussed above. Orthostatic dysregulation may occur in up to 25% patients but is not an early manifestation of the disease [518]. Generally, the approach for treatment of orthostatic dysregulation in patients with MS is as per those in whom the symptoms are attributable to other conditions, and includes maintenance of an adequate fluid volume and sodium content, use of compression stockings, and medication to increase circulating fluid volume and vascular tone, such as fludrocortisone or sympathomimetics. Thermoregulation may also be impaired in patients with MS, and strategies to counter this include cooling prior to exercise (pre-cooling). Licensed medications for the treatment of heat sensitivity in MS are not available, but there are anecdotal reports of 4-aminopyridines being helpful in this context, which require further investigation [519].

7.16 Role of Palliative Care

Life expectancy may be extremely difficult to estimate even in advanced disease and, given that the terminal event is often an acute episode of sepsis, patients frequently die in hospital. However, there is increasing appreciation MS patients may have palliative care needs [520–523], which impact significantly upon both them and their care-givers. Systems to determine how these might be best met are now developing [524–526], but there is recognition that these are likely to involve increased co-ordination between neurological, neurorehabilitative and palliative care services [163, 527–529].

Some patients who retain capacity find it empowering to discuss life-prolonging measures in advance of their requirement, but if a legally binding advance directive is not in place, decisions need to be made on a 'best interest' basis [530].

7.17 Conclusions

Given that MS is a complex, multi-system disease which may cause difficult symptoms in many different systems, the approach to symptom control should be led and co-ordinated by a physician with a specialist interest in MS. Over the course of the disease, a variable degree of input is likely to be required from primary care physicians as well as specialists in a variety of medical specialities including, although not limited to, neurology, neurorehabilitation and palliative care. The role of health professionals in disciplines allied to medicine should not be underestimated and careful attention must be given to patient preference. The needs of care-givers should also be respected and facilitated. In the absence of an available cure for MS, research into improved symptom management should be supported and must include systematic, well-designed clinical trials to evaluate treatments as they emerge.

References

1. Fox RJ, et al. Setting a research agenda for progressive multiple sclerosis: the International Collaborative on Progressive MS. Mult Scler. 2012;18(11):1534–40.
2. Thompson AJ. Neurorehabilitation in multiple sclerosis: foundations, facts and fiction. Curr Opin Neurol. 2005;18(3):267–71.
3. The UN standard rules on the equalization of opportunities for persons with disabilities. Geneva: World Health Organisation; 2001, p. 290.
4. Holper L, et al. Characterization of functioning in multiple sclerosis using the ICF. J Neurol. 2010;257(1):103–13.
5. Kesselring J, et al. Developing the ICF Core Sets for multiple sclerosis to specify functioning. Mult Scler. 2008;14(2):252–4.
6. Clinical Guideline [CG186]. Multiple sclerosis in adults: management. National Institute for Health and Care Excellence; 2014.
7. Principles to promote the quality of life of people with multiple sclerosis. London: Multiple Sclerosis International Federation; 2006.
8. Platform ME, editor. Recommendations on rehabilitation services for persons with multiple sclerosis in Europe. Genova: Associazione Italiana Sclerosi Multipla; 2004.
9. Campbell E, et al. Physiotherapy rehabilitation for people with progressive multiple sclerosis: a systematic review. Arch Phys Med Rehabil. 2016;97(1):141–51. e3
10. Miller D, Rudick RA, Hutchinson M. Patient-centered outcomes: translating clinical efficacy into benefits on health-related quality of life. Neurology. 2010;74(Suppl 3):S24–35.
11. Thompson AJ, Toosy AT, Ciccarelli O. Pharmacological management of symptoms in multiple sclerosis: current approaches and future directions. Lancet Neurol. 2010;9(12):1182–99.
12. Khan F, et al. Multidisciplinary rehabilitation for adults with multiple sclerosis. Cochrane Database Syst Rev. 2007;2:Cd006036.
13. Beier M, et al. Improved physical fitness correlates with improved cognition in multiple sclerosis. Arch Phys Med Rehabil. 2014;95(7):1328–34.
14. Sampson P, et al. Using functional electrical stimulation mediated by iterative learning control and robotics to improve arm movement for people with multiple sclerosis. IEEE Trans Neural Syst Rehabil Eng. 2016;24(2):235–48.
15. Lance JW. Symposium synopsis. In: Spasticity: disordered motor control. Chigago: Year Book; 1980.
16. Pandyan AD, et al. Spasticity: clinical perceptions, neurological realities and meaningful measurement. Disabil Rehabil. 2005;27(1–2):2–6.
17. Rizzo MA, et al. Prevalence and treatment of spasticity reported by multiple sclerosis patients. Mult Scler. 2004;10(5):589–95.
18. Paisley S, et al. Clinical effectiveness of oral treatments for spasticity in multiple sclerosis: a systematic review. Mult Scler. 2002;8(4):319–29.

19. Paty DW, Ebers GC. Clinical features. In: Paty DW, Ebers GC, editors. Multiple Sclerosis. Philadelphia: F. A. Davis; 1998. p. 135–92.
20. Francis HP, et al. Does reducing spasticity translate into functional benefit? An exploratory meta-analysis. J Neurol Neurosurg Psychiatry. 2004;75(11):1547–51.
21. Stevenson VL. Oral medication. In: Stevenson VL, Jarrett L, editors. Spasticity management: a practical multidisciplinary guide. London: Informa Healthcare; 2006. p. 59–70.
22. Paty DW, Hashimoto SA, Ebers GC. Management of multiple sclerosis and interpretation of clinical trials. In: Paty DW, Ebers GC, editors. Multiple Sclerosis. Philadelphia: F. A. Davis; 1998. p. 427–519.
23. Milinis K, Young CA. Systematic review of the influence of spasticity on quality of life in adults with chronic neurological conditions. Disabil Rehabil. 2016;38(15):1431–41.
24. Rosche J, et al. The effects of therapy on spasticity utilizing a motorized exercise-cycle. Spinal Cord. 1997;35(3):176–8.
25. Kakebeeke TH, Lechner HE, Knapp PA. The effect of passive cycling movements on spasticity after spinal cord injury: preliminary results. Spinal Cord. 2005;43(8):483–8.
26. Nuyens GE, et al. Reduction of spastic hypertonia during repeated passive knee movements in stroke patients. Arch Phys Med Rehabil. 2002;83(7):930–5.
27. Schmit BD, Dewald JP, Rymer WZ. Stretch reflex adaptation in elbow flexors during repeated passive movements in unilateral brain-injured patients. Arch Phys Med Rehabil. 2000;81(3):269–78.
28. Katalinic OM, et al. Stretch for the treatment and prevention of contractures. Cochrane Database Syst Rev. 2010;9:CD007455.
29. Gao F, et al. Effects of repeated ankle stretching on calf muscle-tendon and ankle biomechanical properties in stroke survivors. Clin Biomech (Bristol, Avon). 2011;
30. Katalinic OM, Harvey LA, Herbert RD. Effectiveness of stretch for the treatment and prevention of contractures in people with neurological conditions: a systematic review. Phys Ther. 2011;91(1):11–24.
31. White LJ, et al. Resistance training improves strength and functional capacity in persons with multiple sclerosis. Mult Scler. 2004;10(6):668–74.
32. Odeen I, Knutsson E. Evaluation of the effects of muscle stretch and weight load in patients with spastic paraplegia. Scand J Rehabil Med. 1981;13(4):117–21.
33. Bohannon RW. Tilt table standing for reducing spasticity after spinal cord injury. Arch Phys Med Rehabil. 1993;74(10):1121–2.
34. Rietberg MB, et al. Exercise therapy for multiple sclerosis. Cochrane Database Syst Rev. 2005;1:CD003980.
35. Lockley LJ, Buchanan K. Physical management of spasticity. In: Stevenson VL, Jarrett L, editors. Spasticity management: a practical multidisciplinary guide. London: Informa Healthcare; 2006. p. 37–58.
36. Stevenson VL. Rehabilitation in practice: spasticity management. Clin Rehabil. 2010;24(4): 293–304.
37. Dalgas U, et al. Muscle fiber size increases following resistance training in multiple sclerosis. Mult Scler. 2010;16(11):1367–76.
38. Dalgas U, et al. Fatigue, mood and quality of life improve in MS patients after progressive resistance training. Mult Scler. 2010;16(4):480–90.
39. Golzari Z, et al. Combined exercise training reduces IFN-gamma and IL-17 levels in the plasma and the supernatant of peripheral blood mononuclear cells in women with multiple sclerosis. Int Immunopharmacol. 2010;10(11):1415–9.
40. Mori F, et al. Transcranial magnetic stimulation primes the effects of exercise therapy in multiple sclerosis. J Neurol. 2011;
41. Centonze D, et al. Repetitive transcranial magnetic stimulation of the motor cortex ameliorates spasticity in multiple sclerosis. Neurology. 2007;68(13):1045–50.
42. Mori F, et al. Effects of intermittent theta burst stimulation on spasticity in patients with multiple sclerosis. Eur J Neurol. 2010;17(2):295–300.

43. Nielsen JF, Sinkjaer T, Jakobsen J. Treatment of spasticity with repetitive magnetic stimulation; a double-blind placebo-controlled study. Mult Scler. 1996;2(5):227–32.
44. Butefisch CM, et al. Mechanisms of use-dependent plasticity in the human motor cortex. Proc Natl Acad Sci U S A. 2000;97(7):3661–5.
45. Holtmaat A, Svoboda K. Experience-dependent structural synaptic plasticity in the mammalian brain. Nat Rev Neurosci. 2009;10(9):647–58.
46. Cooke SF, Bliss TV. Plasticity in the human central nervous system. Brain. 2006;129(Pt 7):1659–73.
47. Ratchford JN, et al. A pilot study of functional electrical stimulation cycling in progressive multiple sclerosis. NeuroRehabilitation. 2010;27(2):121–8.
48. Barrett CL, et al. A randomized trial to investigate the effects of functional electrical stimulation and therapeutic exercise on walking performance for people with multiple sclerosis. Mult Scler. 2009;15(4):493–504.
49. Everaert DG, et al. Does functional electrical stimulation for foot drop strengthen corticospinal connections? Neurorehabil Neural Repair. 2010;24(2):168–77.
50. Shakespeare DT, Boggild M, Young C. Anti-spasticity agents for multiple sclerosis. Cochrane Database Syst Rev. 2003;4:CD001332.
51. Hobart JC, et al. Rating scales as outcome measures for clinical trials in neurology: problems, solutions, and recommendations. Lancet Neurol. 2007;6(12):1094–105.
52. Otero-Romero S, et al. Pharmacological management of spasticity in multiple sclerosis: systematic review and consensus paper. Mult Scler J. 2016;22(11):1386–96.
53. Summary of Product Characteristics: Baclofen Tablets BP 10 mg, https://www.medicines.org.uk/emc/medicine/23850.
54. Hattab JR. Review of European clinical trials with baclofen. In: Feldman RG, Young RR, Koella WP, editors. Spasticity: disordered motor control. Chicago: Year Book; 1980. p. 71–85.
55. A double-blind, placebo-controlled trial of tizanidine in the treatment of spasticity caused by multiple sclerosis. United Kingdom Tizanidine Trial Group. Neurology. 1994;44(11 Suppl 9):S70–8.
56. Nance PW, et al. Efficacy and safety of tizanidine in the treatment of spasticity in patients with spinal cord injury. North American Tizanidine Study Group. Neurology. 1994;44(11 Suppl 9):S44–51; discussion S51–2.
57. Smith C, et al. Tizanidine treatment of spasticity caused by multiple sclerosis: results of a double-blind, placebo-controlled trial. US Tizanidine Study Group. Neurology. 1994;44(11 Suppl 9):S34–42; discussion S42–3.
58. Groves L, Shellenberger MK, Davis CS. Tizanidine treatment of spasticity: a meta-analysis of controlled, double-blind, comparative studies with baclofen and diazepam. Adv Ther. 1998;15(4):241–51.
59. Summary of Product Characteristics: Tizanidine 2mg Tablets. https://www.medicines.org.uk/emc/medicine/24095.
60. Wagstaff AJ, Bryson HM. Tizanidine. A review of its pharmacology, clinical efficacy and tolerability in the management of spasticity associated with cerebral and spinal disorders. Drugs. 1997;53(3):435–52.
61. Krause T, et al. Dantrolene--a review of its pharmacology, therapeutic use and new developments. Anaesthesia. 2004;59(4):364–73.
62. Summary of Product Characteristics: Dantrium 25 mg Capsules. https://www.medicines.org.uk/emc/medicine/1610.
63. Beard S, Hunn A, Wight J. Treatments for spasticity and pain in multiple sclerosis: a systematic review. Health Technol Assess. 2003;7(40):1–111; p. iii, ix–x.
64. Mueller ME, et al. Gabapentin for relief of upper motor neuron symptoms in multiple sclerosis. Arch Phys Med Rehabil. 1997;78(5):521–4.
65. Cutter NC, et al. Gabapentin effect on spasticity in multiple sclerosis: a placebo-controlled, randomized trial. Arch Phys Med Rehabil. 2000;81(2):164–9.
66. Formica, A., et al., Gabapentin for spasticity: a randomized, double-blind, placebo-controlled trial. Med Clin (Barc), 2005. 124(3): p. 81–5.

67. Summary of Product Characteristics: Gabapentin 100mg Capsules. https://www.medicines.org.uk/emc/medicine/24645.
68. Fink K, et al. Inhibition of neuronal Ca(2+) influx by gabapentin and pregabalin in the human neocortex. Neuropharmacology. 2002;42(2):229–36.
69. Bradley LJ, Kirker SG. Pregabalin in the treatment of spasticity: a retrospective case series. Disabil Rehabil. 2008;30(16):1230–2.
70. Rigo JM, et al. The anti-epileptic drug levetiracetam reverses the inhibition by negative allosteric modulators of neuronal GABA- and glycine-gated currents. Br J Pharmacol. 2002;136(5):659–72.
71. Bedlack RS, et al. Open-label pilot trial of levetiracetam for cramps and spasticity in patients with motor neuron disease. Amyotroph Lateral Scler. 2009;10(4):210–5.
72. Ruegg SJ, Steck AJ, Fuhr P. Levetiracetam improves paroxysmal symptoms in a patient with stiff-person syndrome. Neurology. 2004;62(2):338.
73. Lashch N, Avakian GN. The use of midokalm in patients with multiple sclerosis. Zh Nevrol Psikhiatr Im S S Korsakova. 2000;100(6):24–8.
74. Stamenova P, et al. A randomized, double-blind, placebo-controlled study of the efficacy and safety of tolperisone in spasticity following cerebral stroke. Eur J Neurol. 2005;12(6):453–61.
75. Bresolin N, Zucca C, Pecori A. Efficacy and tolerability of eperisone in patients with spastic palsy: a cross-over, placebo-controlled dose-ranging trial. Eur Rev Med Pharmacol Sci. 2009;13(5):365–70.
76. Bresolin N, Zucca C, Pecori A. Efficacy and tolerability of eperisone and baclofen in spastic palsy: a double-blind randomized trial. Adv Ther. 2009;26(5):563–73.
77. Adams IB, Martin BR. Cannabis: pharmacology and toxicology in animals and humans. Addiction. 1996;91(11):1585–614.
78. Feinstein A, Freeman J, Lo AC. Treatment of progressive multiple sclerosis: what works, what does not, and what is needed. Lancet Neurol. 2015;14(2):194–207.
79. Gaoni Y, Mechoulam R. Isolation, structure and partial synthesis of an active constituent of hashish. J Am Chem Soc. 1964;86:1646–7.
80. Tsou K, et al. Immunohistochemical distribution of cannabinoid CB1 receptors in the rat central nervous system. Neuroscience. 1998;83(2):393–411.
81. Herkenham M, et al. Cannabinoid receptor localization in brain. Proc Natl Acad Sci U S A. 1990;87(5):1932–6.
82. Freund TF, Katona I, Piomelli D. Role of endogenous cannabinoids in synaptic signaling. Physiol Rev. 2003;83(3):1017–66.
83. Van Sickle MD, et al. Identification and functional characterization of brainstem cannabinoid CB2 receptors. Science. 2005;310(5746):329–32.
84. Skaper SD, et al. The ALIAmide palmitoylethanolamide and cannabinoids, but not anandamide, are protective in a delayed postglutamate paradigm of excitotoxic death in cerebellar granule neurons. Proc Natl Acad Sci U S A. 1996;93(9):3984–9.
85. Alger BE. Retrograde signaling in the regulation of synaptic transmission: focus on endocannabinoids. Prog Neurobiol. 2002;68(4):247–86.
86. Kreitzer AC, Regehr WG. Retrograde signaling by endocannabinoids. Curr Opin Neurobiol. 2002;12(3):324–30.
87. Berrendero F, et al. Changes in cannabinoid CB(1) receptors in striatal and cortical regions of rats with experimental allergic encephalomyelitis, an animal model of multiple sclerosis. Synapse. 2001;41(3):195–202.
88. Baker D, et al. Cannabinoids control spasticity and tremor in a multiple sclerosis model. Nature. 2000;404(6773):84–7.
89. Baker D, et al. Endocannabinoids control spasticity in a multiple sclerosis model. FASEB J. 2001;15(2):300–2.
90. Baker D, Pryce G. The endocannabinoid system and multiple sclerosis. Curr Pharm Des. 2008;14(23):2326–36.
91. Chong MS, et al. Cannabis use in patients with multiple sclerosis. Mult Scler. 2006;12(5):646–51.
92. Clark AJ, et al. Patterns of cannabis use among patients with multiple sclerosis. Neurology. 2004;62(11):2098–100.

93. Campbell FA, et al. Are cannabinoids an effective and safe treatment option in the management of pain? A qualitative systematic review. BMJ. 2001;323(7303):13–6.
94. Zajicek JP, et al. Cannabinoids in multiple sclerosis (CAMS) study: safety and efficacy data for 12 months follow up. J Neurol Neurosurg Psychiatry. 2005;76(12):1664–9.
95. Malfitano AM, Proto MC, Bifulco M. Cannabinoids in the management of spasticity associated with multiple sclerosis. Neuropsychiatr Dis Treat. 2008;4(5):847–53.
96. Lakhan SE, Rowland M. Whole plant cannabis extracts in the treatment of spasticity in multiple sclerosis: a systematic review. BMC Neurol. 2009;9:59.
97. Smith PF. New approaches in the management of spasticity in multiple sclerosis patients: role of cannabinoids. Ther Clin Risk Manag. 2010;6:59–63.
98. Wade DT, et al. Meta-analysis of the efficacy and safety of Sativex (nabiximols), on spasticity in people with multiple sclerosis. Mult Scler. 2010;16(6):707–14.
99. Hobart JC, et al. Getting the measure of spasticity in multiple sclerosis: the Multiple Sclerosis Spasticity Scale (MSSS-88). Brain. 2006;129(Pt 1):224–34.
100. Zajicek JP, Apostu VI. Role of cannabinoids in multiple sclerosis. CNS Drugs. 2011;25(3):187–201.
101. Honarmand K, et al. Effects of cannabis on cognitive function in patients with multiple sclerosis. Neurology. 2011;76(13):1153–60.
102. Syed YY, McKeage K, Scott LJ. Delta-9-Tetrahydrocannabinol/cannabidiol (Sativex®): a review of its use in patients with moderate to severe spasticity due to multiple sclerosis. Drugs. 2014;74(5):563–78.
103. Wade DT, et al. Do cannabis-based medicinal extracts have general or specific effects on symptoms in multiple sclerosis? A double-blind, randomized, placebo-controlled study on 160 patients. Mult Scler. 2004;10(4):434–41.
104. Collin C, et al. Randomized controlled trial of cannabis-based medicine in spasticity caused by multiple sclerosis. Eur J Neurol. 2007;14(3):290–6.
105. Collin C, et al. A double-blind, randomized, placebo-controlled, parallel-group study of Sativex, in subjects with symptoms of spasticity due to multiple sclerosis. Neurol Res. 2010;32(5):451–9.
106. Novotna A, et al. A randomized, double-blind, placebo-controlled, parallel-group, enriched-design study of nabiximols* (Sativex((R))), as add-on therapy, in subjects with refractory spasticity caused by multiple sclerosis. Eur J Neurol. 2011;18(9):1122–31.
107. Oreja-Guevara C, et al. Observational safety study of THC: CBD oromucosal spray (Sativex) in multiple sclerosis patients with spasticity. Clin Exp Pharmacol. 2015;5(184):2161–1459.1000184.
108. Fernandez O. THC: CBD in daily practice: available data from UK, Germany and Spain. Eur Neurol. 2016;75(Suppl 1):1–3.
109. Patti F, et al. Efficacy and safety of cannabinoid oromucosal spray for multiple sclerosis spasticity. J Neurol Neurosurg Psychiatry. 2016;87(9):944–51.
110. Lu L, et al. Cost effectiveness of oromucosal cannabis-based medicine (Sativex(R)) for spasticity in multiple sclerosis. PharmacoEconomics. 2012;30(12):1157–71.
111. Slof J, Gras A. Sativex(R) in multiple sclerosis spasticity: a cost-effectiveness model. Expert Rev Pharmacoecon Outcomes Res. 2012;12(4):439–41.
112. Ball S, et al. The Cannabinoid Use in Progressive Inflammatory brain Disease (CUPID) trial: a randomised double-blind placebo-controlled parallel-group multicentre trial and economic evaluation of cannabinoids to slow progression in multiple sclerosis. Health Technol Assess. 2015;19(12):1–187; p. vii–viii, xxv–xxxi.
113. Crabtree BL. Review of naltrexone, a long-acting opiate antagonist. Clin Pharm. 1984;3(3):273–80.
114. Gironi M, et al. A pilot trial of low-dose naltrexone in primary progressive multiple sclerosis. Mult Scler J. 2008;14(8):1076–83.
115. Viganò D, Rubino T, Parolaro D. Molecular and cellular basis of cannabinoid and opioid interactions. Pharmacol Biochem Behav. 2005;81(2):360–8.
116. Dolly JO, Aoki KR. The structure and mode of action of different botulinum toxins. Eur J Neurol. 2006;13(Suppl 4):1–9.

117. Ward AB. Spasticity treatment with botulinum toxins. J Neural Transm. 2008;115(4):607–16.
118. Kabus C, et al. Botulinum toxin in patients with multiple sclerosis. J Neurol. 2006;253(Suppl 1):I26–8.
119. Habek M, et al. The place of the botulinum toxin in the management of multiple sclerosis. Clin Neurol Neurosurg. 2010;112(7):592–6.
120. Giovannelli M, et al. Early physiotherapy after injection of botulinum toxin increases the beneficial effects on spasticity in patients with multiple sclerosis. Clin Rehabil. 2007;21(4):331–7.
121. Borg J, et al. Rationale and design of a multicentre, double-blind, prospective, randomized, European and Canadian study: evaluating patient outcomes and costs of managing adults with post-stroke focal spasticity. J Rehabil Med. 2011;43(1):15–22.
122. Burbaud P, et al. Botulinum toxin treatment in neurological practice: how much does it really cost? A prospective cost-effectiveness study. J Neurol. 2011.
123. Elovic EP, et al. Chemodenervation and nerve blocks in the diagnosis and management of spasticity and muscle overactivity. PM R. 2009;1(9):842–51.
124. Yelnik AP, et al. How to clinically assess and treat muscle overactivity in spastic paresis. J Rehabil Med. 2010;42(9):801–7.
125. Penn RD, et al. Intrathecal baclofen for severe spinal spasticity. N Engl J Med. 1989; 320(23):1517–21.
126. Bensmail D, et al. Effect of intrathecal baclofen on sleep and respiratory function in patients with spasticity. Neurology. 2006;67(8):1432–6.
127. Boviatsis EJ, et al. Functional outcome of intrathecal baclofen administration for severe spasticity. Clin Neurol Neurosurg. 2005;107(4):289–95.
128. Zahavi A, et al. Long term effect (more than five years) of intrathecal baclofen on impairment, disability, and quality of life in patients with severe spasticity of spinal origin. J Neurol Neurosurg Psychiatry. 2004;75(11):1553–7.
129. Rekand T, Gronning M. Treatment of spasticity related to multiple sclerosis with intrathecal baclofen: a long-term follow-up. J Rehabil Med. 2011;43(6):511–4.
130. Schuele SU, et al. Incidence of seizures in patients with multiple sclerosis treated with intrathecal baclofen. Neurology. 2005;64(6):1086–7.
131. Cooper JA, Ridley B. Response of intrathecal baclofen resistance to dose reduction. Neurology. 2006;67(8):1495–6.
132. Kelly RE, Gautier Smith PC. Intrathecal phenol in the treatment of reflex spasms and spasticity. Lancet. 1959;274(7112):1102–5.
133. Maher RM. Relief of pain in incurable cancer. Lancet. 1955;265(6853):18–20.
134. Jarrett L, Nandi P, Thompson AJ. Managing severe lower limb spasticity in multiple sclerosis: does intrathecal phenol have a role? J Neurol Neurosurg Psychiatry. 2002;73(6):705–9.
135. Boop FA. Evolution of the neurosurgical management of spasticity. J Child Neurol. 2001;16(1):54–7.
136. Foerster O. On the indications and results of the excision of posterior spinal nerve roots in men. Surg Gynecol Obstet. 1913;16:463–74.
137. Sherrington C. The integrative action of the central nervous system. London: Archibald Constable; 1906.
138. Gros C, et al. La radicotomie selective posterieure dans le traitement neurochirurgical de l'hypertonie pyramidale. Neurochirurgie. 1967;13:505–18.
139. Salame K, et al. Surgical treatment of spasticity by selective posterior rhizotomy: 30 years experience. Isr Med Assoc J. 2003;5(8):543–6.
140. Maarrawi J, et al. Long-term functional results of selective peripheral neurotomy for the treatment of spastic upper limb: prospective study in 31 patients. J Neurosurg. 2006;104(2):215–25.
141. Sindou M, Mertens P. Selective neurotomy of the tibial nerve for treatment of the spastic foot. Neurosurgery. 1988;23(6):738–44.
142. O'Connor AB, et al. Pain associated with multiple sclerosis: systematic review and proposed classification. Pain. 2008;137(1):96–111.
143. Hirsh AT, et al. Prevalence and impact of pain in multiple sclerosis: physical and psychologic contributors. Arch Phys Med Rehabil. 2009;90(4):646–51.

144. Brichetto G, et al. Symptomatic medication use in multiple sclerosis. Mult Scler. 2003;9(5):458–60.
145. Moulin DE, Foley KM, Ebers GC. Pain syndromes in multiple sclerosis. Neurology. 1988; 38(12):1830–4.
146. Osterberg A, Boivie J, Thuomas KA. Central pain in multiple sclerosis--prevalence and clinical characteristics. Eur J Pain. 2005;9(5):531–42.
147. Vermote R, Ketelaer P, Carton H. Pain in multiple sclerosis patients. A prospective study using the Mc Gill Pain Questionnaire. Clin Neurol Neurosurg. 1986;88(2):87–93.
148. Boneschi FM, et al. Lifetime and actual prevalence of pain and headache in multiple sclerosis. Mult Scler. 2008;14(4):514–21.
149. Solaro C, et al. The prevalence of pain in multiple sclerosis: a multicenter cross-sectional study. Neurology. 2004;63(5):919–21.
150. Hadjimichael O, et al. Persistent pain and uncomfortable sensations in persons with multiple sclerosis. Pain. 2007;127(1–2):35–41.
151. Ehde DM, et al. Chronic pain in a large community sample of persons with multiple sclerosis. Mult Scler. 2003;9(6):605–11.
152. Brochet B, et al. Pain and quality of life in the early stages after multiple sclerosis diagnosis: a 2-year longitudinal study. Clin J Pain. 2009;25(3):211–7.
153. Svendsen KB, et al. Pain in patients with multiple sclerosis: a population-based study. Arch Neurol. 2003;60(8):1089–94.
154. Putzki N, Katsarava Z. Headache in multiple sclerosis. Curr Pain Headache Rep. 2010; 14(4):316–20.
155. Kister I, et al. Tension-type headache and migraine in multiple sclerosis. Curr Pain Headache Rep. 2010;14(6):441–8.
156. Welch KM, et al. Periaqueductal gray matter dysfunction in migraine: cause or the burden of illness? Headache. 2001;41(7):629–37.
157. Knight YE, Goadsby PJ. The periaqueductal grey matter modulates trigeminovascular input: a role in migraine? Neuroscience. 2001;106(4):793–800.
158. Pollmann W, Feneberg W. Current management of pain associated with multiple sclerosis. CNS Drugs. 2008;22(4):291–324.
159. Treede RD, et al. Neuropathic pain: redefinition and a grading system for clinical and research purposes. Neurology. 2008;70(18):1630–5.
160. Grasso MG, et al. Pain in multiple sclerosis: a clinical and instrumental approach. Mult Scler. 2008;14(4):506–13.
161. Attal N, et al. EFNS guidelines on pharmacological treatment of neuropathic pain. Eur J Neurol. 2006;13(11):1153–69.
162. Tan T, et al. Pharmacological management of neuropathic pain in non-specialist settings: summary of NICE guidance. BMJ. 2010;340:c1079.
163. Guidance for the management of MS. In: Multiple sclerosis: national clinical guideline for diagnosis and management in primary and secondary care. London, National Institute for Clinical Excellence; 2004.
164. Multiple sclerosis: management of multiple sclerosis in primary and secondary care. National Institute for Health and Care Excellence (UK). 2014.
165. (UK), C.f.C.P.a.N., Clinical Guideline [CG173]. Neuropathic pain: the pharmacological management of neuropathic pain in adults in non-specialist settings. London: National Institute for Health and Care Excellence (UK); 2013.
166. Rahn EJ, Hohmann AG. Cannabinoids as pharmacotherapies for neuropathic pain: from the bench to the bedside. Neurotherapeutics. 2009;6(4):713–37.
167. Chohan H, et al. Use of cannabinoids for spasticity and pain management in MS. Curr Treat Options Neurol. 2016;18(1):1.
168. Koppel, B.S., et al., Systematic review: efficacy and safety of medical marijuana in selected neurologic disorders: report of the Guideline Development Subcommittee of the American Academy of Neurology. Neurology, 2014. 82(17): p. 1556–1563.

169. Turcotte D, et al. Nabilone as an adjunctive to gabapentin for multiple sclerosis-induced neuropathic pain: a randomized controlled trial. Pain Med. 2015;16(1):149–59.
170. Rowbotham MC, et al. Oral opioid therapy for chronic peripheral and central neuropathic pain. N Engl J Med. 2003;348(13):1223–32.
171. Breuer B, et al. A randomized, double-blind, placebo-controlled, two-period, crossover, pilot trial of lamotrigine in patients with central pain due to multiple sclerosis. Clin Ther. 2007;29(9):2022–30.
172. Kalman S, et al. Morphine responsiveness in a group of well-defined multiple sclerosis patients: a study with i.v. morphine. Eur J Pain. 2002;6(1):69–80.
173. Chitsaz A, et al. Sensory complaints of the upper extremities in multiple sclerosis: relative efficacy of nortriptyline and transcutaneous electrical nerve stimulation. Clin J Pain. 2009;25(4):281–5.
174. Kumar K, Hunter G, Demeria D. Spinal cord stimulation in treatment of chronic benign pain: challenges in treatment planning and present status, a 22-year experience. Neurosurgery. 2006;58(3):481–96; discussion 481–96.
175. Osenbach RK. Motor cortex stimulation for intractable pain. Neurosurg Focus. 2006;21(6):E7.
176. Levy R, Deer TR, Henderson J. Intracranial neurostimulation for pain control: a review. Pain Physician. 2010;13(2):157–65.
177. Patwardhan RV, et al. Neurosurgical treatment of multiple sclerosis. Neurol Res. 2006;28(3):320–5.
178. Sadiq SA, Poopatana CA. Intrathecal baclofen and morphine in multiple sclerosis patients with severe pain and spasticity. J Neurol. 2007;254(10):1464–5.
179. Dahm PO, et al. Long-term intrathecal (i.t.) infusion of bupivacaine relieved intractable pain and spasticity in a patient with multiple sclerosis. Eur J Pain. 1998;2(1):81–5.
180. Andrade C, et al. Stretching the limbs? Tonic spasms in multiple sclerosis. BMJ Case Rep. 2012;2012
181. Spissu A, et al. Anatomic correlates of painful tonic spasms in multiple sclerosis. Mov Disord. 1999;14(2):331–5.
182. Solaro C, Tanganelli P. Tiagabine for treating painful tonic spasms in multiple sclerosis: a pilot study. J Neurol Neurosurg Psychiatry. 2004;75(2):341.
183. Hawker K, Frohman E, Racke M. Levetiracetam for phasic spasticity in multiple sclerosis. Arch Neurol. 2003;60(12):1772–4.
184. Solaro C, et al. Gabapentin is effective in treating nocturnal painful spasms in multiple sclerosis. Mult Scler. 2000;6(3):192–3.
185. Morgan JC, Hess DC, Sethi KD. Botulinum toxin treatment of painful tonic spasms in multiple sclerosis. Neurology. 2004;62(11):2143. author reply 2143.
186. Restivo DA, et al. Botulinum toxin treatment of painful tonic spasms in multiple sclerosis. Neurology. 2003;61(5):719–20.
187. Sakurai M, Kanazawa I. Positive symptoms in multiple sclerosis: their treatment with sodium channel blockers, lidocaine and mexiletine. J Neurol Sci. 1999;162(2):162–8.
188. Putzki N, et al. Prevalence of migraine, tension-type headache and trigeminal neuralgia in multiple sclerosis. Eur J Neurol. 2009;16(2):262–7.
189. Zorro O, et al. Gamma knife radiosurgery for multiple sclerosis-related trigeminal neuralgia. Neurology. 2009;73(14):1149–54.
190. Love S, Gradidge T, Coakham HB. Trigeminal neuralgia due to multiple sclerosis: ultrastructural findings in trigeminal rhizotomy specimens. Neuropathol Appl Neurobiol. 2001;27(3):238–44.
191. Love S, Coakham HB. Trigeminal neuralgia: pathology and pathogenesis. Brain. 2001;124(Pt 12):2347–60.
192. Cruccu G, et al. Trigeminal neuralgia and pain related to multiple sclerosis. Pain. 2009; 143(3):186–91.
193. Espir ML, Millac P. Treatment of paroxysmal disorders in multiple sclerosis with carbamazepine (Tegretol). J Neurol Neurosurg Psychiatry. 1970;33(4):528–31.

194. Solaro C, et al. Antiepileptic medications in multiple sclerosis: adverse effects in a three-year follow-up study. Neurol Sci. 2005;25(6):307–10.
195. Ramsaransing G, Zwanikken C, De Keyser J. Worsening of symptoms of multiple sclerosis associated with carbamazepine. BMJ. 2000;320(7242):1113.
196. Lunardi G, et al. Clinical effectiveness of lamotrigine and plasma levels in essential and symptomatic trigeminal neuralgia. Neurology. 1997;48(6):1714–7.
197. Leandri M, et al. Lamotrigine in trigeminal neuralgia secondary to multiple sclerosis. J Neurol. 2000;247(7):556–8.
198. Solaro C, et al. Low-dose gabapentin combined with either lamotrigine or carbamazepine can be useful therapies for trigeminal neuralgia in multiple sclerosis. Eur Neurol. 2000;44(1):45–8.
199. Khan OA. Gabapentin relieves trigeminal neuralgia in multiple sclerosis patients. Neurology. 1998;51(2):611–4.
200. Solaro C, et al. An open-label trial of gabapentin treatment of paroxysmal symptoms in multiple sclerosis patients. Neurology. 1998;51(2):609–11.
201. Zvartau-Hind M, et al. Topiramate relieves refractory trigeminal neuralgia in MS patients. Neurology. 2000;55(10):1587–8.
202. Solaro C, et al. Topiramate relieves idiopathic and symptomatic trigeminal neuralgia. J Pain Symptom Manag. 2001;21(5):367–8.
203. Misoprostol in the treatment of trigeminal neuralgia associated with multiple sclerosis. J Neurol. 2003;**250**(5): 542–5.
204. Reder AT, Arnason BG. Trigeminal neuralgia in multiple sclerosis relieved by a prostaglandin E analogue. Neurology. 1995;45(6):1097–100.
205. Zakrzewska JM, et al. Patient reports of satisfaction after microvascular decompression and partial sensory rhizotomy for trigeminal neuralgia. Neurosurgery. 2005;56(6):1304–11. discussion 1311–2.
206. Brisman R. Trigeminal neuralgia and multiple sclerosis. Arch Neurol. 1987;44(4):379–81.
207. Eldridge PR, et al. Microvascular decompression for trigeminal neuralgia in patients with multiple sclerosis. Stereotact Funct Neurosurg. 2003;81(1–4):57–64.
208. Athanasiou TC, et al. Some patients with multiple sclerosis have neurovascular compression causing their trigeminal neuralgia and can be treated effectively with MVD: report of five cases. Br J Neurosurg. 2005;19(6):463–8.
209. Broggi G, et al. Operative findings and outcomes of microvascular decompression for trigeminal neuralgia in 35 patients affected by multiple sclerosis. Neurosurgery. 2004;55(4):830–8. discussion 838-9
210. Broggi G, et al. Role of microvascular decompression in trigeminal neuralgia and multiple sclerosis. Lancet. 1999;354(9193):1878–9.
211. Broggi G, et al. Microvascular decompression for trigeminal neuralgia: comments on a series of 250 cases, including 10 patients with multiple sclerosis. J Neurol Neurosurg Psychiatry. 2000;68(1):59–64.
212. Sandell T, Eide PK. The effect of microvascular decompression in patients with multiple sclerosis and trigeminal neuralgia. Neurosurgery. 2010;67(3):749–53. discussion 753–4.
213. Zakrzewska JM, McMillan R. Trigeminal neuralgia: the diagnosis and management of this excruciating and poorly understood facial pain. Postgrad Med J. 2011;87(1028):410–6.
214. Harries AM, Mitchell RD. Percutaneous glycerol rhizotomy for trigeminal neuralgia: safety and efficacy of repeat procedures. Br J Neurosurg. 2011;25(2):268–72.
215. Pickett GE, Bisnaire D, Ferguson GG. Percutaneous retrogasserian Allahglycerol rhizotomy in the treatment of tic douloureux associated with multiple sclerosis. Neurosurgery. 2005;56(3):537–45. discussion 537-45.
216. Kanpolat Y, et al. Percutaneous controlled radiofrequency rhizotomy in the management of patients with trigeminal neuralgia due to multiple sclerosis. Acta Neurochir. 2000;142(6):685–9. discussion 689–90.

217. Verheul JB, et al. Gamma Knife surgery for trigeminal neuralgia: a review of 450 consecutive cases. J Neurosurg. 2010;113(Suppl):160–7.
218. Nurmikko TJ. Pathophysiology of MS-related trigeminal neuralgia. Pain. 2009;143(3):165–6.
219. Minagar A, Sheremata WA. Glossopharyngeal neuralgia and MS. Neurology. 2000;54(6): 1368–70.
220. Al-Araji AH, Oger J. Reappraisal of Lhermitte's sign in multiple sclerosis. Mult Scler. 2005;11(4):398–402.
221. Rudick R, Goodkin D. Multiple sclerosis therapeutics. London: Martin Dunitz Ltd; 1999.
222. Hemmett L, et al. What drives quality of life in multiple sclerosis? QJM. 2004;97(10):671–6.
223. Fowler CJ, Griffiths D, de Groat WC. The neural control of micturition. Nat Rev Neurosci. 2008;9(6):453–66.
224. Betts CD, D'Mellow MT, Fowler CJ. Urinary symptoms and the neurological features of bladder dysfunction in multiple sclerosis. J Neurol Neurosurg Psychiatry. 1993;56(3):245–50.
225. Fowler CJ, et al. A UK consensus on the management of the bladder in multiple sclerosis. J Neurol Neurosurg Psychiatry. 2009;80(5):470–7.
226. de Seze M, et al. The neurogenic bladder in multiple sclerosis: review of the literature and proposal of management guidelines. Mult Scler. 2007;13(7):915–28.
227. Khan F, et al. A randomised controlled trial: outcomes of bladder rehabilitation in persons with multiple sclerosis. J Neurol Neurosurg Psychiatry. 2010;81(9):1033–8.
228. O'Riordan JI, et al. Do alpha-blockers have a role in lower urinary tract dysfunction in multiple sclerosis? J Urol. 1995;153(4):1114–6.
229. Prasad RS, Smith SJ, Wright H. Lower abdominal pressure versus external bladder stimulation to aid bladder emptying in multiple sclerosis: a randomized controlled study. Clin Rehabil. 2003;17(1):42–7.
230. McConnell JD, et al. The long-term effect of doxazosin, finasteride, and combination therapy on the clinical progression of benign prostatic hyperplasia. N Engl J Med. 2003;349(25):2387–98.
231. Infection control. Prevention of healthcare-associated infection in primary andcommunity care. London: National Institute for Health and Clinical Excellence, 2003.
232. Lekka E, Lee LK. Successful treatment with intradetrusor Botulinum-A toxin for urethral urinary leakage (catheter bypassing) in patients with end-staged multiple sclerosis and indwelling suprapubic catheters. Eur Urol. 2006;50(4):806–9. discussion 809–10.
233. Madhuvrata P, et al. Which anticholinergic drug for overactive bladder symptoms in adults. Cochrane Database Syst Rev. 2012;1:CD005429.
234. Ethans KD, et al. Efficacy and safety of tolterodine in people with neurogenic detrusor overactivity. J Spinal Cord Med. 2004;27(3):214–8.
235. Gajewski JB, Awad SA. Oxybutynin versus propantheline in patients with multiple sclerosis and detrusor hyperreflexia. J Urol. 1986;135(5):966–8.
236. van Rey F, Heesakkers J. Solifenacin in multiple sclerosis patients with overactive bladder: a prospective study. Ther Adv Urol. 2011;2011:834753.
237. Amend B, et al. Effective treatment of neurogenic detrusor dysfunction by combined high-dosed antimuscarinics without increased side-effects. Eur Urol. 2008;53(5):1021–8.
238. Pagoria D, O'Connor RC, Guralnick ML. Antimuscarinic drugs: review of the cognitive impact when used to treat overactive bladder in elderly patients. Curr Urol Rep. 2011;12(5):351–7.
239. Kay GG, Ebinger U. Preserving cognitive function for patients with overactive bladder: evidence for a differential effect with darifenacin. Int J Clin Pract. 2008;62(11):1792–800.
240. Weese DL, et al. Intravesical oxybutynin chloride: experience with 42 patients. Urology. 1993;41(6):527–30.
241. Fader M, et al. Intravesical atropine compared to oral oxybutynin for neurogenic detrusor overactivity: a double-blind, randomized crossover trial. J Urol. 2007;177(1):208–13. discussion 213.

242. Jiang YH, Liao CH, Kuo HC. Current and potential urological applications of botulinum toxin A. Nat Rev Urol. 2015;12(9):519–33.
243. Lay AH, Das AK. The role of neuromodulation in patients with neurogenic overactive bladder. Curr Urol Rep. 2012;13(5):343–7.
244. Herschorn S, et al. Efficacy of botulinum toxin a injection for neurogenic detrusor overactivity and urinary incontinence: a randomized, double-blind trial. J Urol. 2011;185(6):2229–35.
245. Khan S, et al. Long-term effect on quality of life of repeat detrusor injections of botulinum neurotoxin-A for detrusor overactivity in patients with multiple sclerosis. J Urol. 2011;185(4):1344–9.
246. Chancellor MB, et al. OnabotulinumtoxinA improves quality of life in patients with neurogenic detrusor overactivity. Neurology. 2013;81(9):841–8.
247. Bosma R, et al. Efficacy of desmopressin in patients with multiple sclerosis suffering from bladder dysfunction: a meta-analysis. Acta Neurol Scand. 2005;112(1):1–5.
248. British National Formulary 61. London: BMJ Group and Pharma Press, 2011.
249. Reynard JM, et al. A novel therapy for nocturnal polyuria: a double-blind randomized trial of frusemide against placebo. Br J Urol. 1998;81(2):215–8.
250. Freeman RM, et al. The effect of cannabis on urge incontinence in patients with multiple sclerosis: a multicentre, randomised placebo-controlled trial (CAMS-LUTS). Int Urogynecol J Pelvic Floor Dysfunct. 2006;17(6):636–41.
251. Brady CM, et al. An open-label pilot study of cannabis-based extracts for bladder dysfunction in advanced multiple sclerosis. Mult Scler. 2004;10(4):425–33.
252. Kavia RB, et al. Randomized controlled trial of Sativex to treat detrusor overactivity in multiple sclerosis. Mult Scler. 2010;16(11):1349–59.
253. Ruggieri MR Sr. Cannabinoids: potential targets for bladder dysfunction. Handb Exp Pharmacol. 2011;202:425–51.
254. Wiart L, et al. The effects of capsaicin on the neurogenic hyperreflexic detrusor. A double blind placebo controlled study in patients with spinal cord disease. Preliminary results. Spinal Cord. 1998;36(2):95–9.
255. Kim JH, et al. Intravesical resiniferatoxin for refractory detrusor hyperreflexia: a multicenter, blinded, randomized, placebo-controlled trial. J Spinal Cord Med. 2003;26(4):358–63.
256. Marinkovic SP, Gillen LM. Sacral neuromodulation for multiple sclerosis patients with urinary retention and clean intermittent catheterization. Int Urogynecol J Pelvic Floor Dysfunct. 2010;21(2):223–8.
257. Tjon Eng Soe SH, et al. Multiple sclerosis patients with bladder dysfunction have decreased symptoms after electro-acupuncture. Mult Scler. 2009;15(11):1376–7.
258. Kabay S, et al. The clinical and urodynamic results of a 3-month percutaneous posterior tibial nerve stimulation treatment in patients with multiple sclerosis-related neurogenic bladder dysfunction. Neurourol Urodyn. 2009;28(8):964–8.
259. Fjorback MV, et al. Event driven electrical stimulation of the dorsal penile/clitoral nerve for management of neurogenic detrusor overactivity in multiple sclerosis. Neurourol Urodyn. 2006;25(4):349–55.
260. Delong J, Tighiouart H, Stoffel J. Urinary diversion/reconstruction for cases of catheter intolerant secondary progressive multiple sclerosis with refractory urinary symptoms. J Urol. 2011;185(6):2201–6.
261. Betts CD, et al. Erectile dysfunction in multiple sclerosis. Associated neurological and neurophysiological deficits, and treatment of the condition. Brain. 1994;117(Pt 6):1303–10.
262. Zorzon M, et al. Sexual dysfunction in multiple sclerosis: a case-control study. I. Frequency and comparison of groups. Mult Scler. 1999;5(6):418–27.
263. Lilius HG, Valtonen EJ, Wikstrom J. Sexual problems in patients suffering from multiple sclerosis. J Chronic Dis. 1976;29(10):643–7.
264. O'Sullivan SS, Hardiman O. Detection rates of sexual dysfunction amongst patients with multiple sclerosis in an outpatient setting--can this be improved? Ir Med J. 2006;99(10):304–6.

265. Zivadinov R, et al. Sexual dysfunction in multiple sclerosis: II. Correlation analysis. Mult Scler. 1999;5(6):428–31.
266. Rees PM, Fowler CJ, Maas CP. Sexual function in men and women with neurological disorders. Lancet. 2007;369(9560):512–25.
267. Darija K-T, et al. Sexual dysfunction in multiple sclerosis: a 6-year follow-up study. J Neurol Sci. 2015;358(1–2):317–23.
268. Giannantoni A, et al. OnabotulinumtoxinA intradetrusorial injections improve sexual function in female patients affected by multiple sclerosis: preliminary results. World J Urol. 2015;33(12):2095–101.
269. Fletcher SG, et al. Sexual dysfunction in patients with multiple sclerosis: a multidisciplinary approach to evaluation and management. Nat Clin Pract Urol. 2009;6(2):96–107.
270. Safarinejad MR. Evaluation of the safety and efficacy of sildenafil citrate for erectile dysfunction in men with multiple sclerosis: a double-blind, placebo controlled, randomized study. J Urol. 2009;181(1):252–8.
271. Fowler CJ, et al. A double blind, randomised study of sildenafil citrate for erectile dysfunction in men with multiple sclerosis. J Neurol Neurosurg Psychiatry. 2005;76(5):700–5.
272. Xiao Y, Wang J, Luo H. Sildenafil citrate for erectile dysfunction in patients with multiple sclerosis. Cochrane Database Syst Rev. 2012;4:CD009427.
273. Pifarre P, et al. Sildenafil (Viagra) ameliorates clinical symptoms and neuropathology in a mouse model of multiple sclerosis. Acta Neuropathol. 2011;121(4):499–508.
274. Pifarre P, et al. Phosphodiesterase 5 inhibition at disease onset prevents experimental autoimmune encephalomyelitis progression through immunoregulatory and neuroprotective actions. Exp Neurol. 2014;251:58–71.
275. Nunes AK, et al. Sildenafil (Viagra(R)) down regulates cytokines and prevents demyelination in a cuprizone-induced MS mouse model. Cytokine. 2012;60(2):540–51.
276. Nunes AK, et al. Phosphodiesterase-5 inhibition promotes remyelination by MCP-1/CCR-2 and MMP-9 regulation in a cuprizone-induced demyelination model. Exp Neurol. 2016;275(Pt 1):143–53.
277. Lombardi G, Macchiarella A, Del Popolo G. Efficacy and safety of tadalafil for erectile dysfunction in patients with multiple sclerosis. J Sex Med. 2010;7(6):2192–200.
278. DasGupta R, Fowler CJ. Bladder, bowel and sexual dysfunction in multiple sclerosis: management strategies. Drugs. 2003;63(2):153–66.
279. Safarinejad MR. Midodrine for the treatment of organic anejaculation but not spinal cord injury: a prospective randomized placebo-controlled double-blind clinical study. Int J Impot Res. 2009;21(4):213–20.
280. Dasgupta R, et al. Efficacy of sildenafil in the treatment of female sexual dysfunction due to multiple sclerosis. J Urol. 2004;171(3):1189–93. discussion 1193.
281. Chia YW, et al. Prevalence of bowel dysfunction in patients with multiple sclerosis and bladder dysfunction. J Neurol. 1995;242(2):105–8.
282. Hinds JP, Eidelman BH, Wald A. Prevalence of bowel dysfunction in multiple sclerosis. A population survey. Gastroenterology. 1990;98(6):1538–42.
283. Sullivan SN, Ebers GC. Gastrointestinal dysfunction in multiple sclerosis. Gastroenterology. 1983;84(6):1640.
284. Hennessey A, et al. Urinary, faecal and sexual dysfunction in patients with multiple sclerosis. J Neurol. 1999;246(11):1027–32.
285. Nortvedt MW, et al. Prevalence of bladder, bowel and sexual problems among multiple sclerosis patients two to five years after diagnosis. Mult Scler. 2007;13(1):106–12.
286. Wiesel PH, et al. Pathophysiology and management of bowel dysfunction in multiple sclerosis. Eur J Gastroenterol Hepatol. 2001;13(4):441–8.
287. Emmanuel A. Managing neurogenic bowel dysfunction. Clin Rehabil. 2010;24(6):483–8.
288. Muller-Lissner SA. Effect of wheat bran on weight of stool and gastrointestinal transit time: a meta analysis. Br Med J (Clin Res Ed). 1988;296(6622):615–7.

289. Wiesel PH, et al. Gut focused behavioural treatment (biofeedback) for constipation and faecal incontinence in multiple sclerosis. J Neurol Neurosurg Psychiatry. 2000;69(2):240–3.
290. McClurg D, et al. Abdominal massage for the alleviation of constipation symptoms in people with multiple sclerosis: a randomized controlled feasibility study. Mult Scler. 2011;17(2):223–33.
291. House JG, Stiens SA. Pharmacologically initiated defecation for persons with spinal cord injury: effectiveness of three agents. Arch Phys Med Rehabil. 1997;78(10):1062–5.
292. Gill KP, et al. Defecography in multiple sclerosis patients with severe constipation. Radiology. 1994;191(2):553–6.
293. Emmanuel A. Review of the efficacy and safety of transanal irrigation for neurogenic bowel dysfunction. Spinal Cord. 2010;48(9):664–73.
294. Preziosi G, Emmanuel A. Neurogenic bowel dysfunction: pathophysiology, clinical manifestations and treatment. Expert Rev Gastroenterol Hepatol. 2009;3(4):417–23.
295. Randell N, et al. Does a colostomy alter quality of life in patients with spinal cord injury? A controlled study. Spinal Cord. 2001;39(5):279–82.
296. Swingler RJ, Compston DA. The morbidity of multiple sclerosis. Q J Med. 1992;83(300):325–37.
297. Alusi SH, et al. A study of tremor in multiple sclerosis. Brain. 2001;124(Pt 4):720–30.
298. Pittock SJ, et al. Prevalence of tremor in multiple sclerosis and associated disability in the Olmsted County population. Mov Disord. 2004;19(12):1482–5.
299. Koch M, et al. Tremor in multiple sclerosis. J Neurol. 2007;254(2):133–45.
300. Deuschl G, et al. The pathophysiology of tremor. Muscle Nerve. 2001;24(6):716–35.
301. Quintern J, et al. Influence of visual and proprioceptive afferences on upper limb ataxia in patients with multiple sclerosis. J Neurol Sci. 1999;163(1):61–9.
302. Feys P, et al. Effects of peripheral cooling on intention tremor in multiple sclerosis. J Neurol Neurosurg Psychiatry. 2005;76(3):373–9.
303. Sandyk R, Dann LC. Weak electromagnetic fields attenuate tremor in multiple sclerosis. Int J Neurosci. 1994;79(3–4):199–212.
304. Dahlin-Webb SR. A weighted wrist cuff. Am J Occup Ther. 1986;40(5):363–4.
305. Aisen ML, et al. The effect of mechanical damping loads on disabling action tremor. Neurology. 1993;43(7):1346–50.
306. Armutlu K, Karabudak R, Nurlu G. Physiotherapy approaches in the treatment of ataxic multiple sclerosis: a pilot study. Neurorehabil Neural Repair. 2001;15(3):203–11.
307. Kalron A, et al. Pilates exercise training vs. physical therapy for improving walking and balance in people with multiple sclerosis: a randomized controlled trial. Clin Rehabil. 2016;
308. Feys P, et al. Assistive technology to improve PC interaction for people with intention tremor. J Rehabil Res Dev. 2001;38(2):235–43.
309. Vergaro E, et al. Adaptive robot training for the treatment of incoordination in Multiple Sclerosis. J Neuroeng Rehabil. 2010;7:37.
310. Spina E, et al. The effects of mechanical focal vibration on walking impairment in multiple sclerosis patients: a randomized, double-blinded vs placebo study. Restor Neurol Neurosci. 2016;34(5):869–76.
311. Paltamaa J, et al. Effects of physiotherapy interventions on balance in multiple sclerosis: a systematic review and meta-analysis of randomized controlled trials. J Rehabil Med. 2012;44(10):811–23.
312. Mills RJ, Yap L, Young CA. Treatment for ataxia in multiple sclerosis. Cochrane Database Syst Rev. 2007;1:CD005029.
313. Henkin Y, Herishanu YO. Primidone as a treatment for cerebellar tremor in multiple sclerosis--two case reports. Isr J Med Sci. 1989;25(12):720–1.
314. Aisen ML, et al. Glutethimide treatment of disabling action tremor in patients with multiple sclerosis and traumatic brain injury. Arch Neurol. 1991;48(5):513–5.
315. Weiss N, et al. Attenuation of cerebellar tremor with implantation of an intrathecal baclofen pump: the role of gamma-aminobutyric acidergic pathways. Case report. J Neurosurg. 2003;99(4):768–71.

316. Schroeder A, et al. Successful treatment of cerebellar ataxia and tremor in multiple sclerosis with topiramate: a case report. Clin Neuropharmacol. 2010;33(6):317–8.
317. Sabra AF, et al. Treatment of action tremor in multiple sclerosis with isoniazid. Neurology. 1982;32(8):912–3.
318. Duquette P, Pleines J, du Souich P. Isoniazid for tremor in multiple sclerosis: a controlled trial. Neurology. 1985;35(12):1772–5.
319. Morrow J, et al. Isoniazid and action tremor in multiple sclerosis. J Neurol Neurosurg Psychiatry. 1985;48(3):282–3.
320. Francis DA, Grundy D, Heron JR. The response to isoniazid of action tremor in multiple sclerosis and its assessment using polarised light goniometry. J Neurol Neurosurg Psychiatry. 1986;49(1):87–9.
321. Koller WC. Pharmacologic trials in the treatment of cerebellar tremor. Arch Neurol. 1984;41(3):280–1.
322. Feys P, et al. The effect of levetiracetam on tremor severity and functionality in patients with multiple sclerosis. Mult Scler. 2009;15(3):371–8.
323. Monaca-Charley C, et al. Double-blind crossover study with dolasetron mesilate, a 5-HT3 receptor antagonist in cerebellar syndrome secondary to multiple sclerosis. J Neurol. 2003;250(10):1190–4.
324. Hallett M, et al. Controlled trial of isoniazid therapy for severe postural cerebellar tremor in multiple sclerosis. Neurology. 1985;35(9):1374–7.
325. Bozek CB, et al. A controlled trial of isoniazid therapy for action tremor in multiple sclerosis. J Neurol. 1987;234(1):36–9.
326. Sechi GP, et al. Treatment of cerebellar tremors with carbamazepine: a controlled trial with long-term follow-up. Neurology. 1989;39(8):1113–5.
327. Rice GP, et al. Ondansetron, a 5-HT3 antagonist, improves cerebellar tremor. J Neurol Neurosurg Psychiatry. 1997;62(3):282–4.
328. Zajicek J, et al. Cannabinoids for treatment of spasticity and other symptoms related to multiple sclerosis (CAMS study): multicentre randomised placebo-controlled trial. Lancet. 2003;362(9395):1517–26.
329. Fox P, et al. The effect of cannabis on tremor in patients with multiple sclerosis. Neurology. 2004;62(7):1105–9.
330. Bittar RG, et al. Thalamotomy versus thalamic stimulation for multiple sclerosis tremor. J Clin Neurosci. 2005;12(6):638–42.
331. Roy HA, Aziz TZ. Deep brain stimulation and multiple sclerosis: therapeutic applications. Mult Scler Relat Disord. 2014;3(4):431–9.
332. Yap L, Kouyialis A, Varma TR. Stereotactic neurosurgery for disabling tremor in multiple sclerosis: thalamotomy or deep brain stimulation? Br J Neurosurg. 2007;21(4):349–54.
333. Johnson RD, et al. Perioperative seizures following deep brain stimulation in patients with multiple sclerosis. Br J Neurosurg. 2010;24(3):289–90.
334. Jahanshahi M, et al. Effects on cognition of stereotactic lesional surgery for the treatment of tremor in multiple sclerosis. Behav Neurol. 2008;20(1–2):1–9.
335. Timmermann L, et al. Deep brain stimulation for tremor in multiple sclerosis: consensus recommendations of the German Deep Brain Stimulation Association. Nervenarzt. 2009;80(6):673–7.
336. Heesen C, et al. Patient perception of bodily functions in multiple sclerosis: gait and visual function are the most valuable. Mult Scler. 2008;14(7):988–91.
337. Goodman AD, et al. Fampridine-SR in multiple sclerosis: a randomized, double-blind, placebo-controlled, dose-ranging study. Mult Scler. 2007;13(3):357–68.
338. Goodman AD, et al. A phase 3 trial of extended release oral dalfampridine in multiple sclerosis. Ann Neurol. 2010;68(4):494–502.
339. Goodman AD, et al. Long-term safety and efficacy of dalfampridine for walking impairment in patients with multiple sclerosis: results of open-label extensions of two Phase 3 clinical trials. Mult Scler. 2015;21(10):1322–31.
340. Allart E, et al. Sustained-released fampridine in multiple sclerosis: effects on gait parameters, arm function, fatigue, and quality of life. J Neurol. 2015;262(8):1936–45.

341. Korsen M, et al. Dalfampridine effects on cognition, fatigue, and dexterity. Brain Behav. 2017;7(1):e00559.
342. Pavsic K, et al. Short-term impact of fampridine on motor and cognitive functions, mood and quality of life among multiple sclerosis patients. Clin Neurol Neurosurg. 2015;139:35–40.
343. Figved N, et al. Caregiver burden in multiple sclerosis: the impact of neuropsychiatric symptoms. J Neurol Neurosurg Psychiatry. 2007;78(10):1097–102.
344. Patten SB, et al. Major depression in multiple sclerosis: a population-based perspective. Neurology. 2003;61(11):1524–7.
345. Chwastiak L, et al. Depressive symptoms and severity of illness in multiple sclerosis: epidemiologic study of a large community sample. Am J Psychiatry. 2002;159(11):1862–8.
346. Harel Y, Barak Y, Achiron A. Dysregulation of affect in multiple sclerosis: new phenomenological approach. Psychiatry Clin Neurosci. 2007;61(1):94–8.
347. Feinstein A. Mood disorders in multiple sclerosis and the effects on cognition. J Neurol Sci. 2006;245(1–2):63–6.
348. Demaree HA, Gaudino E, DeLuca J. The relationship between depressive symptoms and cognitive dysfunction in multiple sclerosis. Cogn Neuropsychiatry. 2003;8(3):161–71.
349. Figved N, et al. Relationship of cognitive impairment to psychiatric symptoms in multiple sclerosis. Mult Scler. 2008;14(8):1084–90.
350. McGuigan C, Hutchinson M. Unrecognised symptoms of depression in a community-based population with multiple sclerosis. J Neurol. 2006;253(2):219–23.
351. Lincoln NB, et al. Evaluation of an adjustment group for people with multiple sclerosis and low mood: a randomized controlled trial. Mult Scler. 2011;
352. Rigby SA, Thornton EW, Young CA. A randomized group intervention trial to enhance mood and self-efficacy in people with multiple sclerosis. Br J Health Psychol. 2008;13(Pt 4):619–31.
353. Dennison L, Moss-Morris R. Cognitive-behavioral therapy: what benefits can it offer people with multiple sclerosis? Expert Rev Neurother. 2010;10(9):1383–90.
354. Thomas PW, et al. Psychological interventions for multiple sclerosis. Cochrane Database Syst Rev. 2006;1:CD004431.
355. Koch MW, et al. Pharmacologic treatment of depression in multiple sclerosis. Cochrane Database Syst Rev. 2011;2:CD007295.
356. Price A, et al. Antidepressants for the treatment of depression in neurological disorders: a systematic review and meta-analysis of randomised controlled trials. J Neurol Neurosurg Psychiatry. 2011;
357. Patten SB, Svenson LW, Metz LM. Psychotic disorders in MS: population-based evidence of an association. Neurology. 2005;65(7):1123–5.
358. Surridge D. An investigation into some psychiatric aspects of multiple sclerosis. Br J Psychiatry. 1969;115(524):749–64.
359. Kosmidis MH, et al. Psychotic features associated with multiple sclerosis. Int Rev Psychiatry. 2010;22(1):55–66.
360. Sechi GP, et al. Dexamethasone-induced schizoaffective-like state in multiple sclerosis: prophylaxis and treatment with carbamazepine. Clin Neuropharmacol. 1987;10(5):453–7.
361. Minden SL, Orav J, Schildkraut JJ. Hypomanic reactions to ACTH and prednisone treatment for multiple sclerosis. Neurology. 1988;38(10):1631–4.
362. Goeb JL, et al. Acute delirium, delusion, and depression during IFN-beta-1a therapy for multiple sclerosis: a case report. Clin Neuropharmacol. 2003;26(1):5–7.
363. Manfredi G, et al. Persistent interferon-ss-1b-induced psychosis in a patient with multiple sclerosis. Psychiatry Clin Neurosci. 2010;64(5):584–6.
364. Feinstein A, du Boulay G, Ron MA. Psychotic illness in multiple sclerosis. A clinical and magnetic resonance imaging study. Br J Psychiatry. 1992;161:680–5.
365. Chong SA, Ko SM. Clozapine treatment of psychosis associated with multiple sclerosis. Can J Psychiatr. 1997;42(1):90–1.
366. Safferman AZ, et al. The use of clozapine in neurologic disorders. J Clin Psychiatry. 1994;55(Suppl B):98–101.

367. Hussain A, Belderbos S. Risperidone depot in the treatment of psychosis associated with multiple sclerosis—a case report. J Psychopharmacol. 2008;22(8):925–6.
368. Davids E, Hartwig U, Gastpar M. Antipsychotic treatment of psychosis associated with multiple sclerosis. Prog Neuro-Psychopharmacol Biol Psychiatry. 2004;28(4):743–4.
369. Schiffer RB, Wineman NM, Weitkamp LR. Association between bipolar affective disorder and multiple sclerosis. Am J Psychiatry. 1986;143(1):94–5.
370. Paparrigopoulos T, et al. The neuropsychiatry of multiple sclerosis: focus on disorders of mood, affect and behaviour. Int Rev Psychiatry. 2010;22(1):14–21.
371. Feinstein A, et al. Prevalence and neurobehavioral correlates of pathological laughing and crying in multiple sclerosis. Arch Neurol. 1997;54(9):1116–21.
372. Pioro EP, et al. Dextromethorphan plus ultra low-dose quinidine reduces pseudobulbar affect. Ann Neurol. 2010;68(5):693–702.
373. Panitch HS, et al. Randomized, controlled trial of dextromethorphan/quinidine for pseudobulbar affect in multiple sclerosis. Ann Neurol. 2006;59(5):780–7.
374. Schiffer RB, Herndon RM, Rudick RA. Treatment of pathologic laughing and weeping with amitriptyline. N Engl J Med. 1985;312(23):1480–2.
375. Iannaccone S, Ferini-Strambi L. Pharmacologic treatment of emotional lability. Clin Neuropharmacol. 1996;19(6):532–5.
376. Nahas Z, et al. Rapid response of emotional incontinence to selective serotonin reuptake inhibitors. J Neuropsychiatr Clin Neurosci. 1998;10(4):453–5.
377. Chiaravalloti ND, DeLuca J. Cognitive impairment in multiple sclerosis. Lancet Neurol. 2008;7(12):1139–51.
378. Portaccio E, et al. Neuropsychological and MRI measures predict short-term evolution in benign multiple sclerosis. Neurology. 2009;73(7):498–503.
379. Potagas C, et al. Cognitive impairment in different MS subtypes and clinically isolated syndromes. J Neurol Sci. 2008;267(1–2):100–6.
380. Amato MP, et al. Cognitive dysfunction in early-onset multiple sclerosis: a reappraisal after 10 years. Arch Neurol. 2001;58(10):1602–6.
381. Denney DR, Sworowski LA, Lynch SG. Cognitive impairment in three subtypes of multiple sclerosis. Arch Clin Neuropsychol. 2005;20(8):967–81.
382. Rao SM, et al. Cognitive dysfunction in multiple sclerosis. II. Impact on employment and social functioning. Neurology. 1991;41(5):692–6.
383. Mitolo M, et al. Cognitive rehabilitation in multiple sclerosis: a systematic review. J Neurol Sci. 2015;354(1–2):1–9.
384. Jennekens-Schinkel A, et al. Cognition in patients with multiple sclerosis after four years. J Neurol Sci. 1990;99(2–3):229–47.
385. Kujala P, Portin R, Ruutiainen J. The progress of cognitive decline in multiple sclerosis. A controlled 3-year follow-up. Brain. 1997;120(Pt 2):289–97.
386. Fischer JS, et al. Neuropsychological effects of interferon beta-1a in relapsing multiple sclerosis. Multiple Sclerosis Collaborative Research Group. Ann Neurol. 2000;48(6):885–92.
387. Patti F, et al. Effects of immunomodulatory treatment with subcutaneous interferon beta-1a on cognitive decline in mildly disabled patients with relapsing-remitting multiple sclerosis. Mult Scler. 2010;16(1):68–77.
388. Pliskin NH, et al. Improved delayed visual reproduction test performance in multiple sclerosis patients receiving interferon beta-1b. Neurology. 1996;47(6):1463–8.
389. Flechter S, et al. Cognitive dysfunction evaluation in multiple sclerosis patients treated with interferon beta-1b: an open-label prospective 1 year study. Isr Med Assoc J. 2007;9(6):457–9.
390. Kappos L, et al. Effect of early versus delayed interferon beta-1b treatment on disability after a first clinical event suggestive of multiple sclerosis: a 3-year follow-up analysis of the BENEFIT study. Lancet. 2007;370(9585):389–97.
391. Weinstock-Guttman B, et al. Additional efficacy endpoints from pivotal natalizumab trials in relapsing-remitting MS. J Neurol. 2012;259(5):898–905.

392. Morrow SA, et al. Evaluation of the symbol digit modalities test (SDMT) and MS neuropsychological screening questionnaire (MSNQ) in natalizumab-treated MS patients over 48 weeks. Mult Scler. 2010;16(11):1385–92.
393. Mattioli F, Stampatori C, Capra R. The effect of natalizumab on cognitive function in patients with relapsing-remitting multiple sclerosis: preliminary results of a 1-year follow-up study. Neurol Sci. 2011;32(1):83–8.
394. Mattioli F, et al. Natalizumab efficacy on cognitive impairment in MS. Neurol Sci. 2011;31(Suppl 3):321–3.
395. Mattioli F, et al. Natalizumab significantly improves cognitive impairment over three years in MS: pattern of disability progression and preliminary MRI findings. PLoS One. 2015;10(7):e0131803.
396. Iaffaldano P, et al. Impact of natalizumab on cognitive performances and fatigue in relapsing multiple sclerosis: a prospective, open-label, two years observational study. PLoS One. 2012;7(4):e35843.
397. Lang C, Reiss C, Maurer M. Natalizumab may improve cognition and mood in multiple sclerosis. Eur Neurol. 2012;67(3):162–6.
398. Portaccio E, et al. Natalizumab may reduce cognitive changes and brain atrophy rate in relapsing-remitting multiple sclerosis—a prospective, non-randomized pilot study. Eur J Neurol. 2013;20(6):986–90.
399. D'Intino G, et al. Cognitive deficit associated with cholinergic and nerve growth factor down-regulation in experimental allergic encephalomyelitis in rats. Proc Natl Acad Sci U S A. 2005;102(8):3070–5.
400. Krupp LB, et al. Multicenter randomized clinical trial of donepezil for memory impairment in multiple sclerosis. Neurology. 2011;76(17):1500–7.
401. Shaygannejad V, et al. Effects of rivastigmine on memory and cognition in multiple sclerosis. Can J Neurol Sci. 2008;35(4):476–81.
402. Villoslada P, et al. Memantine induces reversible neurologic impairment in patients with MS. Neurology. 2009;72(19):1630–3.
403. Lovera JF, et al. Memantine for cognitive impairment in multiple sclerosis: a randomized placebo-controlled trial. Mult Scler. 2010;16(6):715–23.
404. Geisler MW, et al. The effects of amantadine and pemoline on cognitive functioning in multiple sclerosis. Arch Neurol. 1996;53(2):185–8.
405. Lovera J, et al. Ginkgo biloba for the improvement of cognitive performance in multiple sclerosis: a randomized, placebo-controlled trial. Mult Scler. 2007;13(3):376–85.
406. Morrow SA, et al. The effects of L-amphetamine sulfate on cognition in MS patients: results of a randomized controlled trial. J Neurol. 2009;256(7):1095–102.
407. Oleen-Burkey M, Hadjimichael O, Vollmer T. Fatigue characteristics in multiple sclerosis: the North American Research Committee on Multiple Sclerosis (NARCOMS) survey. Health Qual Life Outcomes. 2008;6
408. Krupp L. Fatigue is intrinsic to multiple sclerosis (MS) and is the most commonly reported symptom of the disease. Mult Scler. 2006;12(4):367–8.
409. Lerdal A, et al. A prospective study of patterns of fatigue in multiple sclerosis. Eur J Neurol. 2007;14(12):1338–43.
410. Smith MM, Arnett PA. Factors related to employment status changes in individuals with multiple sclerosis. Mult Scler. 2005;11(5):602–9.
411. Judica E, et al. Impact of fatigue on the efficacy of rehabilitation in multiple sclerosis. J Neurol. 2011;258(5):835–9.
412. Freal JE, Kraft GH, Coryell JK. Symptomatic fatigue in multiple sclerosis. Arch Phys Med Rehabil. 1984;65(3):135–8.
413. Guidelines, F.G.D.P.o.t.M.S.C.f.C.P. Fatigue and multiple sclerosis. Evidence-based management strategies for fatigue in multiple sclerosis. Washington, DC: Paralyzed Veterans of America; 1998.
414. Rudroff T, Kindred JH, Ketelhut NB. Fatigue in multiple sclerosis: misconceptions and future research directions. Front Neurol. 2016;7:122.

415. Braley TJ, Chervin RD. Fatigue in multiple sclerosis: mechanisms, evaluation, and treatment. Sleep. 2010;33(8):1061–7.
416. Flachenecker P, et al. Cytokine mRNA expression in patients with multiple sclerosis and fatigue. Mult Scler. 2004;10(2):165–9.
417. Heesen C, et al. Fatigue in multiple sclerosis: an example of cytokine mediated sickness behaviour? J Neurol Neurosurg Psychiatry. 2006;77(1):34–9.
418. Malekzadeh A, et al. Fatigue in patients with multiple sclerosis: is it related to pro- and anti-inflammatory cytokines? Dis Markers. 2015;2015:758314.
419. Bergh FT, et al. Dysregulation of the hypothalamo-pituitary-adrenal axis is related to the clinical course of MS. Neurology. 1999;53(4):772.
420. Gottschalk M, et al. Fatigue and regulation of the hypothalamo-pituitary-adrenal axis in multiple sclerosis. Arch Neurol. 2005;62(2):277–80.
421. Tellez N, et al. Fatigue in progressive multiple sclerosis is associated with low levels of dehydroepiandrosterone. Mult Scler. 2006;12(4):487–94.
422. Marrie RA, et al. Association of fatigue and brain atrophy in multiple sclerosis. J Neurol Sci. 2005;228(2):161–6.
423. Tartaglia MC, et al. The relationship between diffuse axonal damage and fatigue in multiple sclerosis. Arch Neurol. 2004;61(2):201–7.
424. Roelcke U, et al. Reduced glucose metabolism in the frontal cortex and basal ganglia of multiple sclerosis patients with fatigue: a 18F-fluorodeoxyglucose positron emission tomography study. Neurology. 1997;48(6):1566–71.
425. Filippi M, et al. Functional magnetic resonance imaging correlates of fatigue in multiple sclerosis. NeuroImage. 2002;15(3):559–67.
426. Genova HM, et al. Examination of cognitive fatigue in multiple sclerosis using functional magnetic resonance imaging and diffusion tensor imaging. PLoS One. 2013;8(11):e78811.
427. Rocca MA, et al. Abnormal adaptation over time of motor network recruitment in multiple sclerosis patients with fatigue. Mult Scler. 2016;22(9):1144–53.
428. Tedeschi G, et al. Correlation between fatigue and brain atrophy and lesion load in multiple sclerosis patients independent of disability. J Neurol Sci. 2007;263(1–2):15–9.
429. Giovannoni G. Multiple sclerosis related fatigue. J Neurol Neurosurg Psychiatry. 2006;77(1):2–3.
430. Sumowski JF, Leavitt VM. Body temperature is elevated and linked to fatigue in relapsing-remitting multiple sclerosis, even without heat exposure. Arch Phys Med Rehabil. 2014;95(7):1298–302.
431. Leavitt VM, et al. Elevated body temperature is linked to fatigue in an Italian sample of relapsing-remitting multiple sclerosis patients. J Neurol. 2015;262(11):2440–2.
432. Veauthier C, et al. Fatigue in multiple sclerosis is closely related to sleep disorders: a polysomnographic cross-sectional study. Mult Scler. 2011;17(5):613–22.
433. Kaminska M, et al. Sleep disorders and fatigue in multiple sclerosis: evidence for association and interaction. J Neurol Sci. 2011;302(1–2):7–13.
434. Braley TJ, Boudreau EA. Sleep disorders in multiple sclerosis. Curr Neurol Neurosci Rep. 2016;16(5):50.
435. Lanza G, et al. The impact of drugs for multiple sclerosis on sleep. Mult Scler. 2017;23(1):5–13.
436. Schwartz CE, Coulthard-Morris L, Zeng Q. Psychosocial correlates of fatigue in multiple sclerosis. Arch Phys Med Rehabil. 1996;77(2):165–70.
437. Wood B, et al. Prevalence and concurrence of anxiety, depression and fatigue over time in multiple sclerosis. Mult Scler. 2013;19(2):217–24.
438. Simpson S Jr, et al. Anxiety, depression and fatigue at 5-year review following CNS demyelination. Acta Neurol Scand. 2016;134(6):403–13.
439. Tur C. Fatigue Management in Multiple Sclerosis. Curr Treat Options Neurol. 2016;18(6):26.
440. Rietberg MB, et al. Effects of multidisciplinary rehabilitation on chronic fatigue in multiple sclerosis: a randomized controlled trial. PLoS One. 2014;9(9):e107710.
441. Metz LM, et al. The effect of immunomodulatory treatment on multiple sclerosis fatigue. J Neurol Neurosurg Psychiatry. 2004;75(7):1045–7.

442. Putzki N, et al. Multiple sclerosis associated fatigue during natalizumab treatment. J Neurol Sci. 2009;285(1–2):109–13.
443. Patejdl R, et al. Multiple sclerosis and fatigue: a review on the contribution of inflammation and immune-mediated neurodegeneration. Autoimmun Rev. 2016;15(3):210–20.
444. Yildiz M, Tettenborn B, Putzki N. Multiple sclerosis-associated fatigue during disease-modifying treatment with natalizumab, interferon-beta and glatiramer acetate. Eur Neurol. 2011;65(4):231–2.
445. Sater RA, et al. NAPS-MS: natalizumab effects on parameters of sleep in patients with multiple sclerosis. Int J MS Care. 2016;18(4):177–82.
446. Stephenson JJ, et al. Impact of natalizumab on patient-reported outcomes in multiple sclerosis: a longitudinal study. Health Qual Life Outcomes. 2012;10:155.
447. Wilken J, et al. Changes in fatigue and cognition in patients with relapsing forms of multiple sclerosis treated with natalizumab: the ENER-G Study. Int J MS Care. 2013;15(3): 120–8.
448. Riera R, Porfirio GJ, Torloni MR. Alemtuzumab for multiple sclerosis. Cochrane Database Syst Rev. 2016;4:CD011203.
449. Guidelines, F.G.D.P.o.t.M.S.C.f.C.P. Fatigue and multiple sclerosis. Evidence-based management strategies for fatigue in multiple sclerosis. Washington, DC: Paralyzed Veterans of America; 1998.
450. Branas P, et al. Treatments for fatigue in multiple sclerosis: a rapid and systematic review. Health Technol Assess. 2000;4(27):1–61.
451. Pucci E, et al. Amantadine for fatigue in multiple sclerosis. Cochrane Database Syst Rev. 2007;1:CD002818.
452. Taus C, et al. Amantadine for fatigue in multiple sclerosis. Cochrane Database Syst Rev. 2003;2:CD002818.
453. Stankoff B, et al. Modafinil for fatigue in MS: a randomized placebo-controlled double-blind study. Neurology. 2005;64(7):1139–43.
454. Ford-Johnson L, et al. Cognitive effects of modafinil in patients with multiple sclerosis: a clinical trial. Rehabil Psychol. 2016;61(1):82–91.
455. Rammohan KW, et al. Efficacy and safety of modafinil (Provigil) for the treatment of fatigue in multiple sclerosis: a two centre phase 2 study. J Neurol Neurosurg Psychiatry. 2002;72(2):179–83.
456. Lange R, et al. Modafinil effects in multiple sclerosis patients with fatigue. J Neurol. 2009;256(4):645–50.
457. Moller F et al. HAGIL (Hamburg Vigil Study): a randomized placebo-controlled double-blind study with modafinil for treatment of fatigue in patients with multiple sclerosis. Mult Scler. 2011.
458. Littleton ET, Hobart JC, Palace J. Modafinil for multiple sclerosis fatigue: does it work? Clin Neurol Neurosurg. 2010;112(1):29–31.
459. Weinshenker BG, et al. A double-blind, randomized, crossover trial of pemoline in fatigue associated with multiple sclerosis. Neurology. 1992;42(8):1468–71.
460. Krupp LB, et al. Fatigue therapy in multiple sclerosis: results of a double-blind, randomized, parallel trial of amantadine, pemoline, and placebo. Neurology. 1995;45(11):1956–61.
461. Sheean GL, et al. An open-labelled clinical and electrophysiological study of 3,4 diaminopyridine in the treatment of fatigue in multiple sclerosis. Brain. 1998;121(Pt 5):967–75.
462. Rossini PM, et al. Fatigue in progressive multiple sclerosis: results of a randomized, double-blind, placebo-controlled, crossover trial of oral 4-aminopyridine. Mult Scler. 2001;7(6):354–8.
463. Flet L, et al. 3,4-diaminopyridine safety in clinical practice: an observational, retrospective cohort study. J Neurol. 2010;257(6):937–46.
464. Bennett SE. Fampridine: long-term benefits in walking in multiple sclerosis. Neurology. 2017;
465. Tejani AM, et al. Carnitine for fatigue in multiple sclerosis. Cochrane Database Syst Rev. 2010;2:CD007280.

466. Tomassini V, et al. Comparison of the effects of acetyl L-carnitine and amantadine for the treatment of fatigue in multiple sclerosis: results of a pilot, randomised, double-blind, cross-over trial. J Neurol Sci. 2004;218(1–2):103–8.
467. Ledinek AH, Sajko MC, Rot U. Evaluating the effects of amantadin, modafinil and acetyl-l-carnitine on fatigue in multiple sclerosis—result of a pilot randomized, blind study. Clin Neurol Neurosurg. 2013;115(Supplement 1):S86–9.
468. Kim E, et al. American ginseng does not improve fatigue in multiple sclerosis: a single center randomized double-blind placebo-controlled crossover pilot study. Mult Scler. 2011;
469. van Kessel K, et al. A randomized controlled trial of cognitive behavior therapy for multiple sclerosis fatigue. Psychosom Med. 2008;70(2):205–13.
470. Mathiowetz VG, et al. Randomized controlled trial of an energy conservation course for persons with multiple sclerosis. Mult Scler. 2005;11(5):592–601.
471. Thomas S, et al. A pragmatic parallel arm multi-centre randomised controlled trial to assess the effectiveness and cost-effectiveness of a group-based fatigue management programme (FACETS) for people with multiple sclerosis. J Neurol Neurosurg Psychiatry. 2013;84(10):1092–9.
472. van den Akker LE, et al. Effectiveness of cognitive behavioral therapy for the treatment of fatigue in patients with multiple sclerosis: a systematic review and meta-analysis. J Psychosom Res. 2016;90:33–42.
473. Heesen C, et al. Physical exercise in multiple sclerosis: supportive care or a putative disease-modifying treatment. Expert Rev Neurother. 2006;6(3):347–55.
474. Heine M, et al. Exercise therapy for fatigue in multiple sclerosis. Cochrane Database Syst Rev. 2015;9:125.
475. Heine M, de Groot V. Current evidence does not support exercise therapy for perceived fatigue in multiple sclerosis. Arch Phys Med Rehabil. 2016;97(11):2016–7.
476. Beckerman H, et al. The effectiveness of aerobic training, cognitive behavioural therapy, and energy conservation management in treating MS-related fatigue: the design of the TREFAMS-ACE programme. Trials. 2013;14:250.
477. Syndulko K, et al. Effects of temperature in multiple sclerosis: a review of the literature. J Neurol Rehabilit. 1996;10(1):23–34.
478. Schwid SR, et al. A randomized controlled study of the acute and chronic effects of cooling therapy for MS. Neurology. 2003;60(12):1955–60.
479. White AT, et al. Effect of precooling on physical performance in multiple sclerosis. Mult Scler. 2000;6(3):176–80.
480. Beenakker EA, et al. Cooling garment treatment in MS: clinical improvement and decrease in leukocyte NO production. Neurology. 2001;57(5):892–4.
481. Piatkowski J, Kern S, Ziemssen T. Effect of BEMER magnetic field therapy on the level of fatigue in patients with multiple sclerosis: a randomized, double-blind controlled trial. J Altern Complement Med. 2009;15(5):507–11.
482. Carvalho ML, et al. A randomized placebo-controlled cross-over study using a low frequency magnetic field in the treatment of fatigue in multiple sclerosis. Mult Scler. 2011;
483. Caminero A, Bartolome M. Sleep disturbances in multiple sclerosis. J Neurol Sci. 2011;309(1–2):86–91.
484. Brass SD, et al. Sleep disorders in patients with multiple sclerosis. Sleep Med Rev. 2010;14(2):121–9.
485. Brass SD, Li CS, Auerbach S. The underdiagnosis of sleep disorders in patients with multiple sclerosis. J Clin Sleep Med. 2014;10(9):1025–31.
486. Veauthier C, et al. Treatment of sleep disorders may improve fatigue in multiple sclerosis. Clin Neurol Neurosurg. 2013;115(9):1826–30.
487. Strober LB, Arnett PA. An examination of four models predicting fatigue in multiple sclerosis. Arch Clin Neuropsychol. 2005;20(5):631–46.
488. Ghajarzadeh M, et al. Fatigue, depression and sleep disturbances in Iranian patients with multiple sclerosis. Acta Med Iran. 2012;50(4):244–9.

489. Strober LB. Fatigue in multiple sclerosis: a look at the role of poor sleep. Front Neurol. 2015;6:21.
490. Newman NJ. Multiple sclerosis and related demyelinating diseases. In: Miller NR, Newman NJ, editors. Walsh and Hoyt's Clinical Neuro-Ophthalmology. Baltimore: Williams and Wilkins; 1998. p. 5539–76.
491. Ganley JP. Uveitis and multiple sclerosis: an overview. In: Saari KM, editor. Uveitis update. Amsterdam: Excerpta Medica; 1984. p. 345–9.
492. Rushton D, Cox N. A new optical treatment for oscillopsia. J Neurol Neurosurg Psychiatry. 1987;50(4):411–5.
493. Starck M, et al. Acquired pendular nystagmus in multiple sclerosis: an examiner-blind crossover treatment study of memantine and gabapentin. J Neurol. 2010;257(3):322–7.
494. Leigh RJ, et al. Crossover trial of gabapentin and memantine as treatment for acquired nystagmus. Ann Neurol. 2010;67(5):676–80.
495. Strupp M, et al. Treatment of downbeat nystagmus with 3,4-diaminopyridine: a placebo-controlled study. Neurology. 2003;61(2):165–70.
496. Kalla R, et al. 4-aminopyridine improves downbeat nystagmus, smooth pursuit, and VOR gain. Neurology. 2004;62(7):1228–9.
497. Kalla R, et al. Comparison of 10-mg doses of 4-aminopyridine and 3,4-diaminopyridine for the treatment of downbeat nystagmus. J Neuroophthalmol. 2011;
498. Averbuch-Heller L. Acquired nystagmus. Curr Treat Options Neurol. 1999;1(1):68–73.
499. Menon GJ, Thaller VT. Therapeutic external ophthalmoplegia with bilateral retrobulbar botulinum toxin- an effective treatment for acquired nystagmus with oscillopsia. Eye (Lond). 2002;16(6):804–6.
500. Ruben ST, et al. The use of botulinum toxin for treatment of acquired nystagmus and oscillopsia. Ophthalmology. 1994;101(4):783–7.
501. Adams WE, Leavitt JA, Holmes JM. Strabismus surgery for internuclear ophthalmoplegia with exotropia in multiple sclerosis. J AAPOS. 2009;13(1):13–5.
502. Thomas FJ, Wiles CM. Dysphagia and nutritional status in multiple sclerosis. J Neurol. 1999;246(8):677–82.
503. Giusti A, Giambuzzi M. Management of dysphagia in patients affected by multiple sclerosis: state of the art. Neurol Sci. 2008;29(Suppl 4):S364–6.
504. Alfonsi E, et al. An electrophysiological approach to the diagnosis of neurogenic dysphagia: implications for botulinum toxin treatment. J Neurol Neurosurg Psychiatry. 2010;81(1):54–60.
505. Restivo DA, et al. Botulinum toxin improves dysphagia associated with multiple sclerosis. Eur J Neurol. 2011;18(3):486–90.
506. Marrosu F, et al. Vagal nerve stimulation improves cerebellar tremor and dysphagia in multiple sclerosis. Mult Scler. 2007;13(9):1200–2.
507. Renauld S, Mohamed-Said L, Macoir J. Language disorders in multiple sclerosis: a systematic review. Mult Scler Relat Disord. 2016;10:103–11.
508. Beukelman DR, Kraft GH, Freal J. Expressive communication disorders in persons with multiple sclerosis: a survey. Arch Phys Med Rehabil. 1985;66(10):675–7.
509. Hartelius L, Svensson P. Speech and swallowing symptoms associated with Parkinson's disease and multiple sclerosis: a survey. Folia Phoniatr Logop. 1994;46(1):9–17.
510. Hartelius L, Runmarker B, Andersen O. Prevalence and characteristics of dysarthria in a multiple-sclerosis incidence cohort: relation to neurological data. Folia Phoniatr Logop. 2000;52(4):160–77.
511. Darley FL, Brown JR, Goldstein NP. Dysarthria in multiple sclerosis. J Speech Hear Res. 1972;15(2):229–45.
512. Parker M, et al. Automatic speech recognition and training for severely dysarthric users of assistive technology: the STARDUST project. Clin Linguist Phon. 2006;20(2–3):149–56.
513. Blanco Y, et al. Midbrain lesions and paroxysmal dysarthria in multiple sclerosis. Mult Scler. 2008;14(5):694–7.
514. Marcel C, et al. Symptomatic paroxysmal dysarthria-ataxia in demyelinating diseases. J Neurol. 2010;257(8):1369–72.

515. Valentino P, et al. Lamotrigine therapy for paroxysmal dysarthria caused by multiple sclerosis: a case report. J Neurol. 2011;258(7):1349–50.
516. Goodwin SJ, Carpenter AF. Successful treatment of paroxysmal ataxia and dysarthria in multiple sclerosis with levetiracetam. Mult Scler Relat Disord. 2016;10:79–81.
517. Voiculescu V, Pruskauer-Apostol B, Alecu C. Treatment with acetazolamide of brain-stem and spinal paroxysmal disturbances in multiple sclerosis. J Neurol Neurosurg Psychiatry. 1975;38(2):191–3.
518. Lensch E, Jost WH. Autonomic disorders in multiple sclerosis. Autoimmune Dis. 2011;2011:803841.
519. Davis SL, et al. Thermoregulation in multiple sclerosis. J Appl Physiol. 2010;109(5):1531–7.
520. Higginson IJ, et al. Symptom prevalence and severity in people severely affected by multiple sclerosis. J Palliat Care. 2006;22(3):158–65.
521. O'Brien T. Neurodegenerative disease. In: Addington-Hall JM, Higginson IJ, editors. Palliative care for non-cancer patients. Oxford: Oxford University Press; 2001. p. 44–55.
522. Kumpfel T, et al. Palliative care in patients with severe multiple sclerosis: two case reports and a survey among German MS neurologists. Palliat Med. 2007;21(2):109–14.
523. Strupp J, Voltz R, Golla H. Opening locked doors: integrating a palliative care approach into the management of patients with severe multiple sclerosis. Mult Scler. 2016;22(1):13–8.
524. Higginson IJ, et al. Is short-term palliative care cost-effective in multiple sclerosis? A randomized phase II trial. J Pain Symptom Manag. 2009;38(6):816–26.
525. Edmonds P, et al. Palliative care for people severely affected by multiple sclerosis: evaluation of a novel palliative care service. Mult Scler. 2010;16(5):627–36.
526. Solari A, et al. Home-based palliative approach for people with severe multiple sclerosis and their carers: study protocol for a randomized controlled trial. Trials. 2015;16:184.
527. Golla H, et al. Unmet needs of severely affected multiple sclerosis patients: the health professionals' view. Palliat Med. 2011;
528. Health DO, editor. The National Service Framework for long term conditions. London: DH; 2005.
529. Medicine NCfPCaBSoR, editor. Longterm neurological conditions: management at the interface between neurology, rehabilitation and palliative care. London: Royal College of Physicians; 2008.
530. Campbell CW, Jones EJ, Merrills J. Palliative and end-of-life care in advanced Parkinson's disease and multiple sclerosis. Clin Med. 2010;10(3):290–2.

Chapter 8
Trials of Licenced RRMS DMTs in Progressive MS

Michael Hutchinson and David P.J. Hunt

8.1 Introduction

The success of the phase III randomized controlled trials (RCTs) of disease-modifying therapies (DMTs) in relapsing–remitting multiple sclerosis (RRMS) [1–4] naturally led to exploration of their efficacy in both secondary progressive multiple sclerosis (SPMS) and primary progressive multiple sclerosis (PPMS). This chapter deals with trials of "conventional" disease-modifying therapies (DMTs), by which we mean drugs which are recognised as having therapeutic utility in the treatment of relapsing-remitting multiple sclerosis. These drugs are almost exclusively immunomodulatory, with particular emphasis on restricting the effector functions of T and B cells. Therefore as well as clinical benefit, these clinical trials help identify which pathways drive the poorly understood substrate of disease progression in humans. The bottom line is that almost all of these trials have been unsuccessful at meeting their primary endpoint in a clinically meaningful way. However, much has been learned about trial design and progress towards modest therapeutic activity has been made [5]. The contrast of therapeutic success of these DMTs in RRMS and their failure in progressive forms of disease is a valuable observation in itself. It suggests that transformative therapies in treatment of the progressive MS are unlikely to come from targeting the largely lymphocyte-driven inflammatory process which occurs early in the disease.

Perhaps the most important lesson from trials in relapsing-remitting multiple sclerosis from over the past three decades is that careful selection of the patient

M. Hutchinson
Newman Clinical Research Professor, St. Vincent's University Hospital, University College Dublin, Dublin, Ireland

D.P.J. Hunt (✉)
MRC Institute of Genetics and Molecular Medicine, Anne Rowling Clinic, University of Edinburgh, Edinburgh, UK
e-mail: david.hunt@igmm.ed.ac.uk

A. Wilkins (ed.), *Progressive Multiple Sclerosis*,
https://doi.org/10.1007/978-3-319-65921-3_8

population and use of sensitive imaging biomarkers has been central to the identification of patients who respond to therapy. While patients with SPMS or PPMS are at a different end of the pathophysiological spectrum [6], lessons are being learned on how to identify potentially treatment-responsive from analysis of subgroups of earlier negative progressive MS trials, aided by increasingly sensitive imaging biomarkers. While the primary endpoints in a number of trials were not achieved, many secondary endpoints demonstrated a marked treatment effect, in particular surrogate markers of inflammatory disease activity. Despite the predominantly negative outcomes, the trials described in this chapter have informed the MS research community about the natural history of progressive MS, and have stimulated both expert consensus diagnostic criteria [7–13] and a search for new disability measures. Recognition of the limitations of the most commonly used measure of disability progression, the Expanded Disability Status Scale (EDSS) [14] led to the development of other instruments, including the Multiple Sclerosis Functional Composite (MSFC) [15] and other tools which complement the ambulation-dominated EDSS.

The SPMS and PPMS trials have also contributed to the debate about the nature of the degenerative process in MS; is neurodegeneration in MS a separate primary disorder or simply secondary to an inflammatory process [16]? Central to this question is whether profound suppression of the inflammatory process can prevent neurological progression, with the implication that this phase of disease is secondary to chronic inflammation. The converse hypothesis is that the progressive phase represents the "true" multiple sclerosis and that the inflammatory phase is a reaction to this degenerative disease, as can occur in many other neurological disorders [17]. While debate on this issue continues, it should be acknowledged that our current evidence base of clinical trials in RRMS does not allow this hypothesis to be adequately tested. Clinical trials in RRMS are simply too short to allow meaningful conclusions to be drawn about disease progression, which develops over decades. Well-performed long-term cohort studies of treated patients have, as yet, only been performed on drugs with only weak immunomodulatory activity [18, 19]. However, as we move towards an era where the near-complete suppression of inflammatory activity appears a realistic goal [20], more will be learned of this complex relationship between relapsing-remitting disease and progression.

The practical and ethical constraints of placebo-controlled trials in MS have been discussed elsewhere [21–23]. As in all RCTs of 2–3 years duration, there is a problem with the implied extrapolation of any demonstrated short-term efficacy to a lifelong illness. Apart from an effect on markers of inflammation, it should be recognized that, given the generally negative primary outcome measure of confirmed disability progression, there is no suggestion that presently discussed therapies are effective in altering long-term outcome in SPMS or PPMS.

In this chapter we describe trials in SPMS first, then PPMS. Although there remains some overlap, there is an increasing trend to consider these distinct populations for the purposes of clinical trials.

8.2 SPMS Trials

There were nine major phase III RCTs of DMTs in SPMS and all will be discussed in detail. Prior to the advent of the beta-interferons (IFNB), there were a number of exploratory, observational, phase I and II studies of immunosuppressive therapies, which will be discussed briefly.

A summary of the phase III trials is given in Table 8.1.

Table 8.1 Summary of phase III RCTs in secondary progressive MS

Study	Intervention	Patient population	Study design	Primary endpoint	Secondary endpoint
European Study of Interferon Beta-1b (IFNB-1b) in SPMS	Interferon b	SPMS	Phase III randomised Versus placebo	Time to confirmed progression: Positive	ARR: Positive MRI T2 lesions: Positive
The North American IFNB-1b SPMS Study	Interferon b	SPMS	Phase III randomised Versus placebo	Time to confirmed progression: Negative	ARR: Positive MRI T2 lesions: Positive
SPECTRIMS: IFNB-1a Subcutaneously in SPMS	Interferon b	SPMS	Phase III randomised Versus placebo	Time to confirmed progression: Negative	ARR: Positive MRI T2 lesions: Positive
IMPACT Study	Interferon b	SPMS	Phase III randomised Versus placebo	Change in MSFC: Positive	EDSS: Negative MRI T2 lesions: Positive
Nordic IFNB-1a SPMS Study	Interferon b	SPMS	Phase III randomised Versus placebo	Time to confirmed disability progression: Negative	ARR: Negative
Mitoxantrone in SPMS	Interferon b	SPMS	Phase III randomised Versus placebo	EDSS: Positive	ARR: Positive MRI T2 lesions: Positive
European Intravenous Immunoglobulin (IVIG) in SPMS (ESIMS)	IVIG	SPMS	Phase III randomised Versus placebo	Time to confirmed progression: Negative	MRI T2: Negative

(continued)

Table 8.1 (continued)

Study	Intervention	Patient population	Study design	Primary endpoint	Secondary endpoint
ASCEND	Natalizumab	SPMS	Phase III randomised Versus placebo	Time to confirmed disability progression (EDSS, T25FW, 9HPT): Negative	9HPT: Positive
EXPAND	Siponimod	SPMS	Phase III randomised Versus placebo	Confirmed disability progression at 3 months: Positive	

8.2.1 Interferon-Beta in in the Treatment of SPMS

8.2.1.1 European Study of Interferon Beta-1b (IFNB-1b) in SPMS [24–29]

This was the first phase III RCT in SPMS [24] and followed on the positive results of the RCT of IFNB-1b in RRMS [1]. The European SPMS study was a double-blind, placebo-controlled study of two parallel groups comparing IFNB-1b eight million international units subcutaneously every other day versus placebo in 718 patients over a 3-year period. Secondary progression, as an inclusion criterion, was defined as a period of deterioration, independent of relapses, sustained for at least 6 months, following a period of relapsing–remitting MS. Superimposed relapses were allowed. The primary outcome measure was time to progression in the EDSS score confirmed at 12 weeks by one point when the baseline EDSS was less than 6, or by 0.5 EDSS point when the baseline EDSS was 6.0 or 6.5. The study population was assigned randomly to IFNB-1b in 360 patients and placebo in 358. The study was terminated early when interim analysis, with about 85% of EDSS data collected, indicated a positive outcome.

Primary Endpoint: The time to confirmed progression was significantly different between groups: the placebo group reached the 40% quantile at 549 days and the IFNB-1b group at 893 days ($p = 0.0008$). The probability of remaining progression free was significant after 12 months of treatment and remained significant thereafter. The proportion of patients with confirmed progression over the study period was 49.7% for the placebo group and 38.9% for the IFNB-1b group, a relative reduction of 21.7% ($p = 0.0048$) and an absolute risk reduction of 9.8%. The probability of progression for patients on placebo was 1.6 times that of a patient on IFNB-1b (OR = 0.63, 95% CI: 0.47–0.93). The development of confirmed progression was not influenced by the occurrence or absence of a relapse within 2 years prior to study entry.

Secondary Endpoints: During the trial, annualized relapse rates (ARR) were significantly different between IFNB-1b-treated patients (ARR 0.44 over 3 years) and placebo-treated patients (ARR 0.64 over 3 years; $p = 0.0002$); the median time to first relapse was 644 and 403 days, respectively ($p = 0.003$). Overall, T2 lesion load increased over the 3 years of the study in the placebo group by 15% and decreased by 2% in the IFNB-1b-treated group ($p < 0.0001$) [25]. The proportion of enhancing lesions developing into T1 hypointensities did not differ between the groups and were more likely to form from large than small enhancing lesions [26]. A subgroup of 95 patients (13% of the total cohort of 718) had 6-monthly T1 scans in five centers [27]. Overall, there was no difference between the placebo- and the IFNB-1b-treated patients in relation to atrophy. This disappointing finding was partly ascribed to the small number of patients scanned, but also might relate to the dynamics of cerebral volume change in patients with SPMS. Atrophy may reflect an on-going loss of tissue consequent to inflammatory disease, which occurred in the years prior to entry to the study. Also, paradoxically, a drug with a potent anti-inflammatory effect will cause apparent atrophy (pseudoatrophy) compared to the placebo group because of loss of volume caused by reduced oedema in the cerebrum consequent upon reduced inflammation. This will be most apparent in the first 6–12 months of treatment. This was borne out when a post hoc analysis was performed. Patients with no gadolinium enhancement at baseline (less inflammatory activity) demonstrated a treatment effect on cerebral atrophy with a 5.1% loss of volume in the placebo group and 1.8% loss in the IFNB-1b arm at 36 months ($p = 0.0026$). MRI findings in relation to clinical outcomes were assessed in the subgroup of 125 patients with monthly scans [28]. This study emphasized the weak correlations in SPMS between MRI measures (baseline T2 lesion volume, increase in T2 lesion load, increase in new and enhancing lesions) and clinical measures of disability progression.

8.2.1.2 The North American IFNB-1b SPMS Study [30]

This double-blind phase III RCT of IFNB-1b in SPMS compared, in three arms: IFNB-1b 250 mg; IFNB-1b 160 mg/m^2; and placebo in 939 patients with SPMS over 3 years [30]. The entry criteria differed from the European SPMS study in that the North American study required a documented increase in EDSS score of 1.0 point or more in the 2 years prior to screening or a 0.5-point or more increase for subjects with a screening EDSS score of 6.5. The primary outcome variable was the same as the European study except that disability progression had to be confirmed at 6 months. The trial was terminated prematurely on the recommendation of the independent data and safety monitoring board because it was determined that continuing the study was unlikely to change the results of the primary efficacy outcome. At that time, 75% of the study population had completed the trial.

Primary Endpoint: There was no evidence of any treatment effect on confirmed disability between groups.

Secondary Endpoints: Secondary and tertiary outcomes were positive, indicating a treatment effect on annualized relapse rates, time to first relapse, and MRI measures including T2 lesion load and newly active lesions.

8.2.1.3 Comparing the European and North American IFNB-1b SPMS Trials

The differences between the two trials and the reason why the European study, and not the North American, attained the primary endpoint have been addressed in detail [29]. Differences in the baseline characteristics of the two study populations explain the reason for the divergent results. Patients in the European study at entry were younger, had a shorter disease duration, had a higher pre-study ARR, had more relapses in the preceding 2 years, and had more gadolinium-enhancing lesions at baseline brain MRI than those in the North American study. Seventy percent of European patients but only 45% of North American patients had relapses in the preceding 2 years. Although there were several reasons for the biological heterogeneity of the two study populations, the most important determining factor was the difference in the entry criteria. In both studies, a diagnosis of SPMS was required but, whereas the North American study stipulated an increase in the EDSS by 1.0 point or more, the European study required *either* a one point or more increase in the EDSS or two relapses in the preceding 2 years. How European neurologists differentiated between patients having relapses with resulting accumulating residual disability and those patients with slowly progressive disability and superimposed relapses was left to them. Remarkably, 285 (40%) of the 718 patients entered the European study because of relapse history alone without any required documented pre-study increase in disability. European patients had thus more evidence of an active inflammatory component to their illness than the North American patients and would be more likely to respond to an anti-inflammatory drug.

8.2.1.4 SPECTRIMS: IFNB-1a Subcutaneously in SPMS [31–33]

This phase III RCT Secondary Progressive Efficacy Clinical Trial of Recombinant Interferon-beta-1a in MS (SPECTRIMS) examined the efficacy of IFNB-1a in two doses of 22 and 44 mg subcutaneously three times/week versus placebo in 618 patients with SPMS over 3 years [31]. The primary endpoint was time to progression in the EDSS by one point if the baseline EDSS was <5.5 or by 0.5 point if the baseline EDSS was 5.5 or greater, confirmed at 3 months. Full follow-up data was obtained for 92% of patients.

Primary Endpoint: The primary endpoint, time to confirmed progression in the EDSS, was not significant for either dose of IFNB-1a.

Secondary Endpoints: There was a significant effect on all measures of relapse activity at both doses of IFNB-1a compared to placebo. Neutralising antibodies (Nabs) were more common in the 22 mg dose arm (21% positive) than the 44 mg dose arm (15% positive) and did not seem to affect time to disability progression. In the 44 mg dose cohort, NAbs appeared to negate the effect on relapse suppression. In a further paper, analysis of various ratings of depression in 365 patients during the SPECTRIMS study showed no evidence of an increased risk for depression in patients treated with either dose of IFNB-1a [32]. A significant therapeutic effect on MRI evidence of inflammatory activity was noted with a 70–75% reduction in the T2 active lesions [33]. At baseline, there was a difference in the burden of disease (BOD; total T2 lesion area) with men having a significantly higher BOD than women. As with the clinical outcome measures, a gender difference on therapeutic effect was noted in relation to the percentage change in BOD, which was greater and evident in both 22 and 44 mg doses in women than in men.

8.2.1.5 IMPACT Study: IFNB-1a in SPMS [34]

This was the first phase III RCT to use the Multiple Sclerosis Functional Composite (MSFC) as a primary endpoint *International MS Secondary Progressive Avonex Controlled Trial (IMPACT)* [34]. The MSFC had been devised in an attempt to address the limitations of the ambulatory biased EDSS [15]. The MSFC consists of three items, the timed 25-ft. walk test (T25FWT) as a measure of ambulation, the 9-hole peg test (9-HPT) as a measure of upper limb function, and the paced auditory serial addition test at 3-s intervals (PASAT3), a measure of cognitive processing. The change scores on individual items may be used or the composite.

In the IMPACT study, 217 patients were randomized to treatment with IFNB-1a 60 mg intramuscularly weekly and 219 to placebo and were followed for 24 months. Entry criteria included SPMS *with or without recent relapses,* disease progression over the previous year (not otherwise defined by any definite EDSS change), and an EDSS score of 3.5–6.5.

Primary Endpoint: The primary endpoint was the change in the MSFC from baseline to month 24. In both groups, the mean MSFC worsened over 24 months but the degree of worsening was significantly less in the active treatment group (−0.495) in comparison to the placebo group (−0.362) ($p < 0.033$). The difference between the two groups in the degree of MSFC worsening related mainly to reduced worsening in the 9-HPT ($p < 0.024$) and the PASAT3 ($p < 0.061$) in the group treated with IFNB-1a. The T25FWT showed no significant change.

Secondary Endpoints: The usual disability measure, the EDSS, did not show any significant treatment effect, either assessed as time to confirmed progression or mean change in the EDSS. On a measure of health-related quality of life, the active treatment group showed significant improvement compared to placebo. There was a significant effect of IFNB-1a, compared to placebo, on all MRI end-points, including a 53% reduction of new or enlarging T2 lesions at 12 months.

Comment: This was the first study to use the MSFC and the only SPMS study, other than the European SPMS study, to demonstrate an effect on the primary endpoint. However, the MSFC difference in the two study arms was minimal, and although statistically significant was certainly not clinically important or relevant, and therefore this was essentially a negative study. For the MSFC change, the functional effect of reduced worsening is difficult to judge [35].

8.2.1.6 Nordic IFNB-1a SPMS Study [36]

This phase III RCT examined the effects of a low dose of IFNB-1a, 22 mg subcutaneously, once weekly on disability progression in SPMS [36]. The definition of SPMS was that of progressive increase in disability over at least 6 months with an increase in the EDSS of at least 1.0 point over the last 4 years or 0.5 points if the entry EDSS was 6.0 or 6.5. The EDSS of patients at entry was less than 7.0. The primary efficacy variable was time to deterioration in the EDSS, confirmed at 6 months, by at least one point if the entry EDSS was 5.0 or less or by 0.5 point if the EDSS was 5.5–6.5. After randomization, 186 patients received IFNB-1a subcutaneously and 178 patients received placebo.

Primary Endpoint: There was no difference in the two groups in time to sustained disability progression.

Secondary Endpoints: Confirmed disability progression was found in 41% of the IFNB-1a group and 38% of the placebo patients. There was no effect on annualized relapse rates, time to first relapse, proportion relapse free, or hospitalizations for MS relapses. *Subgroup analyses* in relation to effects of gender or prior disease history showed no significant differences.

Comment: Although trials in early multiple sclerosis using low doses of IFNB had shown therapeutic effects in the clinically isolated syndrome [37, 38], it is clear from the Nordic SPMS study that in established SPMS, such low doses neither affect measures of inflammation nor of disability.

8.2.2 Mitoxantrone in SPMS [39, 40]

The mitoxantrone in MS (MIMS) study was a double-blind phase III study of mitoxantrone in patients with progressive–relapsing MS and included patients with SPMS with or without relapses [39]. There were three arms: mitoxantrone 5 mg/m^2; mitoxantrone 12 mg/m^2; and placebo. The entry criteria were either stepwise progression of disability between clinical relapses (progressive–relapsing multiple sclerosis, also termed worsening relapsing–remitting multiple sclerosis) or gradual progression of disability with or without superimposed clinical relapses (secondary progressive multiple sclerosis), EDSS 3.0–6.0 and no relapse treated with steroids 8 weeks prior to entry. Patients received infusions every 3 months over 2 years of either dose of mitoxantrone or placebo. The primary efficacy outcome consisted of five clinical measures: change from baseline EDSS at 24 months, change from baseline ambulation index at 24 months, number of relapses treated with corticosteroids, time to first treated relapse, and change from baseline standardized neurological status at 24 months. Sixty-three patients were assigned treatment with 12 mg/m^2

mitoxantrone, 66 were assigned to 5 mg/m^2, and 65 were assigned to placebo. One hundred and ninety-one patients received at least one dose of study treatment and 188 underwent at least one clinical assessment and were available for efficacy analyses.

Primary Endpoints: The EDSS worsened by 0.23 in the placebo group over the 2 years of study and improved by a mean of 0.13 in the mitoxantrone 12 mg/m^2 group (p = 0.0194). The number of treated relapses was significantly less in the mitoxantrone 12 mg/m^2 group than placebo (p = 0.0002). First quartile time to first treated relapse was 6.7 months in the placebo group and 20.4 months in the mitoxantrone 12 mg/m^2 group (p = 0.0004). Significant treatment effects were also seen in the Ambulation index change and the standardized neurological status.

Secondary Endpoints: The annualized relapse rate (ARR) was significantly lower in the 12 mg/m^2 mitoxantrone group than in the placebo group for year 1 (0.42 vs. 1.15, $p < 0.0001$) and year 2 (0.27 vs. 0.85, $p = 0.0001$; differences 63% and 68%). Confirmed progression of disability by the EDSS by one point differed between the groups: patients in the 12 mg/m^2 group showed a significant advantage in the analysis of time to confirmed EDSS deterioration at 3 months (p = 0.03) and 6 months (p = 0.03). Significantly fewer patients on 12 mg/m^2 mitoxantrone had enhancing lesions at 24 months compared to those on placebo (none vs. 16%, p = 0.02). The mean increase in the number of T2-weighted lesions was 0.29 in the mitoxantrone group and 1.94 in the placebo group (p = 0.03) [37].

Comment on MIMS Study: On the basis of the results of the MIMS trial, the US Food and Drug Administration approved mitoxantrone 12 mg/m^2 administered intravenously every third month for treatment of worsening relapsing-remitting, progressive-relapsing, and secondary progressive MS. The entry criteria and the baseline characteristics of the patients in this study were very similar to the characteristics of patients who were entered in the European SPMS study of IFNB-1b [24]. Although the authors suggest in their discussion that SPMS patients without relapses might also benefit from treatment with mitoxantrone, they have no evidence to support this (and there has been none since). Other smaller trials and subsequent experience in clinical use would indicate that unless a patient with SPMS has associated relapses and/or gadolinium-enhancing lesions on brain MRI, they are unlikely to benefit from mitoxantrone [41, 42].

Two toxic side effects, cardiomyopathy and, in particular, treatment-related acute leukemia (TRAL), add concern in the use of mitoxantrone in clinical practice. Cardiomyopathy may develop early in the treatment course; patients require regular 3-monthly echocardiography to detect changes in left ventricular ejection fraction (LVEF). An expert review in 2010 suggested a 12% incidence of reduced LVEF and 0.4% of congestive cardiac failure [43].

Although initial studies suggested that TRAL was rare with an incidence of 0.07% [44], the reported incidence of TRAL has been rising; 0.3% in a UK review [45], 0.69% in an Italian series [42], and 0.81% in a recent review by the Therapeutics and Technology Assessment Subcommittee of the American Academy of Neurology [43]. A Cochrane Collaboration review in 2005 concluded that "mitoxantrone has a partial efficacy, but, due to its unclear long-term safety profile, it should be used to treat patients with worsening RR and SPMS with evidence of worsening disability [46]."

8.2.3 European Intravenous Immunoglobulin (IVIG) in SPMS (ESIMS) [47–49]

IVIG had been shown to have effects on reducing disease activity in RRMS when this study in SPMS was planned. This randomized, phase III double-blind, parallel group RCT recruited patients with SPMS to treatment with IVIG 1 g/month (159 patients) or placebo infusions (159 patients), and followed them for 2 years [47]. Secondary progression was defined as continued deterioration of disability for at least 12 months with or without interposed relapses after an initial relapsing–remitting course. Disease activity was defined as a deterioration on the EDSS during the previous 2 years of at least 1.0 if the score at the beginning of that period was less than 6.0, or a deterioration of at least 0.5 if the starting score was 6.0 or higher. The entry criteria were unusual in that the there was provision for inclusion of patients with two relapses combined with worsening on the EDSS of 0.5 points. The primary endpoint was time to confirmed disability progression (at 3 months) by one point in the EDSS for EDSS at baseline less than 5.5 and by 0.5 points in patients with a baseline EDSS 5.5 or more.

Primary Endpoint: There was no difference in time to confirmed progression between the two treatment arms. More patients deteriorated in the IVIG arm (77/159) than the placebo arm (70/159).

Secondary Endpoints: There were no differences between the two treatment arms in relation to performance on the 9-HPT, median increase in the EDSS scores, or on-study relapse rates. Detailed MRI results were published separately and reported no differences in inflammatory disease activity (% enhancing scans, number of enhancing lesions, number of new or enhancing lesions between the two groups) [48]. There was significantly more cerebral volume loss in the placebo group than the IVIG arm (IVIG arm: −0.62% vs. placebo: −0.88%, p = 0.009). Given the extent of inflammatory disease in both groups, this is unlikely evidence of a protective effect of IVIG. The authors postulated that the effect of IVIG on brain atrophy development of these patients might relate to an effect of IVIG on remyelination. However, magnetization transfer (MT) magnetic resonance imaging in a study subgroup found no significant differences between the two arms [49].

8.2.3.1 Summary

This was a completely negative study in that not only was the primary endpoint not achieved but also, in contrast to many of the phase III studies in SPMS, none of the secondary endpoints of inflammatory activity were positive. The authors commented that their study population was more similar to the SPECTRIMS than the European IFNB-1b SPMS study in relation to having fewer preceding relapses and at a more advanced stage of SPMS. There is no evidence that IVIG has any therapeutic effect in SPMS. A Cochrane Review in 2009 came to the same conclusion [50].

8.2.4 Other Immunosuppressants

8.2.4.1 Steroid Therapy [51]

A phase II RCT examined the outcome in 108 SPMS patients randomly assigned to high- or low-dose steroid therapy [51]. Patients in the high-dose arm were given 500 mg of methylprednisolone intravenously for 3 days every 2 months with an oral taper. Patients in the low-dose arm were given 10 mg pulses followed by an oral taper. The primary outcome was a comparison of the proportion of patients in each treatment arm who developed confirmed disability progression (of 1.0 point with an entry EDSS of 4.0–5.0 and of 0.5 point with an entry EDSS of 5.5–6.5). Confirmation of disability progression was made at 5 months or more. Inclusion criteria included patients with SPMS who had deteriorated of 0.5 or more EDSS points sustained for 5 or more months and who had one or more exacerbations with or without recovery to baseline EDSS score during the 2 years preceding study entry.

The primary endpoint was not attained: 29/54 low-dose (53.7%) and 21/54 high-dose (38.9%) recipients met criteria for sustained treatment failure ($p = 0.18$). The secondary endpoint, a log-rank comparison of survival significantly favored the high-dose treatment arm ($p < 0.04$).

Comment: This was a dose comparison study without any placebo arm and suggested that high-dose steroids had a modest effect on disability progression. A Cochrane Collaboration Review found no adequate evidence of an effect of steroid therapy on disability progression in SPMS [52].

A number of other therapies have been examined in SPMS, including total lymphoid irradiation [53], plasma exchange [54], cyclophosphamide [55–57], methotrexate [58], cladribine [59], treosulfan [60], and autologous haematopoietic stem cell transplantation [61, 62] (also see Chap. 9). These studies are not discussed in detail. These nonselective immunosuppressive therapies have generally not shown convincing effects on disability progression and are associated with significant short-term and long-term toxicity or unacceptable mortality [63]. Many of these therapies have shown dramatic effects on the inflammatory process but cerebral atrophy and disability accrual continues.

8.2.5 Natalizumab: The ASCEND Trial

Natalizumab is a recombinant humanized antibody directed to the cell adhesion molecule α4-integrin which prevents lymphocyte trafficking across endothelial cells in the brain [64]. Natalizumab was the first high-efficacy monoclonal antibody licensed for the treatment of relapsing-remitting multiple sclerosis. This has proved an effective strategy for treatment of relapsing-remitting disease, with particular efficacy in patients with highly active disease [64]. However, the focal immune suppression of the brain caused by natalizumab also increases the risk of CNS opportunistic infection, most notably the development of JC virus-associated progressive multifocal leucoencephalopathy [65].

The ASCEND trial was a 2-year phase 3 study (n = 887) comparing natalizumab to placebo in patients with SPMS. At the time of writing, the results have been published in abstract form only [66]. Patients were naïve to natalizumab therapy, with a diagnosis of SPMS for at least 2 years and clinical evidence of progression unrelated to relapses in the year prior to trial entry. Most patients had advanced ambulatory disability at baseline, with 63% of patients with an EDSS score 6–6.5. The active arm (n = 439) received 300 mg natalizumab by intravenous infusion compared to placebo (n = 448). The primary outcome was confirmed disability progression, based on a composite endpoint comprising EDSS, T25FW and 9HPT.

Primary Endpoint: The primary outcome was negative and there was no significant delay in disability progression in the natalizumab-treated group. Natalizumab treated group 44% confirmed progression, versus placebo 48%, adjusted odds ratio = 0.86, 95% CI 0.66–1.13 p = 0.29.

Secondary Endpoints: There was a statistically significant difference favouring treatment with natalizumab, when analyses were performed using upper limb function alone. Confirmed disease progression in the upper limb was 15% in the natalizumab group versus 23% placebo, OR 0.56, p = 0.0012.

Comment: This was one of the first phase III studies of a "high-efficacy" anti-inflammatory monoclonal antibody in SPMS. The results with the primary endpoint were disappointing, but perhaps consistent with earlier data from the pivotal RRMS trials, which suggested that the drug was maximally effective in highly active inflammatory disease, characterized by frequent relapses and high number of gadolinium-enhanced lesions. Preservation of upper limb function is a high priority for patients whose ambulation has been heavily affected, and so may be a relevant secondary outcome of this study, given that the EDSS scores of the majority of enrolled patients was >6.

On a practical clinical note, distinguishing between MS relapse and PML in natalizumab-treated RRMS patients represents a considerable clinical challenge, but is aided by the distinct temporal profile of MS relapses [65]. Distinguishing between PML and progressive MS is a more difficult proposition. When the full spectrum of clinical trials with natalizumab in MS are viewed in their entirety, there is a clear gradient of efficacy, which is maximal for highly active inflammatory MS and minimal for progressive forms with low levels of active inflammation. Given the clearly defined biological role of this drug [64], this allows us to draw the conclusion that the key pivotal step of lymphocyte migration across the cerebral endothelial cells is a key event in mediating clinical disease in RRMS, though likely plays a limited role, if any, in progressive forms of the disease.

8.2.6 Sphingosine-Phosphate Inhibitors: The EXPAND Trial

Fingolimod was the first oral immunosuppressant agent to be approved for the therapy of RRMS and acts via modulation of the sphingosine-1-phosphate receptor, with the result of sequestering circulating lymphocytes within lymph nodes

[67, 68]. Drugs of this class have been tested in both SPMS and PPMS. The results of the negative trial of fingolimod in PPMS are discussed in detail in the next section. More selective sphingosine-1-phosphate modulators have been developed, with efficacy in RRMS, which offer the advantage of avoiding effects on the heart, in particular the well-documented first-dose bradycardia effect. Siponimod (BAF312) is an oral agent which acts on receptor subtypes 1 and 5 [69, 70].

The EXPAND study was a phase 3 (n = 1651), multicenter, double-blind placebo-controlled study in SPMS. Patients aged 18–60 with EDSS 3.0–6.5 and evidence of a progressive increase in disability of >6 months duration were included. Patients were randomized 2:1 to receive 2 mg daily siponimod or placebo.

Primary Endpoint: The primary endpoint was percentage of patients with confirmed disability progression (CDP) at 3 months measured by EDSS. Siponimod reduced confirmed disability progression at 3 months by 21% in the treatment group compared to placebo (p = 0.013) 71, 72]. Full publication of the results of this trial will permit more detailed analysis of these promising results.

8.2.7 Alemtuzumab

In an exploratory phase II study, 25 patients with SPMS were treated with Campath-1H (alemtuzumab) 20 mg daily intravenously for 5 days [73]. Patients at entry had to have SPMS, a deterioration in the EDSS by at least one point in the preceding 12 months and a gadolinium-enhancing lesion on at least one of three MRI scans performed at monthly intervals prior to treatment. Patients were followed for 18 months. There was a significant effect of Campath-1H on suppression of gadolinium-enhancing lesions but EDSS worsened and both cerebral and spinal cord atrophy increased. Reduction in brain volume during the study was predicted by the mean gadolinium-enhancing lesion volume prior to treatment initiation ($r = 0.77$, $p = 0.022$). The authors noted that a key area of MS research is to determine whether early intervention with potent anti-inflammatory therapies would delay or prevent later irreversible atrophy.

8.3 Disease-Modifying Therapies in Primary Progressive Multiple Sclerosis

There are fewer trials in PPMS than SPMS, partly because PPMS forms no more than 15% of the MS population. Other reasons include evidence from MRI of less overt inflammatory disease activity in PPMS and a concept that the pathogenesis of PPMS is more neurodegenerative than RRMS or SPMS. The last 20 years have seen detailed reports from the natural history databases in London, Ontario, Lyon, and British Columbia [74–80] workshops on PPMS [81, 82], numerous MRI studies, and the establishment of uniform diagnostic criteria [9–11]. These are dealt with in detail in other chapters in this book and will not be elaborated further here. The

Table 8.2 Summary of phase III RCTs in primary progressive MS

Study	Intervention	Patient population	Study design	Primary endpoint	Secondary endpoint
IFNB-1a in PPMS	Interferon b	PPMS	Three-arm RCT Versus placebo	Sustained progression in disability: Negative	MRI T2: Positive
IFNB-1b in PPMS	Interferon b	PPMS	Single centre RCT Versus placebo	EDSS progression: Negative	MRI T2: Positive
The PROMiSe Study	Glatiramer	PPMS	Phase III randomised Versus placebo	Disability progression: Negative	MRI T2: Positive
INFORMS	Fingolimod	PPMS	Phase III randomised Versus placebo	3-month confirmed disability progression: Negative	MRI T2: Positive
OLYMPUS	Rituximab	PPMS	Phase III randomised Versus placebo	Confirmed disability progression: Negative	MRI T2: Positive Subgroup analysis (age < 51, Gd+ lesions): Positive
ORATORIO	Ocrelizumab	PPMS	Phase III randomised Versus placebo	3-month confirmed disability progression: Positive	9HPT: Positive

RCTs in PPMS have, as with the SPMS trials, highlighted factors in the characteristics of the patients recruited to these studies, which have illuminated aspects of the natural history, which will be discussed later.

A summary of the phase III trials in PPMS is given in Table 8.2.

8.3.1 *Beta-Interferons in PPMS*

8.3.1.1 IFNB-1a in PPMS [83]

The group at the Institute of Neurology in London recruited 50 patients with PPMS into an exploratory three-arm, double-blind, placebo-controlled RCT studied over a 2-year period [83]. At the time of beginning this study, no agreed diagnostic criteria for PPMS had been established. Patients were recruited on the basis of a progressive history without relapse or remission, at least two typical lesions on MRI brain or spinal cord, and CSF oligoclonal bands, not present in parallel serum, or abnormal visual evoked potentials. The three treatment arms were IFNB-1a 30 mg intramuscularly weekly (15 pts), IFNB-1a 60 mg intramuscularly weekly (15 pts), and placebo (20 pts). Patients were recruited with (1) PPMS of at least 2 years' duration, (2) aged 18–60 years, and (3) EDSS score of 2.0–7.0 inclusive. The primary clinical endpoint was time to sustained progression in disability defined as a 1.0 point or greater increase in EDSS score (confirmed at 3 months) for subjects with a baseline EDSS score equal to or less than 5.0, or a 0.5-point increase for subjects with a baseline EDSS of 5.5 or greater.

Primary Endpoint: There were no significant differences in disease progression between the individual or combined treatment arms and placebo. The primary clinical endpoint was reached in 48% of subjects.

Secondary Endpoints: No treatment effect was seen in the timed 10-m walk or the 9-hole peg test (9-HPT) but there was a lower rate of deterioration in the 9-HPT on the right side in the lower dose of IFNB-1a than the higher dose. There was a trend to a reduction of the increase in the T2 lesion load in both IFNB-1a groups combined versus placebo ($p = 0.075$) and lower rate of increase in the T2 lesion load in the IFNB-1a 30 mg dose group than placebo ($p = 0.025$). No treatment effects were seen in spinal cord atrophy rates, T1 lesion load, or new T2 lesions.

Summary: A negative exploratory study, but it demonstrated the feasibility of RCTs in PPMS. The authors indicated that the change in T2 lesion volume would be a useful MRI marker in PPMS.

8.3.1.2 IFNB-1b in PPMS [84]

This was a single center, double-blind RCT from the Barcelona group which examined the efficacy of IFNB-1b 8 MIU subcutaneously (36 pts) versus placebo (37 pts) in PPMS over 2 years [84]. The recruitment criteria included both patients with a solely progressive course and patients with transitional PPMS which allowed inclusion of patients with a single relapse before or during progression. The main efficacy variable was progression in the EDSS, confirmed at 3 months.

Primary Endpoints: There was no difference between the two groups in EDSS progression.

Secondary Endpoints: Analysis by survival to confirmed disability progression in the EDSS at 6 months did not differ between the two groups. The MSFC or its components and measures of fatigue, cognition, ambulation, and HrQoL did not differ at study end. However at months 18 and 24, there were significant differences in the MSFC favoring the IFNB-1b group. MRI endpoints, which significantly favored the treatment arm included changes in both T1 and T2 lesion load, and lower proportion of patients with active lesions at 24 months ($p = 0.0102$).

Summary: This was a negative study in relation to the primary outcome. However, the MSFC outcomes indicated a minor clinical effect during the second year, which was not sustained at 27 months. The MRI endpoints indicate a significant effect of IFNB-1b on the inflammatory component in PPMS, which did not translate into clinical benefit. A Cochrane review in 2010 noted that limited data on the effect of IFNB treatment on PPMS exists. Larger research studies need to be done in patients with PPMS in order to clarify whether IFNB is effective in this population [85].

8.3.2 Glatiramer Acetate in PPMS [86–89]

Murray Bornstein pioneered the early studies of copolymer-1 (Cop1) in RRMS [90] and performed an exploratory study of progressive MS [86]. The major endpoint, confirmed progression of 1.0 or 1.5 units (depending on baseline disability) on the EDSS, was observed in nine (17.6%) treated and 14 (25.5%) control patients. Progression rates at 12 and 24 months were higher for the placebo group ($p = 0.088$). Two-year progression rates for two secondary endpoints, unconfirmed progression, and progression of 0.5 EDSS units were significant ($p = 0.03$).

8.3.2.1 The PROMiSe Study [87, 89]

The first fully powered phase III RCT of DMTs in PPMS examined the utility of glatiramer acetate 20 mg sc daily versus placebo in 943 patients (randomized in a 2:1 ratio) over 3 years [87]. Eligible patients were between 30 and 65 years of age with an entry EDSS score of 3.0–6.5 inclusive. In particular, patients with a history of any relapses were specifically excluded. All patients were required to have progressive neurological symptoms, including evidence of myelopathy for at least 6 months before the screening visit, with objective evidence of pyramidal damage on neurological examination, including a pyramidal Functional System score of 2 or greater. The primary endpoint was an intention-to-treat analysis of the time to confirmed disease progression, defined as an EDSS change of one point or more sustained for 3 months in patients with an EDSS score at baseline of 3.0–5.0, or a 0.5 point sustained for 3 months in patients with a baseline EDSS score of 5.5–6.5. The clinical characteristics of the two groups did not differ at baseline and were typical of this form of MS: duration of illness 10.9 year, mean EDSS score 4.9, mean 25-ft. walk 12.4 s, and 49% men.

Primary Endpoint: This study was stopped prematurely after a second interim analysis at 2 years by the DMSB; at that time, approximately 60% of the study population had received therapy for 2 years. The primary outcome, delay in disability progression did not differ significantly between the two treatment groups (HR = 0.87, 95% CI: 0.71–1.07, $p = 0.1753$).

Secondary Endpoints: The proportion of patients experiencing disability progression was smaller but not significantly so, in the glatiramer acetate (39.6%) than placebo (45.2%) group. Mean EDSS score increased similarly in the two groups and the MSFC scores did not differ significantly. Gadolinium-enhancing lesions were significantly reduced at 1 year in the glatiramer acetate group compared to placebo ($p = 0.0022$) and borderline significant at year 2 ($p = 0.07$). Increased T2 lesion load was less in the glatiramer acetate group but significant only at year 2 ($p = 0.0026$). No significant differences at year 3 in MRI parameters were noted, which reflected the low numbers in the trial at this time point due to the discontinuation of the study at the second interim analysis. A proton MR spectroscopic imaging sub-study found no difference in *N-acetyl* aspartate/creatine and choline/creatine ratios, between glatiramer acetate-treated and placebo-treated patients [88].

Why Was the Primary Endpoint Not Significant? The outcome of any study is invariably influenced by the behavior of the placebo group. One reason for the non-significant result was that placebo group had progressed more slowly than had been calculated at the stage of study design. Post-hoc analysis showed that there was a treatment effect by gender. Men treated with glatiramer acetate progressed significantly more slowly than men treated with placebo (HR = 0.71, 95% CI: 0.53–0.95, $p = 0.0193$) [89]. For women, there was no treatment effect seen (HR = 1.08, 95% CI: 0.79–1.46, $p = 0.63$). The authors argue cogently that this treatment effect was seen because PPMS progresses faster in men than women; in the London Ontario natural history, cohort time from onset to death was significantly more rapid in men than women [80].

8.3.3 Fingolimod in PPMS: The INFORMS Study

The success of fingolimod in the treatment of RRMS represented a step-change in therapy for relapsing-remitting multiple sclerosis. This was the first oral therapy and showed significant improvement in efficacy compared to interferon-beta [67]. Fingolimod improved almost all metrics of disease activity in relapsing-remitting disease: relapse frequency, some effect on disease progression and reduction of MRI lesion activity. Fingolimod has subsequently been tested as a potential therapy for primary progressive MS in the INFORMS trial. This trial was the first major phase III trial of an oral DMT in the treatment of primary progressive MS.

The trial was a multicenter double-blind (n = 970), placebo-controlled trial of fingolimod for the treatment of primary progressive multiple sclerosis [91]. Patients were recruited across 148 centres and were randomized 1:1 to treatment with fingolimod or placebo for at least 36 months. Patients were initially assigned to a higher dose of fingolimod than licensed in standard clinical practice (1.25 mg), but this was later switched during the trial to 0.5 mg daily, which reflects the dose used to treat RRMS. Overall 483 patients were randomized to receive fingolimod and 487 to receive placebo. The primary endpoint was a composite based on change in EDSS, 25FTW and 9HPT, used to assess time to 3-month confirmed disability progression.

Primary Endpoint: The primary efficacy endpoint was not met. There was no difference between the fingolimod and placebo group in time to 3-month confirmed disability progression (hazard ratio 0.95, 95% CI 0.8–1.12, p = 0.54) Similar conclusions were drawn for 6-month confirmed disability progression. This observation was consistent across individual outcomes measures (EDSS, 9HPT, 25TWT).

Secondary Endpoint: There was no effect of treatment on brain atrophy over 3 years. Despite the negative result for the primary clinical endpoint, patients treated with fingolimod had fewer gadolinium-enhancing lesions and new T2 lesions on brain MRI, consistent with the known anti-inflammatory properties of the drug.

Comment: This trial was negative but notable for a number of reasons. Firstly, a consistent criticism of trials in all forms of MS is that trials are too short, and this trial was longer than most. Secondly, the data showed clear evidence of dissociation between inflammatory MRI outcomes and clinical course. While similar observation had been made in interferon trials, the higher immunomodulatory activity of fingolimod throws this observation into sharper relief. The drug was able to suppress inflammatory MS activity on MRI scans by almost 80%, yet there was no effect on disease progression.

The dosing schedules used here are of interest, since the initial dosing were initially higher than used in relapsing-remitting disease, though earlier clinical trials suggested no added advantage of the higher dose, and this observation is confirmed in this trial. It should be remembered than fingolimod, which was originally developed as an immunosuppressive for non-MS inflammatory disease and transplantation, was used in trials for these diseases at higher doses.

8.3.4 Rituximab in PPMS: The OLYMPUS Study [92]

Rituximab is a chimeric monoclonal antibody which targets the CD20 antigen expressed on B lymphocytes at all stages from the pre-B-cell stage except for the plasma cells. It had been shown, in a phase II study, to be effective in reducing MRI evidence of inflammatory activity in RRMS [93]. Given its evident effect in reducing inflammation, a phase III study in PPMS was performed [92]. The OLYMPUS study was a double-blind, placebo-controlled RCT which recruited 439 patients with PPMS in a 2:1 randomization of rituximab to placebo, and followed them for 96 weeks. Recruitment criteria included a diagnosis of PPMS disease with a duration of >1 year and EDSS baseline between 2.0 and 6.5 points with a pyramidal Functional Systems score of 2.0 or greater and presence of CSF IgG oligoclonal bands. The primary efficacy variable was time to confirmed progression by one point or more on the EDSS sustained for 12 weeks if EDSS was <5.5 at baseline, or 0.5 points if the baseline EDSS was >5.5 or =5.5.

Primary Endpoint: The trial demonstrated no significant difference between the rituximab and placebo groups; confirmed progression rates were 38.5% for the placebo and 30.2% for the rituximab group ($HR = 0.77, p = 0.1442$). Serious adverse events were seen in 16.4% of the rituximab group and 13.6% of the placebo group, the excess was explained by 4.5% infection-associated adverse events in the rituximab group and 0.7% of the placebo group.

Secondary Endpoints: The MSFC timed 25-ft. walk test reached significance at 48 weeks ($p < 0.04$), but was not so at 96 weeks ($p = 0.076$). The overall MSFC change score (and 9-hole peg test and PASAT components individually) showed no difference between groups. In the rituximab group, there was less increase in the T2 lesion volume compared to placebo ($p < 0.001$); the median increase in T2 lesion volume was 301.95 mm^3 for rituximab and 809.5 mm^3 for placebo. Brain volume decrease was similar in both groups ($p = 0.62$).

Subgroup analyses revealed important differences with an additive predictive effect of age and the presence of gadolinium-enhancing lesions at baseline. Patients aged under 51 years with baseline gadolinium-enhancing lesions who were treated with placebo had a three-time higher risk of progression than those treated with rituximab (HR = 0.33, $p = 0.009$). Patients with a shorter disease duration (<3 years) treated with rituximab had a longer time to confirmed progression than those treated with placebo. Age of the patient at study entry seemed to be a more important factor in relation to a treatment effect than duration of illness.

Comment: The trial demonstrated that in patients with PPMS who were younger and who had more active inflammation on baseline MRI (and who tended to have more rapid progression) there was a statistically significant treatment effect. In comparison to PROMiSe there was no effect of gender on the treatment effect. The authors concluded that, while neurological progression in PPMS is mediated by degeneration of demyelinated axons, a sub-group of PPMS patients have inflammatory disease activity, which may be susceptible to amelioration by B-cell depletion. This effect may be particularly seen in younger patients with a shorter duration of illness and with gadolinium enhancement on the baseline MRI brain scan.

8.3.5 Ocrelizumab in PPMS: The ORATORIO Study

While the primary endpoint of the OLYMPUS study was negative, the subgroup analyses seemed to suggest the potential for certain patients to response to therapies which target B-cells. In particular, younger patients with Gd-enhancing lesions appeared to show some evidence of a treatment response, although caution is always need in the interpretation of subgroup analyses. While rituximab is a chimeric antibody, fully humanized antibodies have subsequently been developed. While these may be associated with fewer infusion reactions, it is not clear whether these newer antibodies offer a meaningful improvement in safety profile over the much-used rituximab. This is particularly relevant since it is likely that cheaper biosimilar versions of rituximab will be available in the near future. The fully humanised cell-depleting anti-CD20 antibodies include ocrelizumab and the efficacy of both chimeric and fully humanised anti-CD20 monoclonal antibodies has been demonstrated in relapsing-remitting MS [94, 95]. The efficacy of ocrelizumab in the treatment of primary progressive multiple sclerosis has recently been evaluated in the ORATORIO trial [96].

The design of ORATORIO trial was based in part on subgroup analyses of the rituximab trial described above. As such the patient population was selected to reflect the subgroups which appeared to have some response to rituximab, in particular younger patients (<50 years) with enhancing lesions on MRI.

Primary Endpoint: There was a significant reduction in 3-month confirmed disability progression in the ocrelizumab group compared to placebo by 24% ($p = 0.03$).

Secondary Endpoint: Significant effects were seen on assessments of walking. At week 120, 38.9% of patients treated with ocrelizumab experienced worsening compared to 55.1% with placebo ($p = 0.04$). From a safety perspective, 2.3% of patients treated with ocrelizumab developed neoplasia, compared to 0.8% in the placebo group and infusion reactions and infections were all more common in the treatment group. This highlights an unclear long-term risk benefit profile which will require further clarification.

Comment: The ORATORIO study shows that treatment of PPMS with targeted B-cell therapies might represent a promising therapeutic strategy. However, it should be noted that the very modest efficacy demonstrated in PPMS is in contrast to the much stronger effects in active RRMS [95]. It should also be noted that, by enriching the study population for patients who might be most likely to respond, the study population does not reflect real life populations with PPMS. Therefore, extrapolation of the results to everyday clinical practice represents a challenge. However, despite the modesty of the results, these studies raise important questions as to whether B cells might continue to play a role in the pathogenesis of disease, even in its later stages.

8.4 Conclusions and Future Directions

Taken together these studies allow a number of conclusions to be drawn about the use of licensed DMTs in the treatment of progressive forms of MS:

8.4.1 Therapies Proven to Work for RRMS Are Not Very Effective in the Treatment of Progressive MS

Five years ago, we could be less certain about this conclusion because most large well-conducted trials had used drugs which only modest efficacy in RRMS. However, many of the drugs which have strong anti-inflammatory effects have now been tested in progressive disease, in particular natalizumab and fingolimod. The results of these trials are unequivocal in showing that progressive MS does not respond well to these agents.

8.4.2 There May be a Minor Role for These Therapies in a Limited Subset of Patients

The more promising results from anti-B-cell therapies suggest that there may be subsets of patients with residual inflammatory disease who might potentially benefit from treatment with conventional DMTs. However, extrapolation of these trials to clinical practice is problematic and, even in those patients who respond, the magnitude of benefit is questionable. These therapies carry significant associated risks and the balance of risk-benefit remains to be determined, in particular over the long-term.

8.4.3 Trial Design is Still Being Optimised

It is worth remembering the nihilism which permeated trials for RRMS in the years prior to the interferon trials. The subsequent use of sensitive imaging biomarkers and identification of patient populations who respond well to treatment helped open to the door to a number of effective therapies. In the context of SPMS and PPMS trials, progress has been made in identifying patients and outcome measures which are most sensitive to therapy and this will inform the conduct of future trials.

8.4.4 The Inflammation of Progressive Disease Differs from that of Inflammatory Disease

Inflammation is clearly present in the progressive phase of disease, but many lines of evidence suggest that this differs from the inflammation of the acute inflammatory stage, in terms of cellular and humoral immune effectors and their temporal and spatial distribution. Many currently licensed DMTs target lymphocyte-driven disease arising in the peripheral immune system, either by a cytotoxic effect, or by altering lymphocyte distribution away from the brain. The inflammation of progressive disease may well be more compartmentalized within the CNS and thus less immediately accessible to drug therapy.

8.4.5 If Transformative Therapies for Progressive MS Are to be Delivered, Novel Approaches Will be Needed

Perhaps the most critical finding is that we now know our existing armoury of multiple sclerosis DMTs will likely be insufficient for the treatment of the large numbers of patients with progressive disease. It is important we recognize that the extraordinary progress in RRMS therapies is unlikely to meet the wider needs of people with MS, the majority of whom are experiencing disease progression. As a result, true discovery will be needed at a preclinical and clinical level to deliver the transformative therapies which are so badly needed.

References

1. IFN-(Multiple Sclerosis Study Group). Interferon beta-1b is effective in relapsing-remitting multiple sclerosis. I. Clinical results of a multicenter-randomised, double blind, placebo-controlled trial. Neurology. 1993;43:655–61.
2. Jacobs LD, Cookfair DL, Rudick RA, et al. Intramuscular interferon beta-1a for disease progression in relapsing multiple sclerosis. Ann Neurol. 1996;39:285–94.
3. PRISMS (Prevention of relapses and disability by interferon beta-1a subcutaneously in multiple sclerosis) Study Group. Randomized double-blind placebo controlled study of interferon beta-1a in relapsing/remitting multiple sclerosis. Lancet. 1998;352:1498–504.
4. Johnson KP, Brooks BR, Cohen JA. Extended use of glatiramer acetate (Copaxone) is well tolerated and maintains its clinical effect on multiple sclerosis relapse rate and degree of disability. Copolymer 1 Multiple Sclerosis Study Group. Neurology. 1998;50:701–8.
5. Ontaneda D, Fox RJ, Chataway J. Clinical trials in progressive multiple sclerosis: lessons learned and future perspectives. Lancet Neurol. 2015;14(2):208–23.
6. Mahad DH, Trapp BD, Lassmann H. Pathological mechanisms in progressive multiple sclerosis. Lancet Neurol. 2015;14(2):183–93.
7. Schumacher FA, Beeve GW, Kibler RF, et al. Problems of experimental trials of therapy in multiple sclerosis. Ann N Y Acad Sci. 1965;122:552–68.
8. Poser CM, Paty DW, Scheinberg LC, et al. New diagnostic criteria for multiple sclerosis: guidelines for research protocols. Ann Neurol. 1983;1:227–31.
9. McDonald WI, Compston A, Edan G, et al. Recommended diagnostic criteria for multiple sclerosis: guidelines from the International Panel on the diagnosis of multiple sclerosis. Ann Neurol. 2001;50:121–7.
10. Polman CH, Reingold SC, Edan G, et al. Diagnostic criteria for multiple sclerosis: 2005 revisions to the "McDonald criteria". Ann Neurol. 2005;58:840–6.
11. Polman CH, Reingold SC, Banwell B. Diagnostic criteria for multiple sclerosis: 2010 revisions to the "McDonald criteria". Ann Neurol. 2011;69:292–302.
12. Thompson AJ, Polman CH, Miller DH, et al. Primary progressive multiple sclerosis. Brain. 1997;120:1085–96.
13. Lublin FD, Reingold SC. Defining the clinical course of multiple sclerosis: results of an international survey. National Multiple Sclerosis Society (USA) Advisory Committee on Clinical Trials of New Agents in Multiple Sclerosis. Neurology. 1996;46:907–11.
14. Kurtzke JF. Rating neurologic impairment in multiple sclerosis: an expanded disability status scale (EDSS). Neurology. 1983;33:1444–52.
15. Cutter GR, Baier ML, Rudick RA, et al. Development of a multiple sclerosis functional composite as a clinical trial outcome measure. Brain. 1999;122:871–82.
16. Wilkins A, Scolding N. Protecting axons in multiple sclerosis. Mult Scler. 2008;14:1013–25.
17. Stys PK, et al. Will the real multiple sclerosis please stand up? Nat Rev Neurosci. 2012;13(7):507–14.
18. Boggild M, et al. Multiple sclerosis risk sharing scheme: two year results of clinical cohort study with historical comparator. BMJ. 2009;339:b4677.
19. Palace J, et al. UK multiple sclerosis risk-sharing scheme: a new natural history dataset and an improved Markov model. BMJ Open. 2014;4(1):e004073.
20. Hartung HP, Aktas O. Evolution of multiple sclerosis treatment: next generation therapies meet next generation efficacy criteria. Lancet Neurol. 2011;10(4):293–5.
21. Lublin FD, Reingold SC. Placebo-controlled clinical trials in multiple sclerosis: ethical considerations. National Multiple Sclerosis Society (USA) Task Force on Placebo-Controlled Clinical Trials in MS. Ann Neurol. 2001;49:677–81.
22. McFarland HF, Reingold SC. The future of multiple sclerosis therapies: redesigning multiple sclerosis clinical trials in a new therapeutic era. Mult Scler. 2005;11:669–76.
23. Polman CH, Reingold SC, Barkhof F, et al. Ethics of placebo-controlled clinical trials in multiple sclerosis: a reassessment. Neurology. 2008;70:1134–40.

24. European Study Group on Interferon beta-1b in Secondary Progressive MS. Placebo-controlled multicentre randomized trial of interferon beta-1b in treatment of secondary progressive multiple sclerosis. Lancet. 1998;352:1491–7.
25. Miller DH, Molyneux PD, Barker GJ, et al. Effect of interferon-1b on magnetic resonance imaging outcomes in secondary progressive multiple sclerosis: results of a European multicenter, randomized, double-blind, placebo controlled trial. Ann Neurol. 1999;46:850–9.
26. Brex PA, Molyneux PD, Smiddy P, et al. The effect of IFNbeta-1b on the evolution of enhancing lesions in secondary progressive MS. Neurology. 2001;57:2185–90.
27. Molyneux PD, Kappos L, Polman C. The effect of interferon beta-1b treatment on MRI meaures of cerebral atrophy in secondary progressive multiple sclerosis. European Study Group on Interferon beta-1b in secondary progressive multiple sclerosis. Brain. 2000;123:2256–63.
28. Molyneux PD, Barker GJ, Barkhof F, et al. Clinical-MRI correlations in a European trial of interferon beta-1b in secondary progressive MS. Neurology. 2001;57:2191–7.
29. Kappos L, Weinshenker B, Pozzilli C, et al. Interferon beta-1b in secondary progressive MS: a combined analysis of the two trials. Neurology. 2004;63:1779–87.
30. Panitch H, Miller A, Paty D, Weinshenker B, et al. Interferon beta-1b in secondary progressive MS: results from a 3-year controlled study. Neurology. 2004;63:1788–95.
31. Secondary Progressive Efficacy Clinical Trial of Recombinant Interferon-Beta-1a in MS (SPECTRIMS) Study Group. Randomized controlled trial of interferon-beta-1a in secondary progressive MS: clinical results. Neurology. 2001;56:1496–504.
32. Patten SB, Metz LM. SPECTRIMS Study Group. Interferon beta-1a and depression in secondary progressive MS: data from the SPECTRIMS Trial. Neurology. 2002;59:744–6.
33. Li DK, Zhao GJ, Paty DW, University of British Columbia MS/MRI Analysis Research Group. The SPECTRIMS Study Group. Randomized controlled trial of interferon-beta-1a in secondary progressive MS: MRI results. Neurology. 2001;56:1505–13.
34. Cohen JA, Cutter GR, Fischer JS, et al. Benefit of interferon beta-1a on MSFC progression in secondary progressive MS. Neurology. 2002;59:679–87.
35. Rudick R, Polman C, Cohen J, et al. Assessing disability progression with the Multiple Sclerosis Functional Composite. Mult Scler. 2009;15:984–97.
36. Andersen O, Elovaara I, Farkkila M, et al. Multicentre, randomised, double blind, placebo controlled, phase III study of weekly, low dose, subcutaneous interferon beta-1a in secondary progressive multiple sclerosis. J Neurol Neurosurg Psychiatry. 2004;75:706–10.
37. Comi G, Fillippi M, Barkhof F, et al. Effect of early interferon treatment on conversion to clinically definite multiple sclerosis: a randomized study. Lancet. 2001;357:1576–82.
38. Jacobs L, Beck RW, Simon JH, et al. Intramuscular interferon beta-1a therapy initiated during a first demyelinating event in multiple sclerosis. N Engl J Med. 2000;343:898–904.
39. Hartung HP, Gonsette R, Konig N, et al. Mitoxantrone in progressive multiple sclerosis: a placebo-controlled, double-blind, randomised, multicentre trial. Lancet. 2002;360:2018–25.
40. Krapf H, Morrissey SP, Zenker O, Zwingers T, Gonsette R, Hartung HP, MIMS Study Group. Effect of mitoxantrone on MRI in progressive MS: results of the MIMS trial. Neurology. 2005;65:690–5.
41. Edan G, Miller D, Clanet M, et al. Therapeutic effect of mitoxantrone combined with methylprednisolone in multiple sclerosis: a randomised multicentre study of active disease using MRI and clinical criteria. J Neurol Neurosurg Psychiatry. 1997;62:112–8.
42. Esposito F, Radaelli M, Martinelli V, et al. Comparative study of mitoxantrone efficacy profile in patients with relapsing-remitting and secondary progressive multiple sclerosis. Mult Scler. 2010;16:1490–9.
43. Marriott JJ, Miyasaki JM, Gronseth G, O'Connor PW, Therapeutics and Technology Assessment Subcommittee of the American Academy of Neurology. Evidence Report: the efficacy and safety of mitoxantrone (Novantrone) in the treatment of multiple sclerosis: report of the Therapeutics and Technology Assessment Subcommittee of the American Academy of Neurology. Neurology. 2010;74:1463–70.
44. Ghalie RG, Mauch E, Edan G, Hartung HP, et al. A study of therapy related acute leukaemia after mitoxantrone therapy for multiple sclerosis. Mult Scler. 2002;8:441–5.

45. Ellis R, Boggild M. Therapy-related acute leukaemia with mitoxantrone: what is the risk and can we minimise it? Mult Scler. 2009;15:505–8.
46. Martinelli Boneschi F, Rovaris M, Capra R, Comi G. Mitoxantrone for multiple sclerosis. Cochrane Database Syst Rev. 2005;4:CD002127. Review 83.
47. Hommes OR, Sorensen PS, Fazekas F, et al. Intravenous immunoglobulin in secondary progressive multiple sclerosis: randomised placebo-controlled trial. Lancet. 2004;364:1149–56.
48. Fazekas F, Sorensen PS, Filippi M, et al. MRI results from the European study on intravenous immunoglobulin in secondary progressive multiple sclerosis (ESIMS). Mult Scler. 2005;11:433–40.
49. Filippi M, Rocca MA, Pagani E, et al. European study on intravenous immunoglobulin in multiple sclerosis: results of magnetization transfer magnetic resonance imaging analysis. Arch Neurol. 2004;61:1409–12.
50. Gray O, McDonnell GV, Forbes RB. Intravenous immunoglobulins for multiple sclerosis. Cochrane Database Syst Rev. 2003;3:CD002936. doi:10.1002/14651858.CD002936.
51. Goodkin DE, Kinkel RP, Weinstock-Guttman B. A phase II study of i.v. methylprednisolone in secondary-progressive multiple sclerosis. Neurology. 1998;51:239–45.
52. Ciccone A, Beretta S, Brusaferri F, Galea I, Protti A, Spreafico C. Corticosteroids for the longterm treatment in multiple sclerosis. Cochrane Database Syst Rev. 2008;1:CD006264. doi:10.1002/14651858.CD006264.pub2.
53. Cook SD, Devereux C, Troiano R, et al. Effect of total lymphoid irradiation in chronic progressive multiple sclerosis. Lancet. 1986;1:1405–9.
54. Gordon PA, Carroll DJ, Etches WS, et al. A double-blind controlled pilot study of plasma exchange versus sham apheresis in chronic progressive multiple sclerosis. Can J Neurol Sci. 1985;12:39–44.
55. Perini P, Calabrese M, Tiberio M, Ranzato F, Battistin L, Gallo P. Mitoxantrone versus cyclophosphamide in secondary-progressive multiple sclerosis: a comparative study. J Neurol. 2006;253:1034–40.
56. Perini P, Gallo P. Cyclophosphamide is effective in stabilizing rapidly deteriorating secondary progressive multiple sclerosis. J Neurol. 2003;250:834–8.
57. Schwartzman RJ, Simpkins N, Alexander GM, et al. High-dose cyclophosphamide in the treatment of multiple sclerosis. CNS Neurosci Ther. 2009;15:118–27.
58. Lugaresi A, Caporale C, Farina D, et al. Low-dose oral methotrexate treatment in chronic progressive multiple sclerosis. Neurol Sci. 2001;22:209–10.
59. Rice GP, Filippi M, Comi G. Cladribine and progressive MS: clinical and MRI outcomes of a multicenter controlled trial Cladribine MRI Study Group. Neurology. 2000;54:1145–55.
60. Wiendl H, Kieseier BC, Weissert R. Treatment of active secondary progressive multiple sclerosis with treosulfan. J Neurol. 2007;254:884–9.
61. Mancardi GL, Murialdo A, Rossi P, et al. Autologous stem cell transplantation as rescue therapy in malignant forms of multiple sclerosis. Mult Scler. 2005;11:367–71.
62. Reston JT, Uhl S, Treadwell JR, Nash RA, Schoelles K. Autologous hematopoietic cell transplantation for multiple sclerosis: a systematic review. Mult Scler. 2011;17:204–13.
63. Jeffery DR. The argument against the use of cyclophosphamide and mitoxantrone in the treatment of multiple sclerosis. J Neurol Sci. 2004;223:41–6.
64. Polman CH, et al. A randomized, placebo-controlled trial of natalizumab for relapsing multiple sclerosis. N Engl J Med. 2006;354(9):899–910.
65. Bloomgren G, et al. Risk of natalizumab-associated progressive multifocal leukoencephalopathy. N Engl J Med. 2012;366(20):1870–80.
66. Steiner D, et al. Natalizumab versus placebo in patients with secondary progressive multiple sclerosis (SPMS): results from ASCEND, a Multicenter, Double-blind, Placebo-Controlled, Randomized Phase 3 Clinical Trial. Am Acad Neurol. 2016:P009.
67. Kappos L, et al. A placebo-controlled trial of oral fingolimod in relapsing multiple sclerosis. N Engl J Med. 2010;362(5):387–401.
68. Calabresi PA, et al. Safety and efficacy of fingolimod in patients with relapsing-remitting multiple sclerosis (FREEDOMS II): a double-blind, randomised, placebo-controlled, phase 3 trial. Lancet Neurol. 2014;13(6):545–56.

69. Kappos L, et al. Safety and efficacy of siponimod (BAF312) in patients with relapsing-remitting multiple sclerosis: dose-blinded, randomized extension of the phase 2 BOLD study. JAMA Neurol. 2016;73(9):1089–98.
70. Selmaj K, et al. Siponimod for patients with relapsing-remitting multiple sclerosis (BOLD): an adaptive, dose-ranging, randomised, phase 2 study. Lancet Neurol. 2013;12(8):756–67.
71. Kappos L, Bar-Or A, Cree B, et al. Efficacy and safety of siponimod in secondary progressive multiple sclerosis—Results of the placebo controlled, double-blind, Phase III EXPAND study. ECTRIMS 2016. London, UK: ECTRIMS Online Library; 2016.
72. Kappos L, Bar-Or A, Cree B, Fox R, Giovannoni G, Gold R, Vermersch P, Arnould S, Sidorenko T, Wolf C, Wallström E, Dahlke F. 002—Efficacy of siponimod in secondary progressive multiple sclerosis: results of the phase 3 study. Boston, MA, USA: 69th Annual Meeting of the American Academy of Neurology; 2017.
73. Paolillo A, Coles AJ, Molyneux PD, et al. Quantitative MRI in patients with secondary progressive MS treated with monoclonal antibody Campath1H. Neurology. 1999;53:751–7.
74. Confavreux C, Vukusic S, Moreau T, Adeleine P. Relapses and progression of disability in multiple sclerosis. N Engl J Med. 2000;343:1430–8.
75. Confavreux C, Vukusic S, Adeleine P. Early clinical predictors and progression of irreversible disability in multiple sclerosis: an amnesic process. Brain. 2003;126:770–82.
76. Kremenchutzky M, Rice GP, Baskerville J, Wingerchuk DM, Ebers GC. The natural history of multiple sclerosis: a geographically based study 9: observations on the progressive phase of the disease. Brain. 2006;129:584–94.
77. Koch M, Kingwell E, Rieckmann P, Neurologists THUBCMSC. The natural history of secondary progressive multiple sclerosis. J Neurol Neurosurg Psychiatry. 2010;81:1039–43.
78. Koch M, Kingwell E, Rieckmann P, Tremlett H. The natural history of primary progressive multiple sclerosis. Neurology. 2009;73:1996–2002.
79. Tremlett H, Zhao Y, Devonshire V, UBC Neurologists. Natural history comparisons of primary and secondary progressive multiple sclerosis reveals differences and similarities. J Neurol. 2009;256:374–81.
80. Cottrell DA, Kremenchutzky M, Rice GP, Hader W, Baskerville J, Ebers GC. The natural history of multiple sclerosis: a geographically based study. 6. Applications to planning and interpretation of clinical therapeutic trials in primary progressive multiple sclerosis. Brain. 1999;122:641–7.
81. Montalban X, Thompson AJ. Workshop on primary progressive multiple sclerosis: meeting summary. Mult Scler. 2002;8:177–8.
82. Wolinsky JS. PROMiSe Study Group. The diagnosis of primary progressive multiple sclerosis. J Neurol Sci. 2003;206:145–52.
83. Leary SM, Miller DH, Stevenson VL, et al. Interferon beta-1a in primary progressive MS: an exploratory, randomized, controlled trial. Neurology. 2003;60:44–51.
84. Montalban X, Sastre-Garriga J, Tintore M, et al. A single-center, randomized, double-blind, placebo-controlled study of interferon beta-1b on primary progressive and transitional multiple sclerosis. Mult Scler. 2009;15:1195–205.
85. Rojas JI, Romano M, Ciapponi A, Patrucco L, Cristiano E. Interferon beta for primary progressive multiple sclerosis. Cochrane Database Syst Rev. 2009;1:CD006643. Review. Update in: Cochrane Database Syst Rev. 2010;(1):CD006643.
86. Bornstein MB, Miller A, Slagle S, et al. A placebo-controlled, double-blind, randomized, two-center, pilot trial of Cop 1 in chronic progressive multiple sclerosis. Neurology. 1991;41:533–9.
87. Wolinsky JS, Narayana PA, O'Connor P, et al. Glatiramer acetate in primary progressive multiple sclerosis: results of a multinational, multicenter, double-blind, placebo-controlled trial. Ann Neurol. 2007;61:14–24.
88. Sajja BR, Narayana PA, Wolinsky JS, Ahn CW, PROMiSe Trial MRSI. Group. Longitudinal magnetic resonance spectroscopic imaging of primary progressive multiple sclerosis patients treated with glatiramer acetate: multicenter study. Mult Scler. 2008;14:73–80.
89. Wolinsky JS, Shochat T, Weiss S, Ladkani D. PROMiSe Trial Study Group. Glatiramer acetate treatment in PPMS: why males appear to respond favorably. J Neurol Sci. 2009;286:92–8.

90. Bornstein MB, Miller A, Slagle S, et al. A pilot trial of Cop 1 in exacerbating-remitting multiple sclerosis. N Engl J Med. 1987;317:408–14.
91. Lublin F, et al. Oral fingolimod in primary progressive multiple sclerosis (INFORMS): a phase 3, randomised, double-blind, placebo-controlled trial. Lancet. 2016;387(10023):1075–84.
92. Hawker K, O'Connor P, Freedman MS, OLYMPUS Trial Group. Rituximab in patients with primary progressive multiple sclerosis: results of a randomized double-blind placebo-controlled multicenter trial. Ann Neurol. 2009;66:460–71.
93. Hauser SL, Waubant E, Arnold DL, HERMES Trial Group. B-cell depletion with rituximab in relapsing-remitting multiple sclerosis. N Engl J Med. 2008;358:676–88.
94. Kappos L, et al. Ocrelizumab in relapsing-remitting multiple sclerosis: a phase 2, randomised, placebo-controlled, multicentre trial. Lancet. 2011;378(9805):1779–87.
95. Hauser SL, et al. B-cell depletion with rituximab in relapsing-remitting multiple sclerosis. N Engl J Med. 2008;358(7):676–88.
96. Montalban X, et al. Ocrelizumab versus Placebo in Primary Progressive Multiple Sclerosis. N Engl J Med. 2017;376(3):209–20.

Chapter 9
Trials of Novel Therapies Specifically for Progressive MS

R.S. Nicholas, A. Nandoskar, M. Hutchinson, and T. Friede

9.1 Introduction

Randomised placebo-controlled trials over three decades have attempted to demonstrate slowing of disability accrual in progressive multiple sclerosis (PMS). However, it was not until 2017 that the first drug was licensed, Ocrelizumab for primary progressive MS which was also licensed in relapsing (R)MS [1]. It has been argued over many years that treatments targeting RMS will have an impact on PMS as RMS is a precursor of secondary (S)PMS [2]. In a systematic review and meta-analysis 11 of 43 randomised placebo-controlled trials in PMS utilised treatments licensed for RMS [3]; up until 2017 no treatment principally designed to target RMS, had resulted in a license. There are many reasons for this lack of success including a developing understanding of the pathology, limitations of the outcome measures and an evolution of trial design. Novel molecules and approaches have been a feature of the clinical trials that have been undertaken over the past three decades in PMS. In this review we have restricted our discussion to therapies that have been used in randomised placebo-controlled trials in PMS.

R.S. Nicholas (✉) • A. Nandoskar
Centre for Neuroinflammation and Neurodegeneration, Imperial College London, Hammersmith Campus, Du Cane Road, London W12 0NN, UK
e-mail: r.nicholas@imperial.ac.uk

M. Hutchinson
St Vincent's University Hospital, Dublin, Ireland

Newman Clinical Research, University College Dublin, Dublin, Ireland

T. Friede
Department of Medical Statistics, University Medical Center Göttingen, Humboltallee 32, Göttingen 37073, Germany

A. Wilkins (ed.), *Progressive Multiple Sclerosis*,
https://doi.org/10.1007/978-3-319-65921-3_9

9.2 Changing Placebo Populations in Randomised Controlled Trials in PMS: Help or Hindrance?

A systematic review of randomised placebo-controlled trials in PMS found 43 trials that were reported between 1988 and 2016. The trials were evenly spread with half being published before or in 2002. The majority recruited mixed populations of SPMS/primary (P)PMS. Only five (12%) trials recruited a pure PPMS population starting from 2003 onwards, notably this is where ocrelizumab achieved its license in 2017. As has been widely recognised with RMS trials the characteristics of the study populations have evolved as the environment has changed [4–7]. Similarly the population taking part in PMS trials has also evolved over time. The placebo participants are older with their mean age increasing by roughly 1 year for every three calendar years with a trend towards longer disease duration and increased trial entry level disability with mean EDSS scores increasing over 28 years by over 0.7 points starting from an average of just under 5 points in the early trials. Importantly the on-trial disability accumulation in placebo subjects is changing. Over such a prolonged period with evolving ideas on outcome it was only possible to get a proportion of placebo subjects progressing over 2 years with the majority of results either having unconfirmed disability or confirmed at 3 months. However, over the 28-year study period there was a 21% reduction in the proportion of patients experiencing progression. The use of an outcome, which is known to be impacted by relapses, could indicate the removal of the RMS population consistent with the development of treatment for RMS. There has been some emphasis, at least by European regulators [8], on 6-month confirmation of disease progression. But in fact the population change may have increased the relevance of a 3 month confirmed disability outcome as the majority of those progressing are experiencing true progression rather than relapse driven disability change (Nicholas et al. 2017 in preparation).

9.3 PMS Trials Targeting Inflammation

9.3.1 Antibodies to Interferon Gamma or TNF Alpha

Cytokines upregulating cellular immunity and produced by monocytes (IL1, TNFa) and by Th1 helpers cells (IL2, IFNg, TNFb) are thought to drive the pathological process and tissue injury in MS, whereas cytokines produced by Th2 helper cells (IL4, IL10) have been shown to suppress Th1 helper cells and cell mediated immunity [9]. In a double-blind, placebo-controlled trial, 45 patients with active SPMS were randomized to three groups of 15 patients, each receiving a short course of antibodies to IFNg, TNFa, or placebo. Outcome measures after 12 months were EDSS, lymphocyte subpopulations, cytokine production levels, MRI, and evoked potentials. Only patients who received antibodies to IFNg showed a significant increase in the number of patients without confirmed disability progression versus placebo. MRI also showed a decrease in the number of active lesions with IFNg versus placebo and baseline ($p < 0.05$) [10].

9.3.2 *Azathioprine*

Azathioprine (AZ) is a purine antagonist that impairs DNA replication and reduces T and B lymphocyte function [11]. A Cochrane review of the efficacy of AZ in the treatment of MS included five randomized, double blind, placebo-controlled trials that lasted at least 1 year and had a primary outcome aiming to show that AZ effects on disability progression [12]. A total of 698 MS patients, were included but data from only 87 PMS subjects were available. There was a statistically significant benefit (RR, 95% CI: 0.42 [0.07, 0.64]) favouring AZ therapy at 3 years' follow-up; this result was robust after sensitivity analyses.

The largest trial in the Cochrane review included RRMS and PMS patients, but was not included in the Cochrane review progression analysis. Three hundred and fifty-four patients were randomised to receive either AZ 2.5 mg/kg daily or placebo [13]. After 3 years the mean increase in EDSS was 0.62 with AZ and 0.80 with placebo, a difference of 0.18. There was a non-significant reduction in relapses in the AZ group (average 2.2) compared to the placebo group (average 2.5). The second included PMS study included 98 PPMS and SPMS subjects [14]. The aim was to determine the effect of AZ alone or AZ in combination with methylprednisolone. The "intent-to-treat" analysis of the three treatment groups showed no statistically significant differences in the rates of progression though the AZ treated groups had half the relapse rate of the placebo-treated group. The third included study was [15] a single blind randomised parallel group trial. The trial randomised 185 subjects (74 RR 40%; 111 SPMS 60%): 93 to AZ (2.5 mg/kg/daily) and 92 to placebo. Only 135 (73%) were included in the final analysis (AZ 69; placebo 66). Out of 37 patients with relapsing-progressive disease course in the AZ group 19 improved or were stable in terms of DSS over 18 months (51%) while 25 out of 44 control patients were reported as stable or improved (57%). The fourth included PMS study [16] randomised 40 patients in a double blind trial, 19 received AZ (2 mg/kg daily) and 21 received placebo. The trial lasted 3 years. 47.5% had a relapsing course and 52.5% PMS. Twenty-one patients dropped out of the study (12 AZ and 9 placebo). At the end of the study 82% of the placebo group had deteriorated by one or more points on the EDSS compared with 38% in the AZ group. This was statistically significant ($p = 0.051$).

9.3.3 *B-Cell Depleting Therapies*

The key role of B cells in driving the pathology has emerged from the study of both the pathology and the knowledge gained from clinical trials [17]. Three trials have targeted B cells in PMS, two using Rituximab ([18]; NCT01212094) and one using Ocrelizumab [1].

9.3.3.1 Rituximab

Rituximab is a chimeric mAb of the IgG1j type that targets CD20, which is expressed by more than 95% of B cells [19]. Rituximab has been used in two trials one in PPMS and the other in SPMS. In the PPMS trial 439 subjects were randomised in a 2:1 ratio to either rituximab or placebo. The percentage of patients with confirmed disease progression at 96 weeks was not statistically different between the two groups (38.5% for placebo versus 30.2% for rituximab). A subgroup analysis highlighted that responders may be of younger age with Gd+ lesions [18]. In the second double blind trial it was planned to recruit 80 low-Inflammatory SPMS subjects and randomise them to rituximab given in combination both by intravenous and intrathecal injection versus placebo (RIVITaLISe, NCT01212094). In the treatment arm patients received 25 mg of rituximab into the CSF and 200 mg of rituximab intravenously at Month 0, followed by additional 200 mg rituximab intravenously at month 0.5 and another 25 mg of rituximab into CSF at months 1.5 and 12. The trial involved a 1-year pre-treatment baseline series of visits, followed by a 2-year treatment period. The trial had an adaptive design and all defined outcome measures collected in the first 30 enrolled patients were transformed into z-scores and compared for the robustness of longitudinal change over the coefficient of variation. As a result, the primary outcome measure of this trial was the comparison of individualized rates of brain atrophy progression between the rituximab and placebo groups after 2 years of treatment; unless the predetermined analysis established that one of the secondary outcome measures has a higher z-score. The trial was terminated early as a planned interim analysis for the efficacy of B cell depletion from the intrathecal compartment fitted the criteria for futility: if less than 50% of intrathecal B cells were depleted by active treatment (measured by <25% decrease in CSF CXCL13 and <50% increase in CSF BAFF). At that point 43 subjects had entered the trial. Sixteen subjects did not proceed from year 1 into the treatment phase and nine subjects received placebo and 18 rituximab (https://clinicaltrials.gov/ct2/show/NCT01212094).

9.3.3.2 Ocrelizumab

Ocrelizumab is a second-generation anti-CD20 monoclonal antibody with a humanized IgG1 tail that binds to a different but overlapping epitope to rituximab. It was thought to be less immunogenic than rituximab with a more favourable risk profile [20]. However the development of ocrelizumab has been suspended in rheumatoid arthritis and Systemic Lupus Erthymatosis (SLE) as phase III trials did not demonstrate additional benefit over existing therapies and in fact demonstrated more serious infections in SLE [21]. Seven hundred and thirty-two PPMS subjects were randomised in a 2:1 ratio to receive intravenous ocrelizumab (600 mg) or placebo every 24 weeks for at least 120 weeks and until a prespecified number of confirmed disability progression events had occurred. The primary end point was the percentage of patients with disability progression confirmed at 12 weeks in a time-to-event analysis. The trial was successful with a significant reduction in the percentage of patients with 12 week confirmed disability progression; 32.9% with ocrelizumab versus 39.3% with placebo (hazard ratio, 0.76; 95% CI, 0.59 to 0.98; P = 0.03). This was replicated in the 24 week confirmed disability progression; 29.6% with ocrelizumab versus 35.7% with placebo (hazard ratio, 0.75; 95% CI, 0.58 to 0.98; P = 0.04). By week 120, performance on the timed 25-foot walk worsened by 38.9% with ocrelizumab versus 55.1% with placebo (P = 0.04); the total volume of brain lesions on T2-weighted magnetic resonance imaging (MRI) decreased by 3.4% with ocrelizumab and increased by 7.4% with placebo ($P < 0.001$); and the percentage of brain-volume loss was 0.90% with ocrelizumab versus 1.09% with placebo (P = 0.02). Neoplasms occurred in 2.3% of patients who received ocrelizumab and in 0.8% of patients who received placebo; there was no clinically significant difference between groups in the rates of serious adverse events and serious infections [1]. Ocrelizumab has recently received a license in the USA for PPMS and also RMS (https://www.fda.gov/newsevents/newsroom/pressannouncements/ucm549325.htm).

9.3.4 Cladribine

Cladribine (CL) (2-chlorodeoxyadenosine) is an adenosine deaminase-resistant purine nucleoside chemotherapeutic agent. It produces lymphocyte depletion and long-lasting lymphopenia [22]. Initially, CL was tested intravenously in PMS in a randomized double-blind clinical trial [23] in 51 subjects with PMS with a cross-over to placebo after 1 year. There was a reported favourable influence on both EDSS, Scripps Neurologic Rating Scale (SNRS) scores and the MRI findings in patients treated with CL. In the first year the most striking finding was that while clinical deterioration continued in the placebo-treated patients, the condition of patients who received CL stabilized or even improved slightly [24]. CL was also tested in an oral trial [25] where 159 PMS subjects were randomised to placebo or CL 0.07 mg/kg/day for 5 consecutive days every 4 weeks for either two or six cycles (total dose, 0.7 mg/kg or 2.1 mg/kg, respectively), followed by placebo, for a total of eight cycles. The primary outcome measure was mean change in EDSS. This was not significantly different among the groups at the end of the 12-month double-blind phase. Both CL treatments were superior to placebo those patients who had Gd+ lesions (p = 0.003).

9.3.5 Cyclophosphamide

Cyclophosphamide (CPM) is a widely used alkylating chemotherapeutic agent that forms active metabolites that bind DNA and interferes with mitosis and cell replication [26]. CPM was assessed in a single randomised, placebo-controlled, single-blind study of 168 patients with PMS [27]. Patients were randomised to receive intravenous CPM and oral prednisone (n = 55); daily oral CPM, alternate day prednisone (22 weeks), and weekly plasma exchange (20 weeks) (n = 57); or placebo medications and sham plasma exchange (n = 56). All patients were followed for at least 12 months. There were no significant differences between the groups in this primary analysis; there were 19 [35%] treatment failures with CPM; 18 [32%] with plasma exchange; and 16 [29%] with placebo. Nor were there any differences in the proportions of those improved, stabilised, or worsened at each 6 month assessment or in the mean change in the EDSS at the final assessment (0.81 CPM; 0.69 plasma exchange; 0.69 placebo). CPM was also assessed in a single randomised, placebo-controlled, single-blind study of 42 patients with PMS. Twenty-two subjects received CPM and there was no evidence of disease progression after 1 year in both groups [28].

9.3.6 Cyclosporine

Cyclosporine (CsA) is a neutral lipophilic cyclic undecapeptide that has been widely used for the treatment of allograft rejection and graft-vs.-host disease [29]. CsA inhibits T cell activation by blocking the transcription of cytokine genes, including IL-2 and IL-4 [30]. One trial has used cyclosporine in PMS [31]. Subjects were randomized to receive either CsA (n = 273) or placebo (n = 274) in a 2-year, double-blinded, multicentre trial. The mean increase in EDSS score was 0.39 ± 1.07 with CsA and 0.65 ± 1.08 placebo until the time of early withdrawal or completion (p = 0.002). Of three primary efficacy criteria, CsA delayed the time to becoming wheelchair bound (p = 0.038) but there were no statistically significant effects on time to sustained progression or on a composite score of "activities of daily living". CsA did have a favourable effect on secondary measures including an endpoint analysis of change from baseline EDSS for the patients completing 12 and 24 months, overall clinical assessments by blinded neurologists, and global assessment of change from baseline to 12 and 24 months' completion and comparison of duration of patient follow up in the two study arms. There was a large withdrawal rate for CsA (44% vs. 32% for placebo) mostly due to nephrotoxicity and hypertension, but this did not explain the effect of CsA in delaying disease progression.

9.3.7 Intravenous Immunoglobulin

Intravenous immunglobulin (IVIG) can protect oligodendrocytes against complement-mediated injury and potentially enhance remyelination [32]. In the first study 318 SPMS subjects were randomised to IVIG 1 g/kg/month (n = 159) or placebo (albumin 0.1%; n = 159) for 27 months. Nineteen patients in the IVIG group and 39 in the placebo group terminated study treatment prematurely but were included in the analyses. IVIG treatment had no beneficial effect on time to confirmed EDSS progression (hazard ratio 1.11 [95% CI 0.80–1.53] for IVIG versus placebo) [33]. A second study of 231 subjects stratified for PPMS (n = 34) and

SPMS (n = 197) were randomly assigned to IVIG 0.4 g/kg/month or placebo for 24 months [34]. Analysis of the intention to treat (ITT) population of the total population found the mean time to confirmed progression was 74 weeks in the IVIG versus 62 weeks in the placebo group ($p = 0.041$). When PPMS and SPMS patients were analysed separately as per the primary outcome, the time to confirmed progression was also longer in the IVIG group, but the difference was not significant. In the combined ITT population there were less patients with confirmed progression in the IVIG than in the placebo group ($p = 0.028$). PPMS subjects, but not SPMS subjects showed a slight favourable IVIG effect on the best EDSS score. The difference was significant in PPMS ($p = 0.016$), but not in SPMS. There was a trend for a favourable IVIG effect on the rates of subjects with confirmed progression. In patients with PPMS, this IVIG effect reached significance ($p = 0.036$). There were a large numbers of dropouts; 18 subjects with PPMS and 102 patients with SPMS.

9.3.8 Isoprinosine

Isoprinosine is a physicochemical complex of inosine with the para-acetamidobenzoic acid salt of N,N-dimethylamino-2-propanolol that enhances B lymphocyte activity and it also increases macrophage phagocytosis, release of cytokines increases the action of T cell mitogens. A double-blind placebo trial recruited 52 subjects of whom 26 had PMS. All subjects were given intravenous methylprednisolone prior to randomisation to Isoprinosine (n = 25) or placebo (n = 27). There was no difference in disability between the treated and control groups up to 96 weeks after correcting for multiple comparisons in the whole population and in the PMS group [35].

9.3.9 Linomide

Linomide (quinoline-3-carboxamide) is a synthetic immunomodulator that increases natural killer cell activity [36]. Two studies have used linomide, an initial phase II study [37] that was followed by a phase III study that was stopped due to side effects [38]. A double blind phase II study randomised 30 subjects with SPMS to linomide (2.5 mg) or placebo. Twenty-four patients completed at least 6 months of treatment. At 24 weeks, the mean shift in EDSS was $+0.27 \pm 0.16$ with placebo vs. -0.17 ± 0.17 with linomide ($p = 0.045$). The percentage of patients with evidence of activity on their MRI (new, enlarging, or new Gd+ lesions) throughout the treatment period was 75% with placebo and 33% with linomide ($p = 0.021$). A subsequent trial with linomide was terminated due to serious side effects. The plan for this randomized, double-blind, placebo-controlled trial was to recruit 715 patients with active RRMS (n = 90) or SPMS (n = 625) to receive either linomide (1.0, 2.5, or 7.5 mg) or placebo. The planned primary outcome was the time to the development of confirmed clinical worsening not associated with an acute relapse. The trial was terminated 1 month after it became fully enrolled due to unanticipated life threatening cardiopulmonary toxicities. Significant arthralgia, myalgia, bursitis, and facial and peripheral oedema were common adverse events.

9.3.10 Methotrexate

Methotrexate inhibits dihydrofolic acid reductase, interfering with DNA synthesis, repair, and cellular replication [39]. A Cochrane review identified one trial in PMS [40]. Oral weekly low dose methotrexate 7.5 mg vs. placebo over 2 years was studied in a randomized, double-blinded, placebo-controlled, clinical trial in 60 PMS subjects. Methotrexate had a non-significant trend to reduce sustained EDSS progression and number of relapses. The methotrexate group had significantly less progression of impairment as measured by validated tests of upper-extremity function in the absence of clinically significant toxicity [41].

9.3.11 Mitoxantrone

Mitoxantrone is an anthracenedione cytotoxic agent that inhibits DNA replication, DNA-dependent RNA synthesis and inhibits topoisomerase II activity preventing DNA repair [42]. A Cochrane review looked at mitoxantrone use in PMS and recommended that mitoxantrone should be used in SPMS when there is evidence of persistent inflammatory activity [43]. The data arose from a single phase 3 study where 194 patients with worsening RRMS or SPMS received placebo or mitoxantrone (5 g/m^2 or 12 mg/m^2) every 3 months intravenously [44]. The primary endpoint was a multivariate analysis of five clinical measures. At 24 months, the mitoxantrone group experienced statistically significant benefits compared with the placebo group in the primary outcome (difference 0.30 [95% CI 0.17–0.44]; $p < 0.0001$) and the pre-planned univariate analyses: change in EDSS (0.24 [0.04–0.44]; $p = 0.0194$), change in ambulation index (0.21 [0.02–0.40]; $p = 0.0306$), adjusted total number of treated relapses (0.38 [0.18–0.59]; $p = 0.0002$), time to first treated relapse (0.44 [0.20–0.69]; $p = 0.0004$), and change in standardised neurological status (0.23 [0.03–0.43]; $p = 0.0268$).

9.3.12 Myelin Basic Protein Synthetic Peptides: AG284 and Dirucotide

Antigen-based approaches for the treatment of autoimmune diseases aims to restore immunological tolerance by targeting aberrant activation of T and B cells by particular epitopes. Such approaches have been effective in animal-based models of MS and an immunodominant MS-associated T-cell epitope was identified in the central region of the myelin basic protein (MBP) molecule in patients with HLA haplotype DR2

[45]. AG284 is a solubilized complex of HLA-DR2 with an MBP peptide 84–102 that was administered intravenously to 33 DR2-heterozygous SPMS subjects who received three alternate day IV doses of AG284 or placebo in a double-masked dose escalation study and followed up for 84 days. The formulation was safe at doses of up to 150 mcg/kg but the study was not able to establish that T cells were tolerized by the treatment, and it was not designed to demonstrate clinical efficacy, but no difference in the EDSS was seen [46]. Dirucotide is a synthetic peptide of MBP with a sequence corresponding to amino acid residues 82–98 of human MBP and a molecular replicate of the site of attack that is dominant in MS patients with HLA haplotypes DR2 or DR4. These haplotypes are present in 65–75% of patients [45]. An initial small double-blind, placebo-controlled phase II study of Dirucotide in PMS failed to slow the time to disease progression but post hoc analysis suggested efficacy in a subset of patients with HLA DR2/DR4 [45] as a result a randomized 2-year, double-blind, placebo-controlled study was planned to target in particular this genotype. The trial of 612 SPMS subjects stratified according to baseline EDSS score (3.5–5.0, or 5.5–6.5) and HLA haplotype (DR2+/DR4+, or DR2−/DR4−). Once 100 DR2−/DR4− subjects had been recruited further study enrolment was limited to DR2+/DR4+ subjects. Subjects were randomised to 500 mg MBP8298 or placebo, given by IV injection once every 6 months for 2 years. There were no significant differences between treatment groups in either the primary or secondary endpoints [47].

9.3.13 *Pirfenidone*

TNF-alpha has been implicated in MS pathogenesis and pirfenidone is a known inhibitor of TNF-alpha synthesis. A double blind placebo-controlled trial randomised 43 SPMS subjects to oral pirfenidone ($n = 25$) or placebo ($n = 18$). The dose was titrated up to 2400 mg over 10–14 days and clinical and MRI evaluations were at 6 and 12 months. Seven subjects dropped out of the placebo group and nine dropped out of the pirfenidone group. By 1 month, pirfenidone significantly ($P < 0.05$) improved the SNRS scores, and scores remained significantly improved up to 12 months when compared to the baseline SNRS scores. In contrast, the SNRS scores of patients on oral placebo were not significantly improved up to 12 months of the study, when compared with baseline scores. Oral pirfenidone significantly ($p < 0.04$) reduced the incidence of relapses (27.8% on placebo versus 8.0% on pirfenidone). There was no significant difference in the EDSS between the two groups [48].

9.3.14 *Siponimod*

The non-selective S1P modulator fingolimod was effective in RRMS, reducing brain atrophy, but it was not effective in a double-blind study of 969 PPMS patients with flexible treatment duration [49]. Using fingolimod as an initial lead structure siponimod was developed as a selective S1P1 and S1P5 modulator [50]. Siponimod was effective in a double-blind adaptive dose ranging phase 2 study in RRMS [51, 52], a 24 month extension confirmed effects on MRI and also relapse rate [53, 54]. One thousand six hundred and fifty-one subjects were randomised (2:1) to receive either siponimod or placebo. Eligible patients were randomised to receive either 2 mg of once daily Siponimod following initial dose titration starting at 0.25 mg or matching placebo. The trial was composed of a core and an extension part, with 1363 patients completing the first core phase up to a maximum of 3 years. Eighty-seven percent were followed for at least 1 year, and the median follow-up time was 21 months. Siponimod reduced the risk of 3-month confirmed disability progression by 21% versus placebo (HR [95% CI]: 0.79 [0.65, 0.95]; $p = 0.013$). Point estimates favoured siponimod were consistently observed across predefined subgroups, including patients with no relapses in the 2 years prior to study and those without gadolinium-enhancing lesions at baseline. Siponimod also reduced the risk of 6-month confirmed disability progression by 26% ($p = 0.006$), ARR by 55.5% ($p < 0.0001$), T1 Gd+ lesion number by 86.6% ($p < 0.0001$), and new T2 lesion number by 81% ($p < 0.0001$). Relative difference in change from baseline in T2LV, MSWS-12 and PBVC were 79.1% ($p < 0.0001$), 39.7% ($p = 0.057$) and 23.4% ($p = 0.0002$), respectively, versus placebo. The risk reduction observed for T25FW was 6.2% and not statistically significant ($p = 0.440$) ([53–55], NCT01665144).

9.3.15 *Systemic Lymphoblastoid Interferon*

Interferon beta was the first licensed therapy in RMS whereas systemic lymphoblastoid interferon (IFN) is a combination of primarily alpha with some beta IFN. One hundred PMS subjects were randomised to lymphoblastoid IFN (5×10^6 IU) or placebo daily by subcutaneous injection for 6 months. Sixteen subjects withdrew 15 from the lymphoblastoid IFN group. After 2 years there was no difference between the groups based on EDSS and MRI lesion analysis [56].

9.4 PMS Trials Targeting Principally Non-inflammatory Processes

9.4.1 *Biotin*

Biotin activates acetylCoA carboxylase, a rate-limiting enzyme in myelin synthesis. It is hypothesized that biotin may help to promote remyelination and reduce axonal hypoxia [57]. An uncontrolled non-blinded study of 23 subjects with PPMS and SPMS treated patients with high doses of biotin (100–300 mg/day) from 2–36 months (mean = 9.2 months) [58] showed positive results. A further study recruited 154 PPMS and SPMS subjects. Subjects were randomly assigned to placebo (n = 51) or to oral MD1003 (n = 103) 300 mg/day. About 41% of the treatment group and 55% of the placebo group were also taking fampridine. The primary outcome was improvement at 9 months confirmed at 12 months, using either a change in EDSS score of at least 1 point (if baseline EDSS was 4.5–5.5) and 0.5 point (if baseline EDSS was 6–7) or a decrease in timed 25-foot walk (TW25) of 20% compared to baseline. At the end of the double-blind phase 13 out of 103 patients (12.6%) in the MD1003 group and 0 out of 51 (0%) in the placebo group met the definition of the primary endpoint [59]. In the treatment group, there was a mean EDSS decrease of 0.03 at month 12, compared with a mean increase of 0.13 in the placebo group ($p = 0.014$) (as presented at AAN 2016 by Dr. Tourbah). Biotin has recently been filed for a licence in the European Union.

9.4.2 D-Penicillamine Plus Metacycline

The serine proteinase tissue-type plasminogen activator and the metalloproteinase gelatinase B (MMP-9) are seen in MS lesions. Both enzymes are interconnected in a cascade that can damage the blood brain barrier and cause demyelination. Both enzymes are inhibited by D-penicillamine and Metacycline was shown in in vitro experiments to inhibit gelatinase B. A double-blind placebo-controlled 20 SPMS subjects were randomised to a combination of oral D-penicillamine plus metacycline (n = 10) or placebo (n = 10). The pilot study's objectives was to examine safety with disease progression a secondary endpoint. Over 1 year there was no significant improvement in the EDSS compared to placebo. Toxicity was too high to consider additional trials [60].

9.4.3 Dronabinol

Laboratory evidence has found that cannabinoids have a neuroprotective action [61]. Four hundred and ninety-eight subjects with PPMS or SPMS were randomised (2:1) to dronabinol (Δ (9)-tetrahydrocannabinol) or placebo for 36 months. Maximum dose was 28 mg/day, titrated against bodyweight and adverse effects. Three hundred and twenty-nine subjects received at least one dose of dronabinol and 164 received at least one dose of placebo. One hundred and forty-five patients in the dronabinol group had EDSS score progression (0.24 first progression events per patient-year compared with 73 in the placebo group (0.23 first progression events per patient-year; hazard ratio 0.92, p = 0.57). There was also no significant difference in the Multiple Sclerosis Impact Scale (MSIS-29) physical score between the groups [62].

9.4.4 Erythropoietin

Erythropoietin (EPO) has been shown to promote axonal repair, neurogenesis, and angiogenesis [63] and in an open label study of five PMS subjects treated with high-dose recombinant humanized EPO showed motor and cognitive improvement [64]. A double-blind, placebo-controlled trial randomised 52 subjects with SPMS or PPMS to recombinant EPO (48,000 IU) or placebo, administered intravenously 17 times during 24 weeks. The primary outcome was the change in a composite measure of maximum gait distance, hand dexterity, and cognition from baseline to 24 weeks. There was no difference in the primary outcome between the EPO and the placebo group using the intention-to-treat principle ($p = 0.22$). None of the secondary outcomes showed any significant differences [65].

9.4.5 Fluoxetine

Fluoxetine, a selective serotonin-reuptake inhibitor (SSRI), stimulates glycogenolysis and enhances the production of brain derived neurotrophic factor [66]. After 2 weeks of treatment with fluoxetine a significantly improved cerebral white matter NAA/creatine ratio was found on MRI, suggesting an improvement in axonal mitochondrial energy metabolism [67] and a pilot study in patients with MS with relapses found that a daily dose of 20 mg tended to reduce the formation of new inflammatory lesions [68]. In a double-blind trial 42 PMS subjects were randomised to fluoxetine (40 mg daily, n = 20) or placebo (n = 22). There was no effect on progression with seven subject in both group progressing over 2 years [69].

9.4.6 Lamotrigine

Lamotrigine (LTG) acts via sodium channel blockade and also has antiglutamatergic and neuroprotective actions in several experimental models of inflammatory axonal injury [70]. A double-blind, parallel-group study of 120 SPMS subjects randomised to LTG (target dose 400 mg/day) or placebo for 2 years. The mean change in partial (central) cerebral volume per year was not significant (−3.18 mL (SD −1.25) in LTG; −2.48 mL (−0.97) in the placebo; difference −0.71 mL, 95% CI −2.56 to 1.15; p = 0.40). An exploratory analysis associated LTG with greater partial (central) cerebral volume loss than placebo in the first year (p = 0.04), and volume increased partially after treatment stopped (p = 0.04). This was thought to be as a result of pseudoatrophy. Otherwise LTG treatment reduced the deterioration of the timed 25-foot walk (p = 0.02) but did not affect other secondary clinical outcome measures [71].

9.4.7 Lipoic Acid

Lipoic acid (LA) decreases inflammation and reduces optic nerve and spinal cord atrophy in experimental autoimmune encephalitis [72, 73]. A 2 year, double-blind, randomized controlled trial of 1200 mg daily lipoic acid versus placebo has recently been presented in poster form only [74]. Of the 54 randomized subjects, 51 subjects took at least one dose of study drug and were included in analysis, 27 LA and 24 placebo and four subjects terminated early. There was a baseline difference in whole brain volume with the LA group being significantly larger ($p < 0.004$) however there was a significant reduction in brain volume loss over 96 weeks in the LA group (−0.4+/−0.7) versus placebo (−1.3+/−1.1). None of the secondary outcomes were significant (NCT01188811).

9.4.8 Masitinib

Masitinib is a selective oral tyrosine kinase inhibitor. It inhibits the survival, migration and activity of mast cells [75]. In a randomized, placebo-controlled trial in PMS masitinib was administered orally at 3–6 mg/kg/day for at least 12 months. Thirty-five subjects were randomized to receive masitinib ($n = 27$) or placebo ($n = 8$) [76]. Masitinib had an impact on MS-related impairment for PPMS and relapse-free SPMS subjects with a non-significant improvement in MSFC scores relative to baseline, compared with a worsening MSFC score in placebo; +103% ± 189 versus −60% ± 190 at month 12, respectively. A total of 7/22 (32%) assessable masitinib patients reported a clinical response following 12 months of treatment (according to the modified intent to treat population, observed cases) compared with none in the placebo group. The EDSS remained stable in both treatment groups. This data supported a larger placebo-controlled trial that is recruited and was due to report in 2016 using masitinib (6 mg/kg/day) versus placebo in 450 PMS patients over 2 years (NCT01433497).

9.4.9 Simvastatin

Statins have multiple potentially positive effects but the relevant mechanism of action of statins in MS remains unknown. Simvastatin significant reduced vasculopathy and inhibit matrix metalloproteinases production but also have immune-modulatory effects [77]. A single double-blind, controlled trial randomised 140 SPMS subjects to receive 80 mg of simvastatin or placebo. The primary outcome was annualised rate of whole-brain atrophy. Notably the last MRI was performed 1 month off treatment. Analyses were by intention to treat and per protocol. The mean annualised atrophy rate was significantly lower in patients in the simvastatin group (0.288% per year [SD 0.521]) than in those in the placebo group (0.584% per year [0.498]). The adjusted difference in atrophy rate between groups was −0.254% per year (95% CI −0.422 to −0.087; p = 0.003); a 43% reduction in annualised rate. Simvastatin also showed benefits in both the EDSS and in the MSIS-29 [78]. A phase III study of simvastatin in PMS has received funding and is planned to begin in 2018.

9.5 On-Going and Planned Trials in SPMS and PPMS

9.5.1 Ibudilast (SPRINT-MS; NCT01982942) Fully Recruited in 2016

Ibudilast is a phosphodiesterase inhibitor that on the basis of demonstrating a brain atrophy benefit in RMS [79] is currently being studied in a phase II study in PMS (SPRINT-MS). Patients can be untreated or remain on MS disease modifying therapy. The primary outcome is the covariate-adjusted mean rate of change in brain atrophy over 96 weeks as measured by brain parenchymal fraction. The trial will complete in Summer 2017.

9.5.2 Fluoxetine, Riluzole and Amiloride (MS-SMART; NCT01910259) Fully Recruited in 2016

The MS-Secondary Progressive Multi-Arm Randomisation Trial is a phase IIB double blind placebo-controlled clinical trial comparing the efficacy of three potentially neuroprotective drugs (fluoxetine 20 mg bd, riluzole 50 mg bd or amiloride 5 mg bd) in 440 SPMS subjects. Subjects will be followed up for 96 weeks and the primary outcome is change in brain volume.

9.5.3 Imilecleucel-T Intervention

This phase 2 double-blind, placebo controlled study aims to evaluate the efficacy and safety of Tcelna (imilecleucel-T, autologous T-Cell Immunotherapy) in SPMS. Subjects whose myelin reactive T-cell can be identified by epitope profiling assay will are randomized and provide blood to manufacture Tcelna. Tcelna is an autologous pool of myelin reactive T-cells expanded ex vivo with immunodominant epitopes selected from the three myelin antigens, MBP, proteolipid protein and myelin oligodendrocyte glycoprotein on a per subject basis then attenuated by irradiation to prevent further proliferation before releasing product for administration. Subjects will receive either Tcelna or placebo and will receive five doses in year 1. Subjects will be evaluated for changes in disability and cognitive function every 3 months, and radiographic changes annually (NCT01684761).

9.6 Conclusion

9.6.1 PMS Trials: Where We Are Today

Up to this point there have been 43 placebo-controlled trials that have investigated the effectiveness of treatment in PMS (Nicholas et al. in preparation). Eleven trials have used licensed therapies for RMS, not discussed here. Nine of these 32 trials (28%) were successful in reaching their primary outcome with the first being published in 1990. Yet the first license in PMS has been granted in 2017. This has arisen possibly due to the evolution of a licensing pathway for RMS that has emerged over the last 28 years. This has undoubtedly set expectations of therapy in MS—most importantly that it is not curative. The benefits for people with PMS in the trials of a successful therapy amounts to a slowing of progression of about 20% [1, 55]. Given that both ocrelizumab and siponimod are effective both in RMS and PMS and the evidence that progression starts early in RMS this does mean that to enhance the impact of treatment we should consider starting treatment, certainly for SPMS, in the early relapsing phase to maximise the benefits in PMS for when it becomes clinically evident [2].

9.6.2 PMS Trials: Will Targeting the Immune System be Adequate?

Of the 43 placebo controlled trials in PMS, including the 11 in licensed therapies for RMS, 35 (81%) have used treatments targeting the immune system. Two studies that have been successful recently have used molecules targeting the immune system. This has resulted in the licensing of ocrelizumab for PMS and following on from that success, siponimod has also been successful in a phase 3 trial in SPMS. Like ocrelizumab it has a benefit in RMS though it has not been tested in a phase 3 trial in RMS. Similar molecules to both ocrelizumab and siponimod underwent trials that failed in PMS prior to their development; both rituximab [18] and fingolimod [49] were trialled in PPMS. Fingolimod, a non-selective SP1 antagonist related to siponimod, is licensed in RMS but failed in PMS [49]. The trial was adequately powered but unlike siponimod, fingolimod did not undergo a systematic dose assessment prior to the phase 3 study [51, 52] and was used a lower dose due to safety concerns at the higher dose used initially in the PMS trial [49]. The, as yet unknown, question is whether targeting the immune system is all that will be needed to halt MS progression. Though only 8 of 43 (19%) trials involved molecules which did not target the immune system directly, there have been some notable successes. Biotin is currently being evaluated for a license in PMS and simvastatin, the only other molecule not targeting the immune system that was successful, is starting a phase 3 trial in 2018. These approaches, using neuroprotective therapies, offer some novel insights into MS and need to continue as the imperfect efficacy of purely immune-targeted treatments becomes clear.

9.6.3 PMS Trials: Where Should We Go Next?

For the first time we have trials which have established therapies with modest benefits for PMS. However, much remains to be done to improve the effectiveness with better treatments but also how those treatments are used. It could be argued that an approach, using combined immunomodulatory and neuroprotective therapies, will be needed. We need to design studies that enable us to confirm that we are maximising their effectiveness. This means targeting early in the disease and running potentially longer studies so that we can confirm a long-term treatment regimen is effective with acceptable side effects. The primary endpoint of choice so far has been clinician assessed disability progression. This is now challenged by advances in MR imaging on one end of the spectrum as well as by the development, validation and better understanding of patient reported outcomes on the other. For instance, the patient assessed MSIS-29 physical component has recently be shown to predict survival [80]; this links it to the most unambiguous outcomes of all, which itself could of course only be studied in very long running trials.

References

1. Montalban X, Hemmer B, Rammohan K, Giovannoni G, et al. ORATORIO Clinical Investigators. Ocrelizumab versus placebo in in primary progressive multiple sclerosis. N Engl J Med. 2017;376(3):209–20.
2. Nandoskar A, Raffel J, Scalfari AS, Friede T, Nicholas RS. Pharmacological approaches to the management of secondary progressive multiple sclerosis. Drugs. 2017;77(8):885–910. doi:10.1007/s40265-017-0726-0.
3. Nicholas RS, Han E, Raffel J, Chataway J, Friede T. Temporal changes in placebo populations in progressive multiple sclerosis trials: A systematic review and meta-analysis. In preparation.
4. Inusah S, Sormani MP, Cofield SS, Aban IB, Musani SK, Srinivasasainagendra V, Cutter GR. Assessing changes in relapse rates in multiple sclerosis. Mult Scler. 2010;16(12): 1414–21.
5. Nicholas R, Straube S, Schmidli H, Schneider S, Friede T. Trends in annualized relapse rates in relapsing remitting multiple sclerosis and consequences for clinical trial design. Mult Scler. 2011;17(10):1211–7.

6. Röver C, Nicholas R, Straube S, Friede T. Changing EDSS progression in placebo cohorts in relapsing ms: a systematic review and meta-regression. PLoS One. 2015;10(9):e0137052. doi:10.1371/journal.pone.0137052.
7. Stellmann JP, Neuhaus A, Herich L, Schippling S, Roeckel M, Daumer M, Martin R, Heesen C. Placebo cohorts in phase-3 MS treatment trials—predictors for on-trial disease activity 1990–2010 based on a meta-analysis and individual case data. PLoS One. 2012;7(11):e50347. doi:10.1371/journal.pone.0050347.
8. European Medicines Agency. Guideline on clinical investigation of medicinal products for the treatment of Multiple Sclerosis Committee for Medicinal Products for Human Use. EMA/CHMP/771815/2011, Rev. 2;2015.
9. Cavallo MG, Pozzilli P, Thorpe R. Cytokines and autoimmunity. Clin Exp Immunol. 1994;96(1):1–7.
10. Skurkovich S, Boiko A, Beliaeva I, Buglak A, et al. Randomized study of antibodies to IFN-gamma and TNF-alpha in secondary progressive multiple sclerosis. Mult Scler. 2001;7(5):277–84.
11. Patel AA, Swerlick RA, McCall CO. Azathioprine in dermatology: the past, the present, and the future. J Am Acad Dermatol. 2006;55(3):369–89.
12. Casetta I, Iuliano G, Filippini G. Azathioprine for multiple sclerosis. Cochrane Database Syst Rev. 2007;4:CD003982.
13. Double-masked trial of azathioprine in multiple sclerosis. British and Dutch multiple sclerosis azathioprine trial group. Lancet. 1988;2(8604):179–83.
14. Ellison GW, Myers LW, Mickey MR, Graves MC, et al. A placebo-controlled, randomized, double-masked, variable dosage, clinical trial of azathioprine with and without methylprednisolone in multiple sclerosis. Neurology. 1989;39(8):1018–26.
15. Ghezzi A, Di Falco M, Locatelli C, et al. Clinical controlled randomized trial of azathioprine in multiple sclerosis. In: Consette RE, Delmotte P, editors. Recent advances in multiple sclerosis therapy. Amsterdam: Elsevier; 1989.
16. Milanese CLML, Salmaggi A, Eoli M. A double blind study on azathioprine efficacy in multiple sclerosis: final report. J Neurol. 1993;240:295–8.
17. von Büdingen HC, Palanichamy A, Lehmann-Horn K, Michel BA, Zamvil SS. Update on the autoimmune pathology of multiple sclerosis: B-cells as disease-drivers and therapeutic targets. Eur Neurol. 2015;73(3–4):238–46. doi:10.1159/000377675.
18. Hawker K, O'Connor P, Freedman MS, Calabresi PA, et al. Rituximab in patients with primary progressive multiple sclerosis: results of a randomized double-blind placebo-controlled multicenter trial. Ann Neurol. 2009;66(4):460–71.
19. Maloney DG, Grillo-Lopez AJ, White CA, Bodkin D, et al. IDEC-C2B8 (Rituximab) anti-CD20 monoclonal antibody therapy in patients with relapsed low-grade non-Hodgkin's lymphoma. Blood. 1997;90(6):2188–95.
20. Dörner T, Burmester GR. New approaches of B-cell-directed therapy: beyond rituximab. Curr Opin Rheumatol. 2008;20(3):263–8. doi:10.1097/BOR.0b013e3282f5e08d.
21. Sorensen PS, Blinkenberg M. The potential role for ocrelizumab in the treatment of multiple sclerosis: current evidence and future prospects. Ther Adv Neurol Disord. 2016;9(1):44–52. doi:10.1177/1756285615601933.
22. Comi G, Hartung HP, Kurukulasuriya NC, Greenberg SJ, et al. Cladribine tablets for the treatment of relapsing-remitting multiple sclerosis. Expert Opin Pharmacother. 2013;14(1):123–36.
23. Beutler E, Sipe JC, Romine JS, Koziol JA, et al. The treatment of chronic progressive multiple sclerosis with cladribine. Proc Natl Acad Sci U S A. 1996;93(4):1716–20.
24. Sipe JC, Romine JS, Koziol JA, McMillan R, et al. Cladribine in treatment of chronic progressive multiple sclerosis. Lancet. 1994;344(8914):9–13.
25. Rice GP, Filippi M, Comi G. Cladribine and progressive MS: clinical and MRI outcomes of a multicenter controlled trial. Cladribine MRI Study Group. Neurology. 2000;54(5):1145–55.
26. Kovarsky J. Clinical pharmacology and toxicology of cyclophosphamide: emphasis on use in rheumatic diseases. Semin Arthritis Rheum. 1983;12(4):359–72.

27. The Canadian cooperative trial of cyclophosphamide and plasma exchange in progressive multiple sclerosis. The Canadian Cooperative Multiple Sclerosis Study Group. Lancet. 1991;337(8739):441–6.
28. Likosky WH, Fireman B, Elmore R, Eno G, Gale K, Goode GB, Ikeda K, Laster J, Mosher C, Rozance J, et al. Intense immunosuppression in chronic progressive multiple sclerosis: the Kaiser study. J Neurol Neurosurg Psychiatry. 1991;54(12):1055–60.
29. Borel JF, Feurer C, Magnee C, Stahelin H. Effects of the new anti-lymphocytic peptide cyclosporin A in animals. Immunology. 1977;32(6):1017–25.
30. Granelli-Piperno A. In situ hybridization for interleukin 2 and interleukin 2 receptor mRNA in T cells activated in the presence or absence of cyclosporin A. J Exp Med. 1988;168(5):1649–58.
31. Efficacy and toxicity of cyclosporine in chronic progressive multiple sclerosis: a randomized, double-blinded, placebo-controlled clinical trial. The Multiple Sclerosis Study Group. Ann Neurol. 1990;27(6):591–605.
32. Stangel M, Hartung HP. Intravenous immunoglobulins in multiple sclerosis. Studies and mechanisms of action--an update. Nervenarzt. 2002;73(2):119–24.
33. Hommes OR, Sorensen PS, Fazekas F, Enriquez MM, et al. Intravenous immunoglobulin in secondary progressive multiple sclerosis: randomised placebo-controlled trial. Lancet. 2004;364(9440):1149–56.
34. Pohlau D, Przuntek H, Sailer M, Bethke F, et al. Intravenous immunoglobulin in primary and secondary chronic progressive multiple sclerosis: a randomized placebo controlled multicentre study. Mult Scler. 2007;13(9):1107–17.
35. Milligan NM, Miller DH, Compston DA. A placebo-controlled trial of isoprinosine in patients with multiple sclerosis. J Neurol Neurosurg Psychiatry. 1994;57(2):164–8.
36. Abramsky O, Lehmann D, Karussis D. Immunomodulation with linomide: possible novel therapy for multiple sclerosis. Mult Scler. 1996;2(4):206–10.
37. Karussis DM, Meiner Z, Lehmann D, Gomori JM, et al. Treatment of secondary progressive multiple sclerosis with the immunomodulator linomide: a double-blind, placebo-controlled pilot study with monthly magnetic resonance imaging evaluation. Neurology. 1996;47(2):341–6.
38. Noseworthy JH, Wolinsky JS, Lublin FD, Whitaker JN, et al. Linomide in relapsing and secondary progressive MS: Part I: trial design and clinical results. North American Linomide Investigators. Neurology. 2000;54(9):1726–33.
39. Calabresi P. CBCoND. In: GL S, Gilman A, Rall T, Nies AS, Taylor P, editors. The pharmacological basis of therapeutics. New York: Pergamon Press; 1990. p. 1202–8.
40. Gray O, McDonnell GV, Forbes RB. Methotrexate for multiple sclerosis. Cochrane Database Syst Rev. 2004;2:CD003208.
41. Goodkin DE, Rudick RA, VanderBrug Medendorp S, Daughtry MM, et al. Low-dose (7.5 mg) oral methotrexate reduces the rate of progression in chronic progressive multiple sclerosis. Ann Neurol. 1995;37(1):30–40.
42. Li JM, Yang Y, Zhu P, Zheng F, et al. Mitoxantrone exerts both cytotoxic and immunoregulatory effects on activated microglial cells. Immunopharmacol Immunotoxicol. 2012;34(1):36–41.
43. Martinelli Boneschi F, Vacchi L, Rovaris M, Capra R, et al. Mitoxantrone for multiple sclerosis. Cochrane Database Syst Rev. 2013;5:CD002127.
44. Hartung HP, Gonsette R, Konig N, Kwiecinski H, et al. Mitoxantrone in progressive multiple sclerosis: a placebo-controlled, double-blind, randomised, multicentre trial. Lancet. 2002;360(9350):2018–25.
45. Warren KG, Catz I, Ferenczi LZ, Krantz MJ. Intravenous synthetic peptide MBP8298 delayed disease progression in an HLA Class II-defined cohort of patients with progressive multiple sclerosis: results of a 24-month double-blind placebo-controlled clinical trial and 5 years of follow-up treatment. Eur J Neurol. 2006;13(8):887–95.
46. Goodkin DE, Shulman M, Winkelhake J, Waubant E, Andersson P, Stewart T, Nelson S, Fischbein N, Coyle PK, Frohman E, Jacobs L, Holcenberg J, Lee M, Mocci S. A phase I trial of solubilized DR2:MBP84-102 (AG284) in multiple sclerosis. Neurology. 2000;54(7):1414–20.

47. Freedman MS, Bar-Or A, Oger J, Traboulsee A, et al. A phase III study evaluating the efficacy and safety of MBP8298 in secondary progressive MS. Neurology. 2011;77(16):1551–60.
48. Walker JE, Giri SN, Margolin SB. A double-blind, randomized, controlled study of oral pirfenidone for treatment of secondary progressive multiple sclerosis. Mult Scler. 2005;11(2):149–58.
49. Lublin F, Miller DH, Freedman MS, Cree BA, et al. Oral fingolimod in primary progressive multiple sclerosis (INFORMS): a phase 3, randomised, double-blind, placebo-controlled trial. Lancet. 2016;387(10023):1075–84.
50. Pan S, Gray NS, Gao W, Mi Y, et al. Discovery of BAF312 (Siponimod), a potent and selective S1P receptor modulator. ACS Med Chem Lett. 2013;4(3):333–7.
51. Selmaj K, Li DK, Hartung HP, Hemmer B, et al. Siponimod for patients with relapsing-remitting multiple sclerosis (BOLD): an adaptive, dose-ranging, randomised, phase 2 study. Lancet Neurol. 2013b;12(8):756–67.
52. Selmaj K, Li DK, Hartung HP, Hemmer B, Kappos L, Freedman MS, Stüve O, Rieckmann P, Montalban X, Ziemssen T, Auberson LZ, Pohlmann H, Mercier F, Dahlke F, Wallström E. Siponimod for patients with relapsing-remitting multiple sclerosis (BOLD): an adaptive, dose-ranging, randomised, phase 2 study. Lancet Neurol. 2013a;12(8):756–67. doi:10.1016/S1474-4422(13)70102-9. Erratum in: Lancet Neurol. 2013;12(9):846.
53. Kappos L, Li DK, Stuve O, Hartung HP, et al. Safety and efficacy of siponimod (BAF312) in patients with relapsing-remitting multiple sclerosis: dose-blinded, randomized extension of the phase 2 BOLD study. JAMA Neurol. 2016;73(9):1089–98.
54. Kappos L, Bar-Or A, Cree B, et al. Efficacy and safety of siponimod in secondary progressive multiple sclerosis—Results of the placebo controlled, double-blind, Phase III EXPAND study. ECTRIMS 2016. London, UK: ECTRIMS Online Library; 2016a.
55. Kappos L, Bar-Or A, Cree B, Fox R, Giovannoni G, Gold R, Vermersch P, Arnould S, Sidorenko T, Wolf C, Wallström E, Dahlke F. 002—Efficacy of siponimod in secondary progressive multiple sclerosis: results of the phase 3 study. Boston, MA, USA: 69th Annual Meeting of the American Academy of Neurology; 2017.
56. Kastrukoff LF, Oger JJ, Hashimoto SA, Sacks SL, Li DK, Palmer MR, Koopmans RA, Petkau AJ, Berkowitz J, Paty DW. Systemic lymphoblastoid interferon therapy in chronic progressive multiple sclerosis. I. Clinical and MRI evaluation. Neurology. 1990;40(3 Pt 1): 479–86.
57. Sedel F, Bernard D, Mock DM, Tourbah A. Targeting demyelination and virtual hypoxia with high-dose biotin as a treatment for progressive multiple sclerosis. Neuropharmacology. 2016;110(Pt B):644–53.
58. Sedel F, Papeix C, Bellanger A, Touitou V, et al. High doses of biotin in chronic progressive multiple sclerosis: a pilot study. Mult Scler Relat Disord. 2015;4(2):159–69.
59. Tourbah A, Lebrun-Frenay C, Edan G, Clanet M, et al. MD1003 (high doses of biotin) in progressive multiple sclerosis: subgroup analyses of the MS-SPI trial. ECTRIMS Online Library. 2015;2015:116698.
60. Dubois B, D'Hooghe MB, De Lepeleire K, Ketelaer P, Opdenakker G, Carton H. Toxicity in a double-blind, placebo-controlled pilot trial with D-penicillamine and metacycline in secondary progressive multiple sclerosis. Mult Scler. 1998;4(2):74–8.
61. Hampson AJ, Grimaldi M, Axelrod J, Wink D. Cannabidiol and (-)Delta9-tetrahydrocannabinol are neuroprotective antioxidants. Proc Natl Acad Sci U S A. 1998;95(14):8268–73.
62. Zajicek J, Ball S, Wright D, Vickery J, et al. Effect of dronabinol on progression in progressive multiple sclerosis (CUPID): a randomised, placebo-controlled trial. Lancet Neurol. 2013;12(9):857–65.
63. Cervellini I, Ghezzi P, Mengozzi M. Therapeutic efficacy of erythropoietin in experimental autoimmune encephalomyelitis in mice, a model of multiple sclerosis. Methods Mol Biol. 2013;982:163–73. doi:10.1007/978-1-62703-308-4_10.
64. Ehrenreich H, Fischer B, Norra C, Schellenberger F, Stender N, Stiefel M, Sirén AL, Paulus W, Nave KA, Gold R, Bartels C. Exploring recombinant human erythropoietin in chronic progressive multiple sclerosis. Brain. 2007;130(Pt 10):2577–88.

65. Schreiber K, Magyari M, Sellebjerg F, Iversen P, Garde E, Madsen CG, Börnsen L, Romme Christensen J, Ratzer R, Siebner HR, Laursen B, Soelberg Sorensen P. High-dose erythropoietin in patients with progressive multiple sclerosis: a randomized, placebo-controlled, phase 2 trial. Mult Scler. 2017;23(5):675–85.
66. Allaman I, Fiumelli H, Magistretti PJ, Martin JL. Fluoxetine regulates the expression of neurotrophic/growth factors and glucose metabolism in astrocytes. Psychopharmacology. 2011;216(1):75–84. doi:10.1007/s00213-011-2190-y.
67. Mostert JP, Sijens PE, Oudkerk M, De Keyser J. Fluoxetine increases cerebral white matter NAA/Cr ratio in patients with multiple sclerosis. Neurosci Lett. 2006;402(1–2):22–4.
68. Mostert JP, Admiraal-Behloul F, Hoogduin JM, Luyendijk J, Heersema DJ, van Buchem MA, De Keyser J. Effects of fluoxetine on disease activity in relapsing multiple sclerosis: a double-blind, placebo-controlled, exploratory study. J Neurol Neurosurg Psychiatry. 2008;79(9):1027–31. doi:10.1136/jnnp.2007.139345.
69. Mostert J, Heersema T, Mahajan M, Van Der Grond J, Van Buchem MA, De Keyser J. The effect of fluoxetine on progression in progressive multiple sclerosis: a double-blind, randomized, placebo-controlled trial. ISRN Neurol. 2013;2013:370943. doi:10.1155/2013/370943.
70. Kapoor R, Davies M, Blaker PA, Hall SM, et al. Blockers of sodium and calcium entry protect axons from nitric oxide-mediated degeneration. Ann Neurol. 2003;53(2):174–80.
71. Kapoor R, Furby J, Hayton T, Smith KJ, et al. Lamotrigine for neuroprotection in secondary progressive multiple sclerosis: a randomised, double-blind, placebo-controlled, parallel-group trial. Lancet Neurol. 2010;9(7):681–8.
72. Chaudhary P, Marracci G, Yu X, Galipeau D, et al. Lipoic acid decreases inflammation and confers neuroprotection in experimental autoimmune optic neuritis. J Neuroimmunol. 2011; 233(1–2):90–6.
73. Morini M, Roccatagliata L, Dell'Eva R, Pedemonte E, et al. Alpha-lipoic acid is effective in prevention and treatment of experimental autoimmune encephalomyelitis. J Neuroimmunol. 2004;148(1–2):146–53.
74. Spain RIMC, Horak F, Simon J, et al. P1.373—lipoic acid for neuroprotection in secondary progressive multiple sclerosis. Vancouver, BC, Canada: 68th Annual Meeting of the American Academy of Neurology; 2016.
75. Theoharides TC, Kempuraj D, Kourelis T, Manola A. Human mast cells stimulate activated T cells: implications for multiple sclerosis. Ann N Y Acad Sci. 2008;1144:74–82.
76. Vermersch P, Benrabah R, Schmidt N, Zephir H, et al. Masitinib treatment in patients with progressive multiple sclerosis: a randomized pilot study. BMC Neurol. 2012;12:36.
77. Malfitano AM, Marasco G, Proto MC, Laezza C, et al. Statins in neurological disorders: an overview and update. Pharmacol Res. 2014;88:74–83.
78. Chataway J, Schuerer N, Alsanousi A, Chan D, et al. Effect of high-dose simvastatin on brain atrophy and disability in secondary progressive multiple sclerosis (MS-STAT): a randomised, placebo-controlled, phase 2 trial. Lancet. 2014;383(9936):2213–21.
79. Barkhof F, Hulst HE, Drulovic J, Uitdehaag BM, et al. Ibudilast in relapsing-remitting multiple sclerosis: a neuroprotectant? Neurology. 2010;74(13):1033–40.
80. Raffel J, Wallace A, Gveric D, Reynolds R, Friede T, Nicholas R. The patient-reported outcomes can predict survival in multiple sclerosis. PLOS Medicine. 2017;14(7):e1002346. doi:10.1371/journal.pmed.1002346. eCollection 2017 Jul.

Chapter 10
Rehabilitation in People with Progressive MS

Jennifer Freeman

10.1 Introduction

Managing the progressive phase of MS is widely acknowledged as being challenging for people with MS, their family members and carers, and professionals involved in their care. The hallmark of this phase is a steady accumulation of disability. With limited drug therapy options currently available it is essential that there is a culture of multi-disciplinary team working, which enables participation in targeted neuro-rehabilitation at critical points.

There are many evidence based rehabilitation interventions available to manage the wide ranging and variable symptoms experienced by people with MS [1]. Whilst acknowledging that the evidence has been derived mainly from mixed samples, rather than exclusively of those with progressive disease [2], nevertheless the results demonstrate that significant improvements in activity, participations and quality of life can occur even in people with moderate to severe disability. Despite this, people entering the progressive phase are not always referred on to rehabilitation services. This is highlighted by the findings of qualitative studies that describe people's feelings of "abandonment" by health professionals both during their transition to the progressive phase [3] and when they are more severely disabled [4]. These studies consistently report that people feel they are "left to get on with it" in terms of managing their condition at the very time when they are coming to terms with having a progressive disease, are facing declining mobility and having to readjust to living with disability [3]. Empirical evidence investigating the level of MS service provision further supports these findings [4–6], as do large scale surveys of people affected by MS which highlight unmet need with regard to physical, cognitive and emotional issues [7].

J. Freeman
Health and Human Sciences, School of Health Professions, Plymouth University, Devon, UK
e-mail: jenny.freeman@plymouth.ac.uk

A. Wilkins (ed.), *Progressive Multiple Sclerosis*,
https://doi.org/10.1007/978-3-319-65921-3_10

This chapter provides an overview of the key principles of rehabilitation, describes different models of service delivery, and presents a synopsis of the evidence for a range of rehabilitation interventions. Rather than attempt to cover the full range of symptoms experienced by people with progressive MS that are managed within rehabilitation, it complements Chap. 7 ("Symptomatic management") which discusses the management of key symptoms including spasticity, pain, urogenital symptoms, speech and swallowing problems, psychiatric and cognitive disturbances. Ideally, these two chapters should be read in conjunction with one another to gain a holistic overview. Wherever possible the discussion within this chapter draws on evidence from studies of people with progressive MS, but where this is not available then recommendations are extrapolated from studies of mixed MS samples.

10.2 Key Principles of Rehabilitation

10.2.1 The International Classification of Functioning, Disability and Health

The framework used to describe, plan and provide rehabilitation services is the International Classification of Functioning, Disability and Health (ICF) framework (Fig. 10.1); where impairments (the varied symptoms of MS), activity limitations (e.g. self-care, mobility, continence) and participation restrictions (e.g. paid or unpaid work, driving, leisure activities) interact with contextual factors (environmental, personal) that influence people's performance outcomes [8]. The ICF

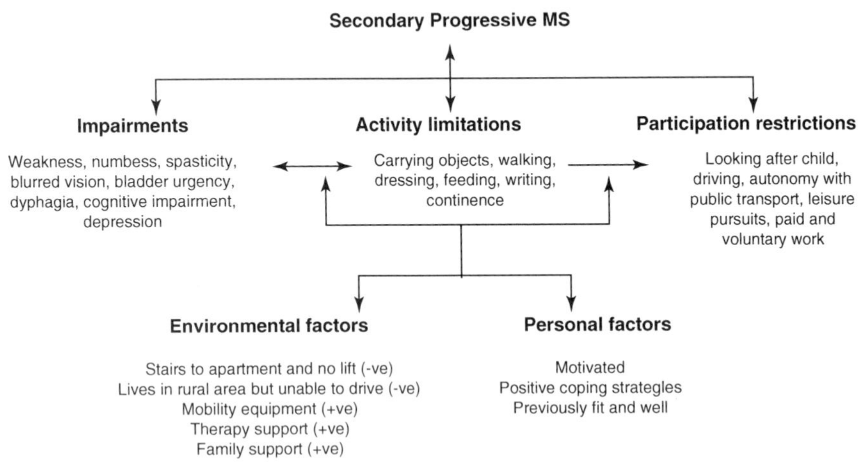

Fig. 10.1 The international classification of functioning, disability and health

terminology is used throughout this chapter. In the progressive phase of MS, rehabilitation often focuses on managing disability and enhancing participation, although not at the exclusion of treating the underlying modifiable impairments.

10.2.2 Collaborative Multi-Disciplinary Approach to Support Self-Management

There are many definitions of rehabilitation; an example being "Rehabilitation is an active process of change by which a person who has become disabled acquires and uses the knowledge and skills necessary for optimal physical, psychological, and social function" [9]. Intrinsic to all of these definitions is the notion that the individual is central to planning and actively participating in the process, with the primary focus being on behavioural change in order to optimise activity and participation.

A strong educational bias is key to successful rehabilitation since the person with MS (and their carer) is constantly having to learn new knowledge and skills so that they can continually adapt and readapt to their circumstances as the disease progresses and disability accumulates. Typically, during the progressive phase the changes experienced are insidious. Provided the person is well informed, actively involved and supported in their rehabilitation management, there can be a gradual accommodation by them to this evolving situation, predominately through self-management. Important to recognise is that effective self-management is a team effort. Maintaining positive behaviours and lifestyle changes over the long term is hard work and requires ongoing support from professionals, family members and friends, particularly in the face of ongoing disease progression.

The neurological consequences of MS can be many and varied and are often interrelated; for example, there can be a combination of motor (weakness, spasticity, ataxia), sensory (proprioceptive and cutaneous loss), visual and vestibular impairments, fatigue, cognitive and emotional factors. Clinical guidelines [10] therefore recommend comprehensive, flexible coordinated multidisciplinary care and appropriate follow-up and support for patients and carers to address limitations in activity and participation levels. Effective targeting of intervention requires individualised assessment and evaluation by the use of appropriate outcome measures [11].

10.2.3 Timely Assessment and Review

With continued advances in healthcare, people with MS are living longer. It is estimated that, on average, people with MS live approximately 6 years fewer than the general population [12], and hence issues related to progressive disability (physical and cognitive), psychosocial adjustment, and social reintegration need to be addressed over long periods. The constantly evolving nature of progressive MS means that assessment cannot be a one-off process; re-evaluation is required for optimal success. A collaborative teamwork approach is required to ensure that the right professional is involved at the right time and in the right place; involving health, social service and third sector organisations where necessary.

The traditional approach to review, wherein the person is re-assessed at set intervals, regardless as to whether or not their situation has changed, is unlikely to meet this need. Self-referral or open access systems, in the form of face-to-face appointments and telephone help lines, offer an alternative model [13]. These systems allow individuals the flexibility to access services when their needs change, thus supporting them to self-manage their condition. To be effective, people with MS and their families need to know how, why and when they should contact services to gain advice and/or assistance in managing problems as they arise. Safety networks should be in place for people with marked cognitive impairment, emotional issues, or those who may struggle to identify problems that may be amenable to change with professional input. Importantly, "crisis management" should be avoided, planned management of disability and deficits should be anticipated (over time), and appropriate mechanisms that accommodate and facilitate functional independence provided [14].

10.2.4 Person Centred, Goal Oriented Approach

A goal-oriented approach aims to encourage individuals to be proactive in setting their own goals and priorities. This is central to rehabilitation. By placing the person at the heart of decision-making it is a useful mechanism for guiding professionals on how to support the individual to best manage their condition in a way that is relevant and meaningful to them, and within the context of their lifestyle. Goal setting is not easy; people with MS, their families and those involved in their care, whilst sharing concerns, also have different perspectives [15]. For example, sometimes people with MS do not wish to expend their energies on therapy and retraining even though the scientific evidence suggests this may provide benefits; family members may disagree on the person's capabilities and desires; and professionals may be tempted to usurp the individual's decision-making power in their enthusiasm to provide "excellent" care. Whilst recognising the complexity of this process, and acknowledging that there remains a need to establish the effectiveness of goal setting in improving activity and participation levels [16], it has been shown that it can provide a useful mechanism for planning and monitoring progress and enhancing team communication. There is also evidence to suggest that patients with increased involvement in goal setting report greater satisfaction with their rehabilitation experience [17].

10.3 Rehabilitation Approaches

The approach to rehabilitation for people with MS can be viewed in three ways. Whilst each provides a different emphasis on management, viewed together they provide a continuum of care throughout the different stages of the disease course.

10.3.1 Health Promotion

The importance of health promotion is increasingly recognised as evidence emerges that the incidence rates of diabetes, hypertension, and hyperlipidemia are rising within the MS population [18]. This is particularly relevant given recent evidence that people with MS are living longer [19]. Optimising brain volume and cognitive reserve is also now being emphasised through the promotion of a 'brain-healthy' lifestyle, for example through encouragement of participation in aerobic exercise, avoidance of smoking and excessive alcohol consumption and weight loss [20]. Whilst this emphasis on "brain-health" has tended to be more prominent for those in the early stages of the disease, this also has relevance for people with progressive MS.

10.3.2 Restorative Rehabilitation

Evidence based Clinical Guidelines recommend early referral for rehabilitation which is targeted at restoring recent functional deterioration and helping people to maintain their usual roles [10, 14]. The strategies implemented are based on a comprehensive assessment of the unique needs of the individual. Where function is being limited by modifiable impairments (such as weakness, spasticity, pain and emotional distress) then this is often the focus of intervention, but where changes in impairments are not possible/limited then improvements can often still be achieved through the acquisition of new skills. For those with complex disability, this may require provision of adaptive equipment and modifications to the environment to restore some functional independence, as well as to reduce the burden of ongoing care in the community.

There is a growing body of evidence, from mixed neurological populations which include people with progressive MS, that specialist inpatient rehabilitation can be highly cost-efficient, producing substantial savings in ongoing care costs, especially in those with more complex disability [21]. Similarly, there a growing evidence-base for many of the other rehabilitation interventions utilised in people with progressive MS; this evidence is presented later in this chapter. Because of the variable nature of the disease course, the benefits gained will generally diminish over time [22]. Rehabilitation therefore cannot be viewed as a "one-off" intervention, and targeted re-referral will be necessary at various time-points throughout the disease course.

10.3.3 Maintenance Rehabilitation

As disability worsens, often over many years, personal and economic costs may soar [23]. During this time, much of the burden of the physical and emotional tasks of caring falls on family members, many of whom become lifelong caregivers [20]. People with severe disabilities may live for many years, enduring co-morbidities and complications such as aspiration pneumonia, urinary tract infections, complications of falls and fractures, and sepsis secondary to pressure ulcers, all of which are major causes of death [24]. Support from health and social care professionals is needed to help manage this. Whilst the physical tasks of caring can be daunting and exhausting, carers have described adjusting to and managing the cognitive impairment of the person with MS as being particularly challenging to deal with [3]. So too is the feeling of loneliness and isolation that can occur, not only for the person with MS, but also for their family and caregivers [25].

It is not uncommon for caregiver support needs to be overlooked [4], and this can be compounded by the fact that carers themselves may reject support offered to them [3]. Key issues to consider include respite, community and/or long-term care, and community mobility. For example, educating carers about how they can best help the person with MS to move, and to achieve comfortable positioning in bed and in the wheelchair can go some way to help to reduce the burden of care. Key too is the provision of equipment to assist with this such as hoists, transfer aids, specialist beds, mattresses and seating [26].

As the disease progresses and disability becomes more advanced, there is an increasing overlap between neuro-rehabilitation and neuro-palliative care. In contrast to typical palliative contexts, coping with disability rather than end-of-life is reported to be the major concern of people with MS and their carers [4], with increasing evidence to support the effectiveness of palliative care in improving symptoms and the quality of life of patients and families [27].

10.4 Organisation of Service Delivery

The nature of progressive MS means that people may have a wide variety of care needs, requiring them to access different pathways of care through a range of services. Reflecting this, rehabilitation is provided by multiple different professionals, within a variety of settings, by a range of services (Table 10.1). Community based rehabilitation closer to home, is particularly important as mobility difficulties arise

Table 10.1 MS service delivery across settings

Hospital outpatient clinics	Inpatient/residential	Community based	Tele-rehabilitation
• Neurology outpatient clinics • Multi-disciplinary clinics: – Spasticity – Foot drop (Functional—Electrical Stimulation; Orthotics) – Vocational rehabilitation • Therapy input, e.g. physiotherapy, occupational therapy	• Specialist inpatient rehabilitation units • General inpatient rehabilitation units • Respite care services • Inpatient hospital stay, e.g. surgical procedures such as intrathecal baclofen pumps, deep brain stimulation for tremor	• General practice • Community rehabilitation: e.g. therapy delivered within the home setting; group based sessions such as fatigue management programmes within local centres • Links with vocational specialist services such as work based assessments, liaison with local employment services • Links with social services providing personal care and home adaptations • Links with local leisure centres, e.g. exercise classes, exercise prescription schemes • Third Sector organisations, such as MS Centres	• Tele-consultations • Video-link consultations with specialist centres • Web-based programmes Telephone advice lines (both NHS and Third sector organisations)

and increased effort and resources may be required to maintain autonomy in aspects such as vocation and transportation.

Close collaboration between the multiple agencies and professions involved is needed to prevent fragmentation and duplication of services. In practice, this is challenging to achieve. For some, the complexity of the system and the number of professionals they have to deal with can be overwhelming. In contrast, others feel they "get lost within the system" or "are left to get on with it", failing to receive the advice and input they need which can lead to minor problems being left unchecked, and a subsequent need for crisis management. Whilst there are no easy solutions, a key-worker system, which provides a single point of contact into the complex array of hospital and community services, can help to enhance communication and channel services to provide input when needed.

Technological advances have begun to enable integration of tele-rehabilitation into some rehabilitation services. In some cases this can provide an alternative approach to face-to-face care, in others it complements existing care [28]. For example, there is some evidence to support the use of web-based programmes in: (1) Education aimed at improving self-efficacy of both the person with MS and their carer; (2) Symptom management, such as fatigue and low mood [29]; and (3) Enhancing long-term behavior change in areas such as physical activity/exercise [30]. These programmes can provide remote access 24 h/day, thereby reducing some barriers to accessing rehabilitation. They potentially enable reach to a larger and broader population. Alongside this, other forms of tele-rehabilitation such as telephone advice lines, tele-consultations, and video link consultations with specialist centres are also being used [31]. Accessing services in this way may be especially relevant to people in the progressive phase because, whilst their complex clinical presentations often require expert advice, they may find it difficult to attend face-to-face clinical appointments because of factors such as transportation difficulties due to their disability, or excessive fatigue. Tele-rehabilitation is a relatively new approach within MS neuro-rehabilitation and whilst promising evidence from small scale RCT's is emerging, definitive evidence is needed to establish clinical and cost effectiveness [28].

10.5 Evidence-Based Rehabilitation Interventions

The evidence base for MS neuro-rehabilitation interventions is steadily increasing, as supported by the findings of a recent umbrella review [1]. This systematic review of 39 systematic reviews provides 'strong' evidence for physical therapy modalities (exercise/physical activities) in terms of functional outcomes such as mobility, muscle strength and aerobic capacity, as well as quality of life. It provides 'moderate' evidence in favour of multi-disciplinary rehabilitation for producing long-term gains at the levels of activity and participation; and comprehensive fatigue management programmes. Psychological interventions such as cognitive behavioural therapy for the treatment of depression is also supported by moderate quality evidence; as is the provision of information for increasing patient's knowledge. The limited number of methodologically robust studies in a number of areas, however, means that evidence currently remains relatively low for interventions including occupational therapy strategies, upper limb rehabilitation programmes, electrical stimulation, interactive video gaming, and robot-assisted training. There is a need for clinical trials in these areas to guide practice.

Numerous rehabilitation interventions are available to treat the wide variety of symptoms experienced by people with MS. A synopsis of the evidence in key areas is provided both here and in Chap. 7 ("Symptomatic management"). As previously highlighted, the vast majority of this evidence is based on mixed MS samples, hence where evidence from studies of people with progressive MS is not available the results have been extrapolated from those with relapse remitting disease.

10.5.1 Mobility, Balance and Falls Management Interventions

By the time that people have reached the progressive phase virtually all have walking difficulties, with an estimated 25% eventually confined to a wheelchair [32]. Mobility impairments frequently restrict participation in work, family, social, vocational, and leisure activities. It is therefore not surprising that surveys of people with MS consistently rank mobility as their highest priority, describing it as their most important yet most challenging daily function [33]. Impaired balance is an important contributor to these mobility difficulties, with evidence demonstrating that balance is more impaired in those with progressive MS [34]. This has important ramifications since impaired balance is associated with falls, with an estimated 70% of ambulant people with progressive MS falling regularly [35]. To date, study samples have excluded people scoring greater than 6.5 on the EDSS, and hence it remains unknown whether falls remain a significant problem for people once they rely almost exclusively on a wheelchair to move about.

A meta-analysis assessing risk factors associated with falls showed that a progressive disease course is associated with a twofold increased risk of falling compared with relapsing remitting disease [36]; at a rate of 26 falls/person/year in those with secondary progressive MS [37]. This is important since more than 10% of falls lead to injuries [38] and people with MS are three times more likely to sustain a fracture then the general population [39]. Crucially, falling and a fear of falling can profoundly affect an individual's quality of life, resulting in a loss of confidence and restriction in activity levels. This in turn can lead to a downward spiral of immobility, deconditioning and disability accumulation [40]. Consequently, the management of safe mobility and falls is an important goal of rehabilitation.

A range of interventions, usually undertaken by physiotherapists, are used to enhance balance and safe mobility including: balance training, functional electrical stimulation, resistance training, aerobic training, gaming technology, robotics and treadmill training. The overall conclusion of the systematic reviews in this area is that physiotherapy has small, but significant, beneficial effects on balance in those with mild to moderate disability [41, 42]. However, when the level of disability increases, evidence to demonstrate the efficacy of physiotherapy is less compelling. With regard to pharmacological treatments, prolonged-release (PR) oral dalfampridine, a voltage-gated potassium channel blocker able to improve action potential conduction in demyelinated axons, is specifically licensed to improve walking in people with MS. Dalfampridine has demonstrated improvements in both walking speed [43] and balance [44], with indications that it may also improve walking distance in some people [45].

Whilst evidence to support the effectiveness of interventions in people with progressive disease remains limited, research is beginning to focus exclusively on this group [46, 47], and there is some encouraging evidence from studies evaluating treadmill training and robot assisted ambulatory training that functional gains can continue to be made even in individuals with more severe disability [48, 49]. To date, the comparative effectiveness of these varied approaches has not been investigated either for those with relapsing and remitting or progressive disease; and duration of follow-up has been limited to the short term. Evidence about cost effectiveness is also needed since these interventions can be particularly resource intensive in people with more severe disability.

It is probable that there is a point at which neural reserve becomes too low for neural plasticity to promote functional change in mobility, although this has yet to be confirmed. Peripheral physiological changes, such as muscle strength and endurance, also impact on balance and mobility status. So too does the ageing process, wherein reintegration of sensory information becomes more difficult and attention demanding for older adults. All of these factors are relevant to people with progressive MS who are typically older and with a higher burden of disability. Nevertheless, it is important to reassure people in the progressive phase, that when balance and gait impairments do not respond to training, compensatory strategies can be used to facilitate mobility. For example assistive devices such as orthotics, walking aids, manual and powered wheelchairs, and scooters can all be used to enhance safety and autonomy, minimise fatigue by energy conservation, and increase occupational performance [50, 51]. It is not unusual for people to express reluctance when first trialling these mobility devices since they can be viewed as a symbol of loss of function, however, it is noteworthy that in addition to the physical benefits gained, many people report increased feelings of competence, adaptability, and self-esteem through the use of this equipment [26].

10.5.2 Enhancing Physical Fitness and Physical Activity

Research demonstrates that even in the early stages of the disease, people with MS are more sedentary than healthy controls and hence at risk of developing adverse health conditions [52]. This is particularly the case for those with progressive MS who are more disabled [53]. As the disease progresses exercise becomes increasingly challenging because of the myriad of symptoms people have to contend with, which may include fatigue, pain, heat-sensitivity, balance and mobility deficits, ataxia, spasticity, weakness, bladder and bowel problems and cognitive impairments [54]. Over time deconditioning occurs, as demonstrated by the close negative association between disease severity and cardiopulmonary fitness [55, 56]. Consequently encouraging people to be less sedentary and to undertake regular physical activity is important since there is evidence that at least some of the disability that occurs after MS is due to this secondary deconditioning from the sedentary lifestyle adopted, not simply CNS damage alone.

The beneficial effects of exercise have been the subject of multiple systematic reviews of mixed samples of MS. Despite methodological problems (e.g. small sample sizes, lack of long-term follow-up), there is now strong evidence that regular exercise can improve aerobic capacity, muscle strength, mobility, balance, and quality of life, with growing evidence that it may benefit fatigue and mood [57, 58]. There is some preliminary evidence that exercise may benefit cognition [59, 60], but replication studies are needed and the best type of exercise needs to be clarified.

Cardiovascular and resistance training have both proven feasible and well tolerated in people with progressive MS, even for those with more severe disability [46, 61]. Neither form of exercise is associated with side effects [62]. There is some evidence to suggest that exercise may influence not just the secondary deconditioning, but may have a positive impact on the CNS damage by reducing inflammation and encouraging neuronal repair [63]. On the basis of evidence from these systematic reviews, it is recommended that people with mild to moderate disability, between 18 and 65 years of age, undertake 30 min of moderate intensity aerobic exercise twice a week (e.g. stationary bicycle, treadmill of rowing machine) and 30 min of moderate intensity strength training for major muscle groups twice a week [57, 58]. It is noteworthy, however, that this evidence is based predominately on people with relapsing and remitting disease, and therefore some caution should be made when extrapolating these results to those in the progressive phase.

Key to sustaining benefits over the longer term is that exercise is incorporated into a person's lifestyle, since it has been repeatedly shown that any benefits gained tail off once exercise is stopped. Because of this, many agree that exercise interventions should incorporate behavioural change techniques, wherein people are provided with skills, resources, and strategies (such as identifying barriers and problem solving), to optimise successful long-term behaviour change [64]; although a recent systematic review showed that many behavioural physical activity interventions also fail to sustain long-term effects [65]. In light of this, it is acknowledged that people also need to have ongoing access to guidance and support from health professionals and/or sports instructors, so that adaptations to the programme and/or equipment can be made as a person's circumstances changes.

10.5.3 Upper Limb Rehabilitation Programmes

Deficits of upper limb function have been reported in up to 75% of people with MS, with a higher prevalence in those with progressive disease [66], and manual dexterity has found to be a key predictor of activity and participation within the community [67]. Despite this relatively little research has been undertaken in this area compared to the lower limb; and this is reflected by the relative lack of attention given to the upper limb in clinical practice.

The emergence of new technologies accessible to rehabilitation, such as robotics, virtual reality and video gaming allows high intensity repetitive training. This has begun to focus people's attention on improving arm and hand functioning, since specificity and intensity of motor training has shown to be important in achieving successful outcomes [68]. Lamers et al. [66] undertook a systematic review of 30 MS studies, half of which specifically targeted the upper limb alone. Most were comprised of mixed MS samples, with just four studies exclusively sampling people in the progressive phase. A wide variety of interventional strategies were investigated, which included strength and endurance training, task-oriented upper limb training, constraint-induced therapy, sensory re-education training, robot-supported training and tele-rehabilitation. Despite the methodological limitations of many of these studies (small sample sizes, lack of randomisation and blinding, lack of long term follow-up) the results show promising benefits in terms of improved upper limb function. Of note, one study that included neuroimaging measures, found that task-oriented upper limb training positively affected the white matter architecture [69]. Thus far, studies have not investigated the comparative effectiveness of these interventions, and there is little evidence to guide practice with regard to the optimal therapy dosage according to the upper limb disability level. It has been postulated, for instance that people in the progressive phase, with more severe upper limb dysfunction, may not be able to tolerate high intensity training due to motor fatigue and reduced neural reserve, and may therefore benefit from longer training duration at low intensity. Further research is required to determine whether this is the case.

10.5.4 Management of Ataxia

Approximately 80% of people with MS experience ataxia [70]. Whilst a range of pharmacological (e.g. isoniazid, pyridoxine, and cannabis), surgical (e.g. stereotactic neurosurgery—thalamotomy or deep-brain stimulation), and rehabilitative treatments are available, this symptom remains particularly challenging to manage effectively and reviews in this area highlight that the evidence base available to guide choice of intervention remains limited [70–73]. To date, no studies have focused specifically on people with progressive MS.

Rehabilitation interventions utilised for ataxia can be either compensatory or restorative in their approach. Restorative strategies aim at treating the underlying co-ordination impairment. These typically involve the use of intensive balance and co-ordination exercises, or balance and ocular exercises delivered as part of a physiotherapy programme [74]. More recently, novel methods have been trialled, for example using adaptive robot therapy to deliver highly repetitive, interactive activity with some improvements demonstrated in manual dexterity and co-ordination of the upper limbs [75]. Biofeedback linked to computer games that require balance and multi-segment coordination has also been used with some success to improve balance and falls [76].

Compensatory strategies are commonly taught to people when disability levels are greater. This approach includes the provision of equipment such as walking aids (typically wheeled frames) to help improve posture, balance, and mobility; and adaptive appliances to help with independence in daily functional tasks such as eating and drinking (e.g. neater eaters which dampen tremor, wheelchair mounted cup holders with steady straw systems), use of computers (e.g. adaptive key boards, voice recognition software) and household activities (such as kettle tippers). Different techniques can also be taught to minimise the interference of tremor and ataxia when moving. These may include: breaking movement patterns into simpler single joint movements; using visual and verbal cues to help walking speed and stride length; and biofeedback through virtual reality or electromyography [71, 72]. Interventions that increase inertia by loading the limbs or trunk with weights demonstrate variable success [73]. More recently, lycra garments have been used to reduce ataxia/tremor by improving trunk stability and function, with some preliminary evidence to support their success [77].

10.5.5 *Fatigue Management*

Fatigue has been defined as a decrease in physical and/or mental performance that results from changes in central, psychological, and/or peripheral factors [78]. Estimated to occur in approximately 80% of people with MS, fatigue is more common in progressive than in relapsing-remitting disease [79]. Fatigue impacts negatively on functional performance in daily life, societal participation and quality of life [80] and hence it is unsurprising that two-thirds of people with MS report this as one of their most troubling symptoms [81]. Despite being such a commonly experienced symptom, research about its characteristics, mechanisms and therapeutics is hampered by the difficulty in clearly defining and measuring fatigue [82]. Table 10.2 provides a summary of the contributors to fatigue, which are broadly divided into primary and secondary factors (Table 10.2).

Given that both the causes and consequences of MS fatigue are multidimensional, multidisciplinary intervention is usually necessary for successful management. Clinical practice guidelines suggest medication in conjunction with rehabilitation strategies for managing fatigue [10], however, these recommendations are based on relatively little scientific evidence, which is from studies of mixed samples, and variable methodological quality.

The most commonly used pharmacological treatments for MS related fatigue include amantadine, modafinil, and pemoline, and whilst systematic reviews provide some evidence to support their use [83, 84] the results of these studies are mixed. Two systematic reviews and meta-analyses of a broad range of interventions, including medication, exercise, energy conservation treatment, vestibular rehabilitation, and educational strategies which incorporate advice on healthy living (nutritional diet, regular sleeping patterns), suggest that rehabilitation should be the initial treatment choice for those who are reporting disabling fatigue [85, 86]. The effectiveness of exercise [87] in reducing fatigue has also been supported by a recent systematic reviews and meta-analysis; although few of the studies explored people with severe fatigue. Randomised controlled trials of patient education programmes,

Table 10.2 Contributors to fatigue in MS

Primary factors	Secondary factors
• Nervous system damage leading to increased energy exertion • Decreases in brain metabolism • Dysregulation of the immune system • Dysregulation of the endocrine system	• Lack of physical conditioning • Interrupted sleep (because of sleep apnoea, restless legs, pain, bladder/bowel problems, alcohol/caffeine use) • Pain • Psychological factors such as anxiety, depression, chronic stress • Drugs used to treat MS (such as interferon therapies, muscle relaxants, analgesics, sedatives, anti-depressants, anti-convulsants) • Poor diet

that incorporate a cognitive behavioural approach have also demonstrated to be beneficial [88]. The vast majority of research to date in this area has been in mixed samples, and hence caution should be taken when extrapolating the conclusions to the progressive phase. However, it is encouraging that in the few small-scale studies of energy conservation techniques or exercise that have focused solely on progressive MS [61, 89], short term benefits have been shown.

10.5.6 Emotional Support

The availability of psychological support is viewed by many people with MS as an important deficit in available services [90]. Evidence from qualitative studies suggest that the transition to secondary progressive MS appears to be a particular 'fear-point' in the disease course, often triggering a significant emotional reaction [3]. Clinicians have described the patient's experience of receiving confirmation of the onset of secondary progressive MS as similar to 'being diagnosed again' [90]. At this time point, the person is not only having to come to terms with the uncertainties related to having a progressive disease in which they face declining mobility, physical and cognitive function, but may also find that they are discontinued from disease modifying interventions [91]. Alongside this, they may experience a reduction in follow-up reviews by the neurology team [3]. It is common at this stage for people to feel abandoned and unclear about future options. Emotional support and information provision is therefore particularly important at this time to help people to develop coping strategies such as being positive, accessing support and taking each day as it comes [92]; at times this may require professional input.

Relationships with health care providers and the patterns of communication within these relationships is of critical importance to people with MS [93]. Not only can it shape how they feel about their experiences of health care but it also influences their ongoing ability to manage their illness in the context of their daily lives. Reassuring individuals that rehabilitation interventions/symptomatic treatments of demonstrable benefit are available to help manage physical, cognitive and emotional problems as they arise may go some way to help alleviate their fears that they will be "left to get on with it" by themselves. Follow-up mechanisms should be set in place so that problems can be addressed as they arise. For example, the availability of MS Clinical Specialist Nurses, Therapists, and the use of self-referral systems/telephone helplines can facilitate timely access to services as required [13]. Signposting to appropriate information and local support groups can also be helpful, with encouragement to continue to engage in physical and social activity. Taking the time to communicate with people about their situation and to provide clear and honest information is viewed as important by people with MS and their carers who want to know what progressive MS means for them and what they could be doing to help themselves. There is evidence that people with MS do not want information to be 'sugar-coated', and that they can feel betrayed or patronised if they believe that clinicians have chosen to withhold information [93]. By providing honest explanations in a sensitive manner, professionals can support people to self-manage and give them confidence that health professionals will form part of a supportive network for the future [3].

Alongside the provision of emotional support, the diagnosis and management of depression and anxiety is important, since these symptoms impact significantly on the quality of peoples' lives and their ability to engage in rehabilitation [94]. A recent systematic review identified the lifetime prevalence for major depression or anxiety as approximately 30% [95], which is significantly more common than in healthy individuals. Pharmacological and rehabilitation interventions to help manage depression, as well as other neuropsychiatric disorders, has been described in Chap. 7 on symptomatic management and so will not be elaborated on here.

10.6 MS Rehabilitation and Brain Plasticity

It has been suggested that the main goal of rehabilitation therapy is to facilitate adaptation and reorganization within the CNS, in other words "applied neuroplasticity." [96]. Neuroplasticity is the ability of the nervous system to respond to intrinsic or extrinsic stimuli by reorganizing its structure, function and connections [97]. Recent research with advanced MRI techniques demonstrate that neuroplastic changes are present in people with MS; with differences in functional organisation of the brain, and increased brain activation compared to healthy controls on both passive and active motor tasks [98, 99] and cognitive tasks [100]. Particularly relevant to people with progressive MS is that this brain activation pattern appears to increase with increasing diffuse brain injury and increasing disability [101, 102].

In his recent review of current scientific evidence relating to neuroplasticity and non-invasive, non-pharmacological, MS rehabilitation interventions, Flachenecker [103] provides evidence from a (limited) number of studies to support the hypothesis that compensatory adaptive changes in brain activation and functional connectivity may account, at least in part, for the motor and cognitive recovery seen following rehabilitation [104, 105]. These studies demonstrated that clinical improvements correlated with neural plasticity in the CNS (increased fMRI activity), even in patients with a high burden of pathology. There was some indication that the changes in patterns of cerebral activation and connectivity are maintained over the longer term [106]. Of significance, however, it has been shown that neuroplasticity can also be maladaptive and thus contribute to or sustain disability [101, 107]. It is therefore key to validate those specific rehabilitation interventions that are associated with positive adaptive neuroplasticity and associated functional gains. Whilst many of these studies have targeted those people in the relapsing/remitting phase, and have tapped into brain recovery processes in the earlier stages of MS, this remains relevant in the progressive phase, with encouraging evidence that the capacity for neuroplasticity and motor learning seems to continue even in those with more severe disability [108, 109].

Non-invasive neuro-modulatory therapies such as repetitive transcranial magnetic stimulation and transcranial direct current stimulation (amongst others) provide information on motor cortex excitability and plasticity and offer a method for evaluating the efficacy of rehabilitation interventions [102]. They have also been used to directly modulate cortical excitability, with some promising results for example in reducing fatigue [109, 110], spasticity [111] and pain [112]; and have been trialled for people with MS in neuro-rehabilitation settings as an add-on treatment [113], with benefits shown. In their review of techniques used to modulate plasticity in MS, Houdayer and colleagues [102] highlight the potential importance of these in helping to personalise treatments for people with MS, whilst recognising that their therapeutic value is yet to be established.

10.7 Conclusion

Progressive MS is challenging to manage, both for people with MS and those involved in their care. No disease modifying therapy has yet shown robust benefits, and so rehabilitation strategies in combination with symptomatic therapy are the mainstay of clinical practice. People in the progressive phase should not be "left to get on with it". Person centred management, based on an assessment of the individual's needs, and provided in a co-ordinated and timely manner by members of the multi-disciplinary team is essential to best manage the wide ranging and interacting physical, cognitive and emotional symptoms that people may face on a daily basis, and which can impact significantly on the quality of their lives.

The lack of robust evidence for many of the existing rehabilitation treatments for patients with progressive MS means that clinical decisions currently rely on extrapolating evidence from those with relapse remitting MS and other neurological conditions. Large, high quality, multicentre clinical trials and innovative studies targeting people with progressive MS are needed to establish benefit and guide management. Encouragingly, an improved understanding of brain plasticity is beginning to inform the development of new and potentially effective rehabilitation approaches. This together with advances in technology has the potential to improve outcomes for people with progressive MS, including those with significant disability.

References

1. Khan F, Amatya B. Rehabilitation in multiple sclerosis: a systematic review of systematic reviews. Arch Phys Med Rehabil. 2017;98(2):353–67.
2. Feinstein A, Freeman J, Lo AC. Treatment of progressive multiple sclerosis: what works, what does not, and what is needed. Lancet Neurol. 2015;14(2):194–207.
3. Davies F, Edwards A, Brain K, Edwards M, Jones R, Wallbank R, et al. 'You are just left to get on with it': qualitative study of patient and carer experiences of the transition to secondary progressive multiple sclerosis. BMJ Open. 2015;5(7):e007674.

4. Borreani C, Bianchi E, Pietrolongo E, Rossi I, Cilia S, et al. Unmet needs of people with severe multiple sclerosis and their carers: qualitative findings for a home-based intervention. PLoS One. 2014;9(10):e109679.
5. Freeman JA, Thompson AJ. Community services in multiple sclerosis: still a matter of chance. J Neurol Neurosurg Psychiatry. 2000;69(6):728–32.
6. Ronning OM, Tornes KD. Need for symptomatic management in advanced multiple sclerosis. Acta Neurol Scand. 2016;135(5):529–32. doi:10.1111/ane.12631.
7. Lonergan R, Kinsella K, Fitzpatrick P, Duggan M, Jordan S, Bradley D, et al. Unmet needs of multiple sclerosis patients in the community. Mult Scler Relat Disord. 2015;4(2):144–50.
8. Coenen M, Cieza A, Freeman J, Khan F, Miller D, Weise A, et al. The development of ICF Core Sets for multiple sclerosis: results of the International Consensus Conference. J Neurol. 2011;258(8):1477–88.
9. Disability committee of the royal college of physicians. London: HMSO; 1981.
10. National Institute for Clinical Excellence (NICE). Multiple sclerosis: management of multiple sclerosis in primary and secondary care. Clinical Guidelines -8, NICE. 2014. http://www.nice.org.uk.
11. Thompson AJ, et al. J Neurol Neurosurg Psychiatry. 2001;71(suppl 2):ii22–i7.
12. Kaufman DW, Reshef S, Golub HL, Peucker M, Corwin MJ, Goodin DS, et al. Survival in commercially insured multiple sclerosis patients and comparator subjects in the U.S. Mult Scler Relat Disord. 2014;3(3):364–71.
13. Zajicek J, Freeman JA, Porter B. Multiple sclerosis care: a practical manual. Oxford: Oxford University Press; 2007. ISBN: 13: 9780198569831.
14. National Institute for Clinical Excellence (NICE). Multiple sclerosis: management of multiple sclerosis in primary and secondary care. Clinical Guidelines -8, NICE. 2003. ISBN: 1842574426, http://www.nice.org.uk.
15. Audulv A, Asplund K, Norbergh KG. Who's in charge? The role of responsibility attribution in self-management among people with chronic illness. Patient Educ Couns. 2010;81(1):94–100.
16. Levack WMM, Weatherall M, Hay-Smith EJC, Dean SG, McPherson K, Siegert RJ. Goal setting and strategies to enhance goal pursuit for adults with acquired disability participating in rehabilitation. Cochrane Database Syst Rev. 2015;7:CD009727. doi:10.1002/14651858.CD009727.pub2.
17. Holliday RC, Cano S, Freeman JA, Playford ED. Should patients participate in clinical decision making? An optimised balance block design controlled study of goal setting in a rehabilitation unit. J Neurol Neurosurg Psychiatry. 2007;78(6):576–80.
18. Marrie RA, Cohen J, Stuve O, Trojano M, Sorensen PS, Reingold S, et al. A systematic review of the incidence and prevalence of comorbidity in multiple sclerosis: overview. Mult Scler. 2015;21(3):263–81.
19. Mackenzie IS, Morant SV, Bloomfield GA, MacDonald TM, O'Riordan J. Incidence and prevalence of multiple sclerosis in the UK 1990–2010: a descriptive study in the General Practice Research Database. J Neurol Neurosurg Psychiatry. 2014;85:76–84.
20. Giovannoni G, Butzkueven H, Dhib-Jalbut S, Hobart J, Kobelt G Pepper G et al. MS brain health: time matters. ISBN 978-1-903539-13-2. www.msbrainhealth.org.
21. Turner-Stokes L, Williams H, Bill A, Bassett P, Sephton K. Cost-efficiency of specialist inpatient rehabilitation for working-aged adults with complex neurological disabilities: a multicentre cohort analysis of a national clinical data set. BMJ Open. 2016;6(2):e010238.
22. Freeman JA, Langdon DW, Hobart JC, Thompson AJ. Inpatient rehabilitation in multiple sclerosis: do the benefits carry over into the community? Neurology. 1999;52(1):50.
23. Ernstsson O, Gyllensten H, Alexanderson K, Tinghög P, Friberg E, Norlund A. Cost of Illness of multiple sclerosis—a systematic review. PLoS One. 2016;11(7):e0159129.
24. Higginson I, Hart S, Silber E, Burman R, Edmonds P. Symptom prevalence and severity in people severely affected by multiple sclerosis. J Palliat Care. 2006;22(3):158–65.
25. Beal CC, Stuifbergen A. Loneliness in women with multiple sclerosis. Rehabil Nurs. 2007;32(4):165–71.

26. Souza A, Kelleher A, Cooper R, Cooper RA, Iezzoni LI, Collins DM. Multiple sclerosis and mobility-related assistive technology: systematic review of literature. J Rehabil Res Dev. 2010;47(3):213.
27. Oliver DJ, Borasio GD, Caraceni A, de Visser M, Grisold W, Lorenzl S, et al. A consensus review on the development of palliative care for patients with chronic and progressive neurological disease. Eur J Neurol. 2016;23(1):30–8.
28. Amatya B, Galea MP, Kesselring J, Khan F. Effectiveness of telerehabilitation interventions in persons with multiple sclerosis: a systematic review. Mult Scler Relat Disord. 2015;4(4):358–69.
29. Ghahari S, Packer T. Effectiveness of online and face-to-face fatigue self-management programmes for adults with neurological conditions. Disabil Rehabil. 2012;34(7):564–73.
30. Dlugonski D, Motl RW, McAuley E. Increasing physical activity in multiple sclerosis: replicating Internet intervention effects using objective and self-report outcomes. J Rehabil Res Dev. 2011;48(9):1129–36.
31. Porter B, Thompson A. Connecting to the future-the promise of telecare. Mult Scler. 2012; 18(4):384–6.
32. Noseworthy JH, Lucchinetti C, Rodriguez M, Weinshenker BG. Multiple sclerosis. N Engl J Med. 2000;343(13):938–52.
33. Heesen C, Bohm J, Reich C, Kasper J, Goebel M, Gold SM. Patient perception of bodily functions in multiple sclerosis: gait and visual function are the most valuable. Mult Scler. 2008;14(7):988–91.
34. Soyuer F, Mirza M, Erkorkmaz U. Balance performance in three forms of multiple sclerosis. Neurol Res. 2006;28:555–62.
35. Gunn H, Creanor S, Haas B, Marsden JF, Freeman J. Risk factors for falls in multiple sclerosis: an observational study. Mult Scler. 2013;19:1913–22.
36. Gianni C, Prosperini L, Jonsdottir J, Cattaneo D. A systematic review of factors associated with accidental falls in people with multiple sclerosis: a meta-analytic approach. Clin Rehabil. 2014;28(7):704–16.
37. Gunn H, Creanor S, Haas B, Marsden J, Freeman J. Frequency, characteristics and consequences of falls in multiple sclerosis: findings from a cohort study. Arch Phys Med Rehabil. 2014; 95:538–45.
38. Peterson EW, Cho CC, von Koch L, Finlayson ML. Injurious falls among middle aged and older adults with multiple sclerosis. Arch Phys Med Rehabil. 2008;89:1031–7.
39. Bazelier MT, van Staa T-P, Uitdehaag BMJ, Cooper C, Leufkens HGM, Vestergaard P, et al. Risk of fractures in patients with multiple sclerosis: a population-based cohort study. Neurology. 2012;78:1967–73.
40. Peterson EW, Cho CC, Finlayson ML. Fear of falling and associated activity curtailment among middle aged and older adults with multiple sclerosis. Mult Scler. 2007;13(9):1168–75.
41. Paltamaa J, Sjogren T, Peurala SH, Heinonen A. Effects of physiotherapy interventions on balance in multiple sclerosis: a systematic review and meta-analysis of randomized controlled trials. J Rehabil Med. 2012;44(10):811–23.
42. Campbell E, Coulter EH, Mattison PG, Miller L, McFadyen A, Paul L. Physiotherapy rehabilitation for people with progressive multiple sclerosis: a systematic review. Arch Phys Med Rehabil. 2016;97(1):141–51.
43. Goodman AD, Brown TR, Edwards KR, Krupp LB, Schapiro RT, Cohen R, et al. A phase 3 trial of extended release oral dalfampridine in multiple sclerosis. Ann Neurol. 2010;68(4):494–502.
44. Prosperini L, Gianni C, Fortuna D, Marchetti MR, et al. Oral dalfampridine improves standing balance detected at static posturography in multiple sclerosis. Mult Scler Int. 2014;2014:802307. doi:10.1155/2014/802307.
45. Pickering H, Murray J, Lin CS, Cormack C, Martin A, Kiernan MC, et al. Fampridine treatment and walking distance in multiple sclerosis: a randomised controlled trial. Clin Neurophysiol. 2017;128(1):93–9.
46. Skjerbaek AG, Naesby M, Lutzen K, Moller AB, Jensen E, Lamers I, et al. Endurance training is feasible in severely disabled patients with progressive multiple sclerosis. Mult Scler. 2014;20(5):627–30.

47. Freeman JA, Hendrie W, Creanor S, Jarrett L, Barton A, Green C, et al. Standing up in multiple sclerosis (SUMS): protocol for a multi-centre randomised controlled trial evaluating the clinical and cost effectiveness of a home-based self-management standing frame programme in people with progressive multiple sclerosis. BMC Neurol. 2016;16:62.
48. Swinnen E, Beckwee D, Pinte D, Meeusen R, Baeyens JP, Kerckhofs E. Treadmill training in multiple sclerosis: can body weight support or robot assistance provide added value? A systematic review. Mult Scler Int. 2012;2012:240274.
49. Straudi S, Fanciullacci C, Martinuzzi C, Pavarelli C, Rossi B, Chisari C, et al. The effects of robot-assisted gait training in progressive multiple sclerosis: a randomized controlled trial. Mult Scler J. 2016;22(3):373–84.
50. Finlayson M, Guglielmello L, Liefer K. Describing and predicting the possession of assistive devices among persons with multiple sclerosis. Am J Occup Ther. 2001;55(5):545–51.
51. Stevens V, Goodman K, Rough K, Kraft GH. Gait impairment and optimizing mobility in multiple sclerosis. Phys Med Rehabil Clin N Am. 2013;24(4):573–92.
52. Backus D. Increasing physical activity and participation in people with multiple sclerosis: a review. Arch Phys Med Rehabil. 2016;97(9 Suppl):S210–7.
53. Motl RW, Arnett PA, Smith MM, Barwick FH, Ahlstrom B, Stover EJ. Worsening of symptoms is associated with lower physical activity levels in individuals with multiple sclerosis. Mult Scler. 2008;14(1):140–2.
54. Beckerman H, de Groot V, Scholten MA, Kempen JC, Lankhorst GJ. Physical activity behavior of people with multiple sclerosis: understanding how they can become more physically active. Phys Ther. 2010;90(7):1001–13.
55. Langeskov-Christensen M, Heine M, Kwakkel G, Dalgas U. Aerobic capacity in persons with multiple 4 sclerosis: a systematic review and meta-analysis. Sports Med. 2015;45(6):905–23.
56. Heine M, Wens I, Langeskov-Christensen M, Verschuren O, Eijnde BO, Kwakkel G, et al. Cardiopulmonary fitness is related to disease severity in multiple sclerosis. Mult Scler. 2016;22(2):231–8.
57. Latimer-Cheung AE, Pilutti LA, Hicks AL, Martin Ginis KA, Fenuta AM, MacKibbon KA, et al. Effects of exercise training on fitness, mobility, fatigue, and health-related quality of life among adults with multiple sclerosis: a systematic review to inform guideline development. Arch Phys Med Rehabil. 2013;94(9):1800–28. e3
58. Latimer-Cheung AE, Martin Ginis KA, Hicks AL, Motl RW, Pilutti LA, Duggan M, et al. Development of evidence-informed physical activity guidelines for adults with multiple sclerosis. Arch Phys Med Rehabil. 2013;94(9):1829–36. e7
59. Kierkegaard M, Lundberg IE, Olsson T, Johansson S, Ygberg S, Opava C, et al. High-intensity resistance training in multiple sclerosis—An exploratory study of effects on immune markers in blood and cerebrospinal fluid, and on mood, fatigue, health-related quality of life, muscle strength, walking and cognition. J Neurol Sci. 2016;362:251–7.
60. Kalron A, Zeilig G. Efficacy of exercise intervention programs on cognition in people suffering from multiple sclerosis, stroke and Parkinson's disease: a systematic review and meta-analysis of current evidence. NeuroRehabilitation. 2015;37(2):273–89.
61. Briken S, Gold SM, Patra S, Vettorazzi E, Harbs D, Tallner A, et al. Effects of exercise on fitness and cognition in progressive MS: a randomized, controlled pilot trial. Mult Scler. 2014;20(3):382–90.
62. Pilutti LA, Platta ME, Motl RW, Latimer-Cheung AE. The safety of exercise training in multiple sclerosis: a systematic review. J Neurol Sci. 2014;343(1–2):3–7.
63. Dalgas U, Stenager E. Exercise and disease progression in multiple sclerosis: can exercise slow down the progression of multiple sclerosis? Ther Adv Neurol Disord. 2012;5(2):81–95.
64. Geidl W, Semrau J, Pfeifer K, et al. Disabil Rehabil. 2014;36(24):2091–100. 9
65. Sangelaji B, Smith CM, Paul L, Sampath KK, Treharne GJ, Hale LA. The effectiveness of behaviour change interventions to increase physical activity participation in people with multiple sclerosis: a systematic review and meta-analysis. Clin Rehabil. 2016;30(6):559–76.
66. Lamers I, Maris A, Severijns D, Dielkens W, Geurts S, Van Wijmeersch B, et al. Upper limb rehabilitation in people with multiple sclerosis: a systematic review. Neurorehabil Neural Repair. 2016;30(8):773–93.

67. Kierkegaard M, Einarsson U, Gottberg K, von Koch L, Holmqvist LW. The relationship between walking, manual dexterity, cognition and activity/participation in persons with multiple sclerosis. Mult Scler. 2012;18(5):639–46.
68. Spooren AI, Timmermans AA, Seelen HA. Motor training programs of arm and hand in patients with MS according to different levels of the ICF: a systematic review. BMC Neurol. 2012;12(1):49.
69. Bonzano L, Tacchino A, Brichetto G, et al. Upper limb motor rehabilitation impacts white matter microstructure in multiple sclerosis. NeuroImage. 2014;90:107–16.
70. Mills RJ, Yap L, Young CA. Treatment for ataxia in multiple sclerosis. Cochrane Database Syst Rev. 2007;1:CD005029.
71. Marsden J, Harris C. Cerebellar ataxia: pathophysiology and rehabilitation. Clin Rehabil. 2011;25:195–216.
72. Marquer A, Barbieri G, Perennou D. The assessment and treatment of postural disorders in cerebellar ataxia: a systematic review. Ann Phys Rehabil Med. 2014;57(2):67–78.
73. Fonteyn EM, Keus SH, Verstappen CC, Schols L, de Groot IJ, van de Warrenburg BP. The effectiveness of allied health care in patients with ataxia: a systematic review. J Neurol. 2014;261(2):251–8.
74. Armutlu K, Karabudak R, Nurlu G. Physiotherapy approaches in the treatment of ataxic multiple sclerosis: a pilot study. Neurorehabil Neural Repair. 2001;15:203–11.
75. Vergaro E, Squeri V, Brichetto G, et al. Adaptive robot training for the treatment of incoordination in multiple sclerosis. J Neuroeng Rehabil. 2010;7:37.
76. Baram Y, Miller A. Virtual reality cues for improvement of gait in patients with multiple sclerosis. Neurology. 2006;66(2):178–81.
77. Betts L. Dynamic movement lycra orthosis in multiple sclerosis. Br J Neurosci Nurs. 2015;11(2):60–4.
78. Rudroff T, Kindred JH, Ketelhut NB. Fatigue in multiple sclerosis: misconceptions and future research directions. Front Neurol. 2016;7:122.
79. Induruwa I, Constantinescu CS, Gran B. Fatigue in multiple sclerosis—a brief review. J Neurol Sci. 2012;323(1–2):9–15.
80. de Groot V, Beckerman H, Twisk JW, Uitdehaag BM, Hintzen RQ, Minneboo A, et al. Vitality, perceived social support and disease activity determine the performance of social roles in recently diagnosed multiple sclerosis: a longitudinal analysis. J Rehabil Med. 2008;40(2):151–7.
81. Branas P, Jordan R, Fry-Smith A, Burls A, Hyde C. Treatments for fatigue in multiple sclerosis: a rapid and systematic review. Health Technol Assess. 2000;4(27):1–62.
82. Schwid SR, Covington M, Segal BM, Goodman AD. Fatigue in multiple sclerosis: current understanding and future directions. J Rehabil Res Dev. 2002;39(2):211–24.
83. Pucci E, Branas P, D'Amico R, Giuliani G, Solari A, Taus C. Amantadine for fatigue in multiple sclerosis. Cochrane Database Syst Rev. 2007;1:CD002818.
84. Tejani AM, Wasdell M, Spiwak R, Rowell G, Nathwani S. Carnitine for fatigue in multiple sclerosis. Cochrane Database Syst Rev. 2010;2:CD007280.
85. Asano M, Finlayson ML. Meta-analysis of three different types of fatigue management interventions for people with multiple sclerosis: exercise, education, and medication. Mult Scler Int. 2014;2014:798285.
86. Blikman LJ, Huisstede BM, Kooijmans H, Stam HJ, Bussmann JB, van Meeteren J. Eff ectiveness of energy conservation treatment in reducing fatigue in multiple sclerosis: a systematic review and meta-analysis. Arch Phys Med Rehabil. 2013;94:1360–76.
87. Heine M, van de Port I, Rietberg MB, van Wegen EE, Kwakkel G. Exercise therapy for fatigue in multiple sclerosis. Cochrane Database Syst Rev. 2015;9:CD009956.
88. Thomas S, Thomas PW, Kersten P, Jones R, Green C, Nock A, et al. A pragmatic parallel arm multi-centre randomised controlled trial to assess the effectiveness and cost-effectiveness of a group-based fatigue management programme (FACETS) for people with multiple sclerosis. J Neurol Neurosurg Psychiatry. 2013;84(10):1092–9.

89. Vanage SM, Gilbertson KK, Mathiowetz V. Effects of an energy conservation course on fatigue impact for persons with progressive multiple sclerosis. Am J Occup Ther. 2003;57(3):315–23.
90. Deibel F, Edwards M, Edwards A. Patients', carers' and providers' experiences and requirements for support in self-management of multiple sclerosis: a qualitative study. Eur J Pers Cent Healthc. 2013;1:457–67.
91. Gajofatto A, Benedetti MD. Treatment strategies for multiple sclerosis: when to start, when to change, when to stop? World J Clin Cases. 2015;3(7):545–55.
92. Soundy A, Benson J, Dawes H, et al. Understanding hope in patients with multiple sclerosis. Physiotherapy. 2012;98:344–50.
93. Thorne S, Con A, McGuinness L, McPherson G, Harris SR. Health care communication issues in multiple sclerosis: an interpretive description. Qual Health Res. 2004;14(1):5–22.
94. Feinstein A, Magalhaes S, Richard J-F, Audet B, Moore C. The link between multiple sclerosis and depression. Nat Rev Neurol. 2014;10(9):507–17.
95. Marrie RA, Reingold S, Cohen J, Stuve O, Trojano M, Sorensen PS, et al. The incidence and prevalence of psychiatric disorders in multiple sclerosis: a systematic review. Mult Scler. 2015;21(3):305–17.
96. Zeller D, Rocca MA. Editorial: Plasticity in multiple sclerosis: from molecular to system level, from adaptation to maladaptation. Front Neurol. 2015;6:265.
97. Cramer SC, Sur M, Dobkin BH, et al. Harnessing neuroplasticity for clinical applications. Brain. 2011;134:1591–609.
98. Reddy H, Narayanan S, Arnoutelis R, Jenkinson M, Antel J, Matthews PM, et al. Evidence for adaptive functional changes in the cerebral cortex with axonal injury from multiple sclerosis. Brain. 2000;123:2314–20.
99. Reddy H, Narayanan S, Woolrich M, Mitsumori T, La Pierre Y, Arnold DL, et al. Functional brain reorganization for hand movement in patients with multiple sclerosis: defining distinct effects of injury and disability. Brain. 2002;125:2646–57.
100. Staffen W, Mair A, Zauner H, Unterrainer J, Niederhofer H, Kutzelnigg A, et al. Cognitive function and fMRI in patients with multiple sclerosis: evidence for compensatory cortical activation during an attention task. Brain. 2002;125(Pt 6):1275–82.
101. Chiaravalloti ND, Genova HM, DeLuca J. Cognitive rehabilitation in multiple sclerosis: the role of plasticity. Front Neurol. 2015;6:67.
102. Houdayer E, Comi G, Leocani L. The neurophysiologist oerspective into MS plasticity. Front Neurol. 2015;6:193.
103. Flachenecker P. Clinical implications of neuroplasticity: the role of rehabilitation in multiple sclerosis. Front Neurol. 2015;6:36.
104. Sastre-Garriga J, Alonso J, Renom M, Arevalo MJ, Gonzalez I, Galan I, et al. A functional magnetic resonance proof of concept pilot trial of cognitive rehabilitation in multiple sclerosis. Mult Scler. 2011;17:457–67.
105. Cerasa A, Gioia MC, Valentino P, Nistico R, Chiri aco C, Pirritano D, et al. Computer-assisted cognitive rehabilitation of attention deficits for multiple sclerosis: a randomized trial with fMRI correlates. Neurorehabil Neural Repair. 2013;27:284–95.
106. Parisi L, Rocca MA, Mattioli F, Copetti M, Capra R, Valsasina P, et al. Changes of brain resting state functional connectivity predict the persistence of cognitive rehabilitation effects in patients with multiple sclerosis. Mult Scler. 2014;20(6):686–94.
107. Lipp I, Tomassini V. Neuroplasticity and motor rehabilitation in multiple sclerosis. Front Neurol. 2015;6:59.
108. Tomassini V, Johansen-Berg H, Leonardi L, et al. Preservation of motor skill learning in patients with multiple sclerosis. Mult Scler. 2011;17:103–15.
109. Ferrucci R, Vergari M, Cogiamanian F, Bocci T, Ciocca M, Tomasini E, et al. Transcranial direct current stimulation (tDCS) for fatigue in multiple sclerosis. NeuroRehabilitation. 2014;34:121–7.
110. Tecchio F, Cancelli A, Cottone C, Ferrucci R, Vergari M, Zito G, et al. Brain plasticity effects of neuromodulation against multiple sclerosis fatigue. Front Neurol. 2015;6:141.

111. Leocani L, Nuara A, Formenti A, Rossi P, Zangen A, Comola M, et al. Deep rTMS with H-coil associated with rehabilitation enhances improvement of walking abilities in patients with progressive multiple sclerosis: randomized, controlled, double blind study. Neurology. 2012;78:7–49.
112. Mori F, Codecà C, Kusayanagi H, Monteleone F, Buttari F, Fiore S, et al. Effects of anodal transcranial direct current stimulation on chronic neuropathic pain in patients with multiple sclerosis. J Pain. 2010;11:436–42.
113. Mori F, Ljoka C, Magni E, Codecà C, Kusayanagi H, Monteleone F, et al. Transcranial magnetic stimulation primes the effects of exercise therapy in multiple sclerosis. J Neurol. 2011;258:1281–7.

Chapter 11
Future Therapies for Progressive Multiple Sclerosis

Neil Scolding

11.1 Introduction

The vast majority of interested clinicians and scientists, and probably even more people affected by multiple sclerosis, would surely agree that the absence of any useful disease-modifying treatments for progressive disability in multiple sclerosis is one of the most important remaining challenges in this disease. As preceding chapters have indicated, symptomatic therapies for progressive MS can have an enormous impact on many of the major problems associated with longstanding disease—perhaps particularly incontinence, pain, spasticity and mood disturbance. No less dramatically, there has been a sea change in our ability to prevent relapses in MS over the past four decades—from no useful treatments at all, to a dozen or more licensed relapse-reducing agents (and more on the way), including monoclonal antibodies capable of preventing up to 80% relapses. However, stopping relapses does not stop disease progression. Indeed, one major beneficial side-effect of the numerous, large scale and high quality clinical trials of relapse-preventing immunotherapies for MS has been to inform our understanding of this disease, and to illustrate that the link between relapses and disability progression is not direct, and that successfully treating the first may have no effect on the second.

The last decade has consequently seen a serious re-orientation of therapeutic research in MS, both within the pharmaceutical industry and in academic centres, with the realisation that the problems of progressive disability and its treatment, in both secondary and primary progressive disease, need to be addressed separately and distinctly from the problem of preventing relapses. The question

N. Scolding
Institute of Clinical Neurosciences, University of Bristol, Second Floor,
Learning and Research, Southmead Hospital, Westbury-on-Trym, Bristol BS10 5NB, UK
e-mail: n.j.scolding@bris.ac.uk

A. Wilkins (ed.), *Progressive Multiple Sclerosis*,
https://doi.org/10.1007/978-3-319-65921-3_11

now is whether the next few decades will see the same level of success in developing disease-modifying treatments for progressive MS as the last two have seen in therapies for relapsing-remitting disease. Some might argue that the omens are not good, and the problems of progression are much greater than those of relapse—in the 1980s, there were already available a large number of prescribable drugs available for other inflammatory conditions that could significantly suppress or alter immune function, whereas at present there are no drugs that can modify neuronal or axonal loss in any progressive neurodegenerative disorder. However, the pace and scale of therapeutic research in recent years, the extraordinary advances in stem cell science, and the remarkable changes in molecular medicine—but above all the single fact that at least we have identified and are attempting to address the right question, that of halting (or, better, reversing) progressive neurodegeneration in MS rather than focussing exclusively on inflammatory relapses—all this must give grounds for cautious but reasonable and realistic optimism.

11.2 Rationale and Scientific Background to Repair and Neuroprotection in Multiple Sclerosis

There are essentially two aspects to treatment strategies for established progressive MS—neuroprotective therapies, aiming to stop further progression, and reparative therapies, aiming to reverse neurological disability by repairing tissue in the brain or spinal cord.

The distinction is far less clear than it might first appear. As outlined in the previous chapters, despite the complex relationship between relapse and progression (in secondary progressive disease), inflammatory relapses can directly cause a certain amount of residual axon damage. Therefore, the currently available successful immune therapies, in preventing relapses, clearly have *some* neuroprotective activity. Also, the central nervous system has a remarkable capacity for endogenous repair, and so successful immune therapy (preventing further inflammatory damage), and successful neuroprotection would both, by stabilising the CNS environment, be expected to facilitate, or rather permit, endogenous repair, so helping to bring about a degree of clinical improvement rather than just stability. Precisely the same pertains in relation to CNS plasticity—both immunotherapeutic and neuroprotective treatments, by stabilizing the environment should maximize any beneficial effects of plasticity, so again allowing improvement, not just arresting progression.

Nonetheless, there is a consensus, partly for simplicity, that neuroprotective therapies are considered to be those aimed primarily and directly at preserving axons and neurons (and excluding those treatments aimed primarily at the immune system); while reparative therapies are those aimed primarily at stimulating or supplementing CNS repair. We will therefore consider each, separately.

11.3 Neurotrophins for Neuroprotection

There is, as discussed in previous chapters, a consensus that progressive axonal and neuronal damage and loss represent the principal pathophysiological substrate for disability in chronic progressive multiple sclerosis (in both primary and secondary progressive disease). If a neuroprotective therapy is to help prevent this, the cause of such axon loss needs to be understood, but at present this knowledge remains very partial. The inflammatory processes responsible for acute relapse in multiple sclerosis undoubtedly contribute to axon loss—'primary demyelination', the term emphasising the targeted nature of damage to myelin and oligodendrocytes in acute inflammatory lesions, is an accurate description, but indicates relative, not absolute selectivity of tissue injury. But inflammatory damage to axons in acute demyelinating lesions does not appear to represent the principal cause of steadily accumulating disability in progressive MS. In other words, relentlessly progressive axon and neuron loss does not inevitably result from inflammatory demyelination. Relapses do not govern time to [1] or rate of [2] disease progression; and treatments that have profound effects in preventing relapse do not affect progression [3].

This by no means implies that immune processes can play no role in neurodegeneration: rather, if they do, they are different to those that cause relapses. Smouldering low grade inflammation, sequestered within the CNS, with microglial activation and accompanying oxygen free radical damage, impaired mitochondrial function and disrupted axonal transport are postulated [4–9]. These help justify past and current continuing attempts—thus far unsuccessful—to influence primary progressive MS using immune therapies [10–13] (notwithstanding the possibility of modest benefit from CD20 blockade in progressive patients with MRI evidence of inflammatory episodes [14]; and see preceding chapters).

However, other non-immunological causes of neuronal and axonal loss are also likely to contribute. One, suggested by several lines of evidence, is that, since several myelin and oligodendrocyte-derived factors constitutively support axons, their loss contributes to axon loss [15, 16]. Autopsy neuropathological studies suggest that chronic axon loss does not correlate either with inflammatory cells or pro-inflammatory molecules (tumour necrosis factor or nitric oxide expression), or demyelinating activity, but can be linked with overall extent of established myelin loss [17, 18]. Axon loss is rare in remyelinated lesions [18]. Axon loss as a consequence of persistent demyelination, long known to occur in the peripheral nervous system, has been shown to occur in the CNS [19]. A variety of mechanisms are responsible for axon loss, including sustained (demyelination-induced) conduction block and electrical silence [20], increased vulnerability of the exposed axon to injurious agents [21], or the loss of oligodendrocyte-derived trophic support [22–24] and/or the lack of specific myelin proteins [25, 26].

This implies that remyelination, and effective remyelination therapies, could themselves be neuroprotective, so providing an important link between reparative and axon- and neuro- protective therapies; and that remyelination protects axons is clearly shown [27]. In addition, these considerations have stimulated a search for potentially therapeutic molecules—biological agents—that might directly (i.e., aside from any pro-remyelinating activity) help protect axons and neurons.

The search for such therapeutically useful neurotrophic factors, acting irrespective of the nature of the neurological disease or injurious process, has a long and unfruitful history. Clinical trials in disorders ranging from stroke and motor neuron disease to sensory neuropathy have all failed, invariably proving either intolerable or ineffective. A small pilot study of a directly infused neurotrophic factor, GDNF, in Parkinson's disease showed highly promising clinical and (in one case) autopsy benefit [28, 29], but a later multicentre study failed to confirm this [30] (though possibly for reasons of neurosurgical technical and statistical trial design [31, 32]).

Nonetheless, we do have an increasing understanding of those growth factors offering neurotrophic support to axons and neurons, and therapeutic approaches are being pursued based on this knowledge. Various growth factors and neurotrophins are synthesised by oligodendrocytes [33]. GDNF and IGF-1 are implicated in the trophic support provided for axons by oligodendrocytes [24, 34, 35]; these might be predicted to be deficient in MS and so potentially represent therapeutically useful axon-protective agents. GDNF in particular is produced by mature, differentiated oligodendrocytes, but not oligodendrocyte precursor cells, and improves axon survival in vitro [24]. Of these growth factors, IGF-1 has been explored in early phase clinically studies [36] (without success), but there remains considerable interest both in the research community and in the pharmaceutical industry for exploring small molecule approaches to neurotrophic therapeutics [37, 38].

11.4 More Conventional Pharmacological Approaches to Neuroprotection

The only neuroprotective agent currently in clinical use is riluzole, for motor neuron disease (though the extent to which this drug's efficacy is indeed mediated through neuroprotection, as opposed to other additional mechanisms, is uncertain). Riluzole has shown beneficial effects in EAE [39], and has been tested clinically (without success) in a phase II trial in patients with multiple sclerosis [40]. Riluzole inhibits glutamate transmission; and excitotoxicity and oxidative stress in multiple sclerosis are increasingly considered as therapeutic targets [41].

Cannabinoids have attracted much recent attention as neuroprotectants. They may at least in part act through limiting excitotoxicity, [42] though other mechanisms are postulated—interactions with Toll-like receptors, for example [43]. Both cell culture paradigms and MS disease models suggest relevant neuroprotective effects [44–46]. Following the first successfully executed multicentre randomised controlled trial of cannabis in MS [47], a large scale study of cannabinoids as protective agents in MS was undertaken (the MRC CUPID trial—*Cannabinoid Use in Progressive Inflammatory Disease)*, but in the primary outcome measure did not show a positive result [48].

Sodium channel blockade is a further mechanism by which axons could possibly be protected in multiple sclerosis [49]. The intracellular accumulation of sodium is associated with reversal of sodium/calcium pump activity, and this results in toxic levels of calcium within the axon. Reducing intra-axonal sodium levels may therefore be protective. Sodium channel blockade using various agents has reduced axonal injury in EAE [50–53], and a trial of lamotrigine as a neuroprotective agents aiming to prevent the accumulation of disability in progressive MS followed—but was unsuccessful [54]. A phase II controlled trial of phenytoin has also been completed, with encouraging results in terms of OCT measurements [55]—though interpreting OCT results is complex [56]. A study of topiramate is also underway (http://clinicaltrials.gov/ct2/show/NCT00217295).

Minocycline is a tetracycline antibacterial, but has many additional biological activities, including anti-inflammatory activity and, more pertinently, direct neuroprotectant properties *in vivo* and *in vitro* [57, 58]. Minocycline increases levels of phosphorylated neurofilament within axons exposed to both inflammatory mediators and withdrawal of trophic support, leading to improved survival of axons [59]. Pilot studies and larger controlled trials have begun to investigate the drug in MS, though these have perhaps concentrated more on its anti-inflammatory effects [60, 61]. One recent trial showed there to be no significant benefit when minocycline was added to sub-cutaneous IFN β-1a therapy [62].

Erythropoietin is another molecule whose primary role has been long understood, but whose additional and unexpected neuroprotective properties are now emerging [63]. Rodent model studies have indicated benefit in inflammatory demyelination [64, 65]; early trials of erythropoietin have been completed in MS [66], though more recent studies of high dose erythropoietin have been disappointing [67]. Other bone marrow-stimulating agents also have neuroprotective activities [68, 69].

Lastly, statins, primarily used as cholesterol-lowering agents, are also now recognised to have unexpectedly potent anti-inflammatory and neuroprotective effects [70, 71], and their potential in multiple sclerosis was quickly recognised [72]. There followed a flurry of trials in (though again concentrating more on their immune effects than on neuroprotection, and looking almost exclusively at relapsing remitting MS), but no great evidence of efficacy emerged [73–76]—indeed there has been some suggestion that disease activity might be adversely affected by such agents [77–80]. Certainly a Cochrane review, and subsequent further trialling suggested no benefit [81, 82], though speculation concerning putative benefits in progression continues [83], gaining support from phase II study suggesting a slowing in the rate of increase in brain atrophy [84].

11.5 Repairing Tissue in Progressive MS

11.5.1 Cell Therapy for MS: The Background and the Problems

Three ground-breaking observations, starting over 50 years ago, laid the foundation of virtually every consideration concerning the possibility of cell therapy for multiple sclerosis. First, Dick and Mary Bunge and colleagues showed that

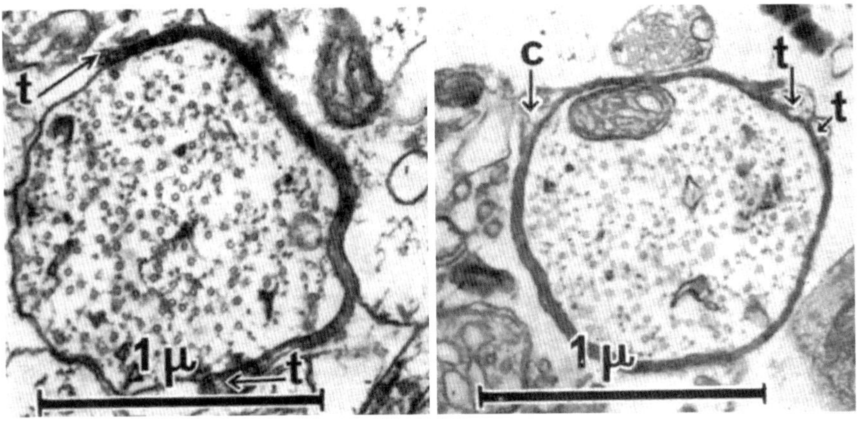

Fig. 11.1 The first electron microscopic images showing what the authors termed 'abortive remyelination'—spontaneous myelin repair—at the edge of a multiple sclerosis plaque [86]

spontaneous remyelination could and did follow experimental myelin damage in the adult mammalian central nervous system [85]. Secondly, Perier and Gregoire in Paris provided evidence that such spontaneous remyelination was indeed found in patients with multiple sclerosis [86]. Finally, 40 years ago, Bill Blakemore showed in a remarkable study, funded in part by the UK MS Society, that transplanted exogenous myelinating cells (Schwann cells in this instance), injected into a demyelinated lesion in the rodent CNS, could indeed achieve successful remyelination [87] (Fig. 11.1).

These and subsequent studies offered vital proof of principle for remyelinating cell therapy for patients with MS; and various other considerations further suggested that, of all neurological diseases, MS might be particularly suitable and realistic as a test bed for developing reparative cell therapy. The presumed autoimmune process appeared highly targeted and specific—only one single cell type, the oligodendrocyte appeared to be damaged and so needed to be replaced. The ability to disclose lesions using MRI scans would allow cells to be injected directly and accurately into a damaged area—where, the hope was, they would generate new myelin, restoring normal impulse conduction and with that, improved neurological function. Finally, axons appeared largely spared, so the insurmountably complex challenge of 're-connecting' circuitry, a problem central to many if not most other CNS diseases—did not apply in MS. Repair therapies therefore 'only' need to reinvest axons with myelin.

So by the 1990s, it was rather optimistically thought that only two key hurdles remained: identifying an appropriate (safe and effective) source of remyelinating cells, and means of monitoring the effect of implantation [88]. To the first problem, the emergence of embryonic stem cells and their potential oligodendrocyte progeny, and then later induced pluripotent stem cells, appeared offer a clear potential solution.

It might have been predicted during the 1990s that the rapidly increasing appreciation of the importance of axon loss in MS in generating progressive disability should seriously undermine the rationale for remyelinating cell therapy as a means of treating primary or secondary progressive disease. It did not, for several reasons [15]. First, although axon loss clearly occurred earlier in the course of MS than previously believed, neither experimental, imaging nor neuropathological studies challenged the concept that disease processes in MS are primarily directed against oligodendrocytes and/or myelin: it 'remains' a demyelinating disease, and most axons are *relatively* spared until late in its course [89, 90]. Secondly, despite the importance of axon loss, the likelihood remained that some portion of progressive disability might still depend on demyelination *per se* [91, 92]. Finally and perhaps most importantly, the trophic effects of oligodendrocytes mentioned above, and the ability of newly laid down myelin to stabilise and protect axons and so prevent axon loss, in fact provided an added imperative for remyelinating cell therapy [27, 93]: the restoration of a more normal cellular and molecular environment was not only likely to improve conduction, but represented a powerful approach to neuroprotection. Accordingly, a number of approaches to remyelinating cell therapy continue to be explored.

11.5.2 Cell Therapy [1]: Repairing Myelin

Given the experimental background outlined above, a number of approaches were taken towards addressing the key remaining challenge of identifying a usable (i.e., transplantable) source of remyelinating cells. Several candidates have been explored.

(a) Myelinating cells derived from outside the CNS.

Counterintuitive as this might initially appear, non-CNS derived cells may carry two clear and potentially very important advantages over sources of oligodendrocytes: accessibility, and likely resistance to MS-related disease processes. Three types of cells have been considered:

Schwann cells have long been known to contribute to endogenous myelin repair in multiple sclerosis, particularly in the spinal cord [94–96]. Initially it was thought that these cells invaded the CNS from outside, but it is now clear that endogenous neural stem cells produce Schwann cells as well as oligodendrocytes during the process of spontaneous experimental myelin repair [97]. From a practical perspective, techniques for preparing cell cultures of human Schwann cells from peripheral nerve biopsies, and for purifying and expanding the cells in vitro to generate large populations of highly enriched Schwann cells, are well established [98, 99]. Additionally, experimental models clearly confirm the functionally useful repair of CNS myelin by exogenous, implanted Schwann cells (including those of human origin) or their precursors [100–106]. Even in primates, large scale remyelination can be achieved by transplanted expanded autologous Schwann cells in the demyelinated macaque spinal cord [107].

However, other studies of expanded human Schwann cells transplanted into the rodent spinal cord have shown by contrast substantial fibroblast overgrowth with axon destruction, [105], and earlier transplantation experiments with rodent Schwann cells immortalised by growth factor expansion showed tumour formation *in vivo* [108]. The inhibitory effect of astrocytes on Schwann cell migration and remyelination in CNS [109–111] offers another potential problem for the use of Schwann cells in remyelination therapy—though genetic engineering of Schwann cells to increase surface expression of PSA on NCAM can help address this problem, at least *in vitro* [112].

One clinical study of intracerebral implantation of autologous non-cultured (or purified or expanded) Schwann cells in patients with chronic MS, the first of its kind, was undertaken in the USA in 2001 [113]. No identifiable peer-reviewed publication of the results has emerged; it has been suggested that three patients were treated and the study then stopped.

Olfactory ensheathing cells (OECs) [114].

OECs represent a special class of glial cell, exhibiting some properties similar to those of Schwann cells, and others more typical of CNS glia [115]. They can myelinate CNS axons, forming peripheral-type myelin sheaths, but unlike Schwann cells, their migration within the CNS (e.g., after transplantation) is not impeded by astrocytes—perhaps because of their effects on astrocyte expression of chondroitin sulfate proteoglycans [116, 117]. Human OECs can be relatively easily obtained per-nasally, where they traverse the cribriform plate.

OEC also synthesise of a number of neurotrophic factors [118]; and may additionally exert potentially valuable effects by augmenting endogenous repair [119]. Early phase clinical trials of OEC implantation in patients with spinal cord injury are already underway [120–123]. Not least for practical reasons of autologous transplantation, probably safety, and accessibility, there is much interest in their future therapeutic potential [124, 125].

Haemapoietic precursors and other cells isolated from bone marrow.

It was initially suggested that certain sub-populations of bone marrow derived cells—haemapoeitic stem cells (HSCs) and mesenchymal stem cells (MSCs) in particular—can transdifferentiate into myelinating glia [126–129]. This stimulated much interest in the possible therapeutic transplantation of these cells to replace myelinating glia in MS. However, many other authors have not found such transdifferentiation [130], and the observation of cell fusion of (for example) MSCs with neuronal cells was taken to offer an alternative explanation for at least some reports of apparent transdifferentiation, and to imply that transdifferentiation might not necessarily occur *in vivo* [131]. The current consensus appears to be that while such cells may be induced to express neural and glia antigens, they may not be able to form myelin-elaborating glia (or, for that matter, neurons). Interest in their potential as implantable, myelinating cells therefore waned—though this is more than matched by an increase in interest in the therapeutic potential of such cells acting through other mechanisms, including fusion (see below).

Meanwhile, reports that mesenchymal stem cells may in fact originate from the neural crest [132], and that there are populations of neural crest derived stem cells persisting post-natally within bone marrow that are capable of generating neural progeny [133] have re-kindled interest in bone marrow as a source of both remyelinating cells and neurons.

(b) CNS myelinating cells—oligodendrocytes and their progenitors.

Far more experimental effort has been expended on studying oligodendrocytes and their precursors, including stem cells, as a source of transplantable myelin-producing cells, than on Schwann cells or olfactory glia, despite the practical advantages of the latter. The theoretical attraction is plain: oligodendrocytes are the 'normal' myelinating and remyelinating cells of the CNS.

Many potential sources of myelinating oligodendrocyte s have been explored, and almost all have shown experimental success. (None, however, has yet been tested clinically, in patients.) Their potential for remyelination appears very much to depend on the degree of differentiation and maturation. Fully mature, terminally differentiated oligodendrocytes are poor at re-myelination [134]. Oligodendrocyte progenitors are more efficient, whether of rodent [134, 135] or human origin [136]. Both adult and foetally-derived cells repair myelin—indeed oligodendrocyte progenitors from adult human brain may be rather more efficient [136]. The translational difficulty, however, of using adult cells, despite the advantage of being autologous, would be the need for a brain biopsy to obtain and expand the multiple sclerosis patient's own cells—neither without risk, nor a practical option for any large scale treatment.

Concerning embryonic cells, numerous protocols for yielding oligodendrocyte progenitors, often in extremely high purity, from human embryonic stem cells or from embryonic neural precursors, have been developed; and these cells myelinate *in vivo* in a variety of myelin disease paradigms [137–145]. Whilst there is no serious doubt therefore about the potential remyelinating capacity of such cells, concerns remain about the practicalities and safety of using embryonic stem cells (or rather, committed oligodendrocyte progenitors derived from them) in patients. The principal questions are those of immune rejection, potential tumorigenesis, and possible infection (including non-screenable disorders such as prion diseases, and zoonoses derived from the cell culture constituents) [142, 146–148]. There are of course also ethical issues regarding the source of the cells.

Induced pluripotent stem cells—adult somatic cells reprogrammed to a status near-identical to embryonic stem cells—bypass several of these hurdles, including rejection (since autologous cells would be used), many sources of cross-infection, and the major ethical issues. The potential question of tumour formation, however, remains [149]. The hope has always been that implanting terminally differentiated cells, rather than proliferative stem cells themselves, would solve this question, but there is good experimental evidence that the potential for phenotypic instability and undifferentiated expansion remains even after neuronal differentiation [150, 151].

This risk has—tragically but unsurprisingly—been confirmed to be real rather than theoretical by various and continuing case reports often related to so-called 'stem cell tourism'—for example, a child developing multiple donor-derived intracranial tumours following implantation of embryonic neural stem cells [152]. Whether the cells injected in this instance were neural stem cells or not has been questioned [153] (and defended) [154], but other cases of tumour formation following transplant of some form of embryonic neural cells have also been reported [153, 155]. A clinical trial using human embryonic stem cell derived oligodendrocytes in patients has nonetheless commenced—not in multiple sclerosis, but in spinal cord injury, though not without controversy [156–158].

11.5.3 Cell Therapy [2]: Beyond Remyelination

11.5.3.1 Questions Regarding the Classical Remyelinating Cell Therapy Approach

In recent years, a number of changes in our understanding of various aspects of multiple sclerosis have challenged the rationale of pursuing cell transplantation for the purpose of achieving remyelination [159–161]. Neuropathological studies of MS-affected CNS tissue have shown that oligodendrocyte progenitors are present in lesions—and are found not sparsely, as first thought [162], but in significant numbers [163–167]. This superficially counter-intuitive finding casts doubt on the need for or value of adding further precursors [159]. Furthermore, although there are no specific markers for endogenous neural stem cells, studies using the best available approaches suggest that these cells too—the precursors of (oligodendrocyte) precursors—also respond to disease processes in MS, and achieve increased numbers in lesions [168]. The same point is emphasised: adding stem cells 'therapeutically' when significant numbers are already present does not seem logical.

The extent and pathophysiological significance of remyelination in chronic, progressive multiple sclerosis also requires further clarification. As mentioned above, it has been known since the 1960s that a certain amount of spontaneous myelin repair occurred in MS [86]. Initially, this was considered partial, and sparse, or 'abortive'. Later studies suggested, however, that spontaneous remyelination in MS is far more widespread, and successful, than previously thought [169, 170]. This raises the question of whether, since spontaneous myelin repair is so successful, attempts to augment the process are as likely to yield any therapeutic dividend as first thought.

Commensurate with these findings, but moving from neuropathology towards pathophysiology, it remains the case that inflammatory demyelinating lesions are commonly agreed to provide the pathophysiological substrate for relapses. However, chronic progressive disability in MS is more closely correlated with neuronal and axonal damage in the brain and spinal cord than to demyelinated lesions. No less importantly, neuro-axonal damage *outside* individual lesions, and of a more diffuse (rather than multifocal) nature, may be the principal generator of progression

[171–174]. It is therefore quite possible that repairing discrete lesions might not usefully affect chronic progressive disability.

To summarise the above in a rather extreme way, the conventional cell therapeutic approach in MS has proposed to add neural stem or myelinating cells to lesions that (a) already have stem cells, (b) already have oligodendrocyte precursors, (c) may already have myelin, and (d) make little contribution to neurological functional impairment.

11.5.3.2 Novel Cell Therapy Approaches

An alternative conclusion of the foregoing would be that many very different studies over the last decade have yielded findings in multiple sclerosis that were surprising and often counter-intuitive: they raised more (and/or deeper) questions than they answered. We still have much to learn—there are more 'known unknowns' than a decade ago—concerning the cell biology and the clinical and pathological physiology of MS.

One obvious and very rational implication might be to postpone any thought of clinical exploration of cell therapy in MS until we understand the disease better. An alternative argument can, however, be offered. While securing a full understanding of disease processes before making efforts towards clinical translation is plainly ideal, it is hardly (if ever) realistic. There are few diseases whose mechanisms have been completely dissected. Taking the example of MS itself, our comprehension of the immune disturbance is not remotely complete, and indeed neither do we have any real idea of what, biologically and immunologically, beta-interferon (to take just one example) actually does in MS patients—but of course neither of these patches of partial but serious ignorance prevented clinical trials of interferon in MS.

What these changes in our perception of MS processes do mean, however, is that our intentions and designs in exploring cell therapy must evolve, and our demands of the 'therapeutic' cell to be used in particular are different and more complex.

Stopping inflammation in patients with progressive disease did not have the hoped-for downstream effect of stopping progression (or by implication neurodegeneration). Similarly, even if demyelination could be fully repaired, we cannot assume that axonal degeneration will necessarily be halted (still less reversed). Therefore, an idealised reparative cell therapy in MS would have distinct and separate beneficial actions on each and all of the damaging disease processes. The perfect MS cell therapy would (1) modulate immune processes both systemically and inside the CNS, and so dampen inflammation in the brain and spinal cord; (2) have remyelinating activity (unrelated to suppressing immune damage); and (3) have separate axon- and neuroprotective and/or reparative effects. What is more, we would need to demand of our cell that it be capable of exhibiting these effects in both white matter and grey, and both within and between lesions.

Whether or not this is a realisable 'shopping list' of desirable properties, it is arguably a more realistic place to start than the classical 'injecting myelinating cells into lesions' paradigm. It does seem highly unlikely that any one single cell type could successfully and entirely meet every one of these demands. However, rapid recent advances in our knowledge of some reparative cell types—perhaps particularly bone marrow-derived mesenchymal stem cells—indicates that multifunctionality may be the rule rather than the exception. Also, the best should not be the enemy of the good: a cell therapy that might only partially ameliorate some of these pathophysiological processes would be better than no cell therapy at all (and better than any current pharmacological options).

Bone marrow-[BM] derived stem cells are attractive candidates for cell therapies in a wide range of diseases (neurological and otherwise) not least because the normal function of some BM cell sub-populations, mesenchymal stem cells [MSCs] having perhaps been most carefully studied, is to do with spontaneous tissue repair [175, 176]. Furthermore, they execute this function through multiple and very varied reparative mechanisms [176, 177]. While the true biological 'stem-ness' of mesenchymal stem cells remains open to question, it seems likely (if paradoxical) that trans-differentiation into oligodendrocytes is actually the least important amongst their properties in the context of chronic progressive MS. Here, as outlined above, replacing myelinating cells to regenerate myelin may well no longer be the core aim.

What are these other properties? First, MSCs exhibit pronounced immune modulating and immune suppressive properties, with both local and systemic effects relevant to MS [178–181].

Secondly, both mixed, unseparated, bone marrow cells and isolated MSCs, have been shown to promote myelin repair following experimental demyelination—and significantly, such pro-remyelinating activity is seen not just in experimental inflammatory demyelination (where the beneficial remyelinating effects might well be secondary to their immune-suppressive functions), but in toxic or chemical, non-immune experimental demyelination [182, 183]. The mechanisms of this effect remain uncertain. Initially it was thought that trans-differentiation into myelinating cells was responsible [126–129, 184, 185], but as mentioned above, trans-differentiation of MSCs into functional, myelin-elaborating oligodendrocytes is seriously questioned [186, 187] (though not entirely settled [132, 133]). Alternative, indirect pro-remyelination effects may be more likely—stimulating the proliferation of endogenous neural stem cells [188, 189] and directing their differentiation along oligodendrocyte pathways [190–192], for example.

Other properties could also be important. MSCs can reduce gliotic scar formation—and gliosis is considered a major barrier to spontaneous repair in MS [192–195]. MSCs have powerful neuroprotective properties [196–200], again independent of their anti-inflammatory activity, although protection against oxidative stress applies to both immune and non-immune tissue damage [201, 202]. Also, and again as a distinct property, fusion of MSCs with some cell types (perhaps particularly cerebellar Purkinje cells) may represent a further mechanism by which MSCs may offer protection [203–207] and restore function.

Aside from the notable exception of MSCs' systemic effects on immunity, these potentially valuable therapeutic capacities of MSCs could have no value in multiple sclerosis unless the cells gained close proximity to areas of tissue damage, and this is where a further crucial property of MSCs becomes relevant. Circulating MSCs 'home' specifically to areas of tissue damage or inflammation [175, 208–210]. This applies not only to endogenous cells released from the marrow in health and disease, but also to exogenous cells, delivered intravenously, which successfully infiltrate the brain and spinal cord, and migrate towards those cytokines known to be expressed in MS lesions [211, 212].

Two further points should be emphasised. These studies of potential therapeutic mechanisms of action concentrate on bone marrow MSCs. However, it is firstly the case that other tissues—indeed, probably all adult tissues—also harbour MSCs [213], and some (adipose tissue, for example) may also serve as a source of therapeutic cells [214]. No less important, other sub-populations of bone marrow cells can similarly contribute to and promote tissue repair, also by utilising a wide variety of effector mechanisms. This includes haematopoetic stem cells (HSCs) [128, 215–219], Stro-1 positive cells [220–225], CD133+ve cells [226–229], MAPCs and others [132, 133, 230–234]. Many of these sub-types have so far not been as intensively studied as MSCs, but may yet prove as interesting and potentially valuable. Finally, MSCs themselves are not likely to be a single, homogenous cell type: sub-varieties are probable [176, 235, 236].

Remarkably, there is powerful *in vivo* evidence in humans of the capacities of migration into the CNS, and successful functional differentiation and integration of bone marrow derived cells. Various tissues from bone marrow transplant recipients who happened to receive cells from sex-mismatched donors as treatment for leukaemias and related conditions have been examined in carefully executed and highly informative autopsy studies for the presence of donor-derived (i.e., 'wrong' sex) cells. Such studies reveal that intravenously-delivered bone marrow cells do indeed infiltrate throughout the human CNS, apparently remain in place for years if not decades [237, 238], and are identifiable as highly differentiated neuronal and glial phenotypes fully integrated into the host brain. Such studies do not shed information on which particular bone marrow cell type(s) yielded these CNS-resident cells, or explain the mechanism of integration—but they do attest to its success and longevity.

The possible hazards of using embryonic (and likewise embryonic-like)-derived cells in patients have been mentioned above [149], but it would be wrong to assume that adult stem cells, simply through not being embryonic, were necessarily hazard-free [239]. Safety must remain paramount: MS is a chronic but non-fatal disease, making therapies with significant and predictable risks far less acceptable than in, say, cancer treatments, or even in serious cardiac disease. The repeated cell cycling and expansion required to prepare purified, selected MSCs (or other sub-populations) may induce unwelcome genetic instability [149, 240–243]—and can also compromise differentiation and repair capacities [244–248]. However, malignant, donor-derived tumours have not been reported in patients receiving MSCs, including the now several hundred treated in trials for various cardiac diseases [249]. Nonetheless, a recent report does indicate that MSCs directly injected intra-ventricularly can form non-proliferating cellular mass lesions [250, 251]; other studies have not found the same, though one reported axon-damaging effects (and no beneficial consequences) of direct intra-parenchymal injection of MSCs in rodents [252].

The use of non-selected, non-expanded bone marrow cells would eliminate the potentially unwanted effects of cell culture and expansion (and would be far easier and cheaper to adopt and apply widely and in relatively non-specialist units, with no requirement for a sterile GMP cell growth or selection facility). This approach also bypasses the question of choosing one specific BM stem cell sub-type to study clinically—cell selection obviously excludes the majority of cell types, and as mentioned above there is no good reason to exclude any specific BM stem cell sub-population. Using unselected BM cells is an increasingly common approach, successfully explored not just in experimental models of stroke [253] and spinal cord injury [254], but also clinically, in patients with myocardial infarction [255, 256], liver disease [257] and peripheral vascular disease [258], and more recently stroke [259, 260]. Indeed in some circumstances, unfiltered cells have been directly compared with purified MSCs and shown to better reparative potential [261, 262]. Certainly, in MS, this approach would mimic the relatively unselected mononuclear cell population that proved beneficial in the original therapeutic studies in rodent demyelinating models [182, 263]. For these and other reasons, non-selected mononuclear cells were used in the Bristol safety and feasibility study of bone marrow cell therapy in MS [264], though intravenously and intrathecally delivered mesenchymal stem cells were used in a more recently published early phase trial [265]. Both studies confirmed safety, but no less relevantly, helping to justify the further clinical exploration of reparative bone marrow cell therapy in large trials in patients with progressive multiple sclerosis [186, 266].

References

1. Scalfari A, Neuhaus A, Degenhardt A, et al. The natural history of multiple sclerosis: a geographically based study 10: relapses and long-term disability. Brain. 2010;133(Pt 7):1914–29.
2. Confavreux C, Vukusic S, Moreau T, Adeleine P. Relapses and progression of disability in multiple sclerosis. N Engl J Med. 2000;343(20):1430–8.
3. Coles AJ, Wing MG, Molyneux P, et al. Monoclonal antibody treatment exposes three mechanisms underlying the clinical course of multiple sclerosis. Ann Neurol. 1999;46(3):296–304.
4. Campbell GR, Ziabreva I, Reeve AK, et al. Mitochondrial DNA deletions and neurodegeneration in multiple sclerosis. Ann Neurol. 2011;69(3):481–92.
5. Lassmann H. Mechanisms of neurodegeneration shared between multiple sclerosis and Alzheimer's disease. J Neural Transm. 2011;118(5):747–52.
6. Witherick J, Wilkins A, Scolding N, Kemp K. Mechanisms of oxidative damage in multiple sclerosis and a cell therapy approach to treatment. Autoimmune Dis. 2010;2011:164608.
7. Kemp K, et al. Oxidative injury in multiple sclerosis cerebellar grey matter. Brain Res. 2016;1642:452–60. doi:10.1016/j.brainres.2016.04.027.
8. Hares K, et al. Axonal motor protein KIF5A and associated cargo deficits in multiple sclerosis lesional and normal-appearing white matter. Neuropathol Appl Neurobiol. 2017;43:227–41. doi:10.1111/nan.12305.
9. Rajda C, Pukoli D, Bende Z, Majlath Z, Vecsei L. Excitotoxins, mitochondrial and redox disturbances in multiple sclerosis. Int J Mol Sci. 2017;**18**(2):E353. doi:10.3390/ijms18020353.

10. Rojas JI, Romano M, Ciapponi A, Patrucco L, Cristiano E. Interferon Beta for primary progressive multiple sclerosis. Cochrane Database Syst Rev. 2010;1:CD006643.
11. Hawker K, O'Connor P, Freedman MS, et al. Rituximab in patients with primary progressive multiple sclerosis: results of a randomized double-blind placebo-controlled multicenter trial. Ann Neurol. 2009;66(4):460–71.
12. Wolinsky JS, Narayana PA, O'Connor P, et al. Glatiramer acetate in primary progressive multiple sclerosis: results of a multinational, multicenter, double-blind, placebo-controlled trial. Ann Neurol. 2007;61(1):14–24.
13. Lublin F, et al. Oral fingolimod in primary progressive multiple sclerosis (INFORMS): a phase 3, randomised, double-blind, placebo-controlled trial. Lancet (London, England). 2016;387:1075–84. doi:10.1016/s0140-6736(15)01314-8.
14. Montalban X, et al. Ocrelizumab versus placebo in primary progressive multiple sclerosis. N Engl J Med. 2017;376:209–20. doi:10.1056/NEJMoa1606468.
15. Scolding N, Franklin R. Axon loss in multiple sclerosis. Lancet. 1998;352(9125):340–1.
16. Rodriguez M. A function of myelin is to protect axons from subsequent injury: implications for deficits in multiple sclerosis. Brain. 2003;126(Pt 4):751–2.
17. Bitsch A, Schuchardt J, Bunkowski S, Kuhlmann T, Bruck W. Acute axonal injury in multiple sclerosis. Correlation with demyelination and inflammation. Brain. 2000; 123(Pt 6):1174–83.
18. Kornek B, Storch MK, Weissert R, et al. Multiple sclerosis and chronic autoimmune encephalomyelitis: a comparative quantitative study of axonal injury in active, inactive, and remyelinated lesions. Am J Pathol. 2000;157(1):267–76.
19. Wilkins A, et al. Slowly progressive axonal degeneration in a rat model of chronic, nonimmune-mediated demyelination. J Neuropathol Exp Neurol. 2010;69:1256–69. doi:10.1097/NEN.0b013e3181ffc317.
20. Lipton SA. Blockade of electrical-activity promotes the death of mammalian retinal ganglion-cells in culture. Proc Natl Acad Sci U S A. 1986;83:9774–8.
21. Raine CS, Cross AH. Axonal dystrophy as a consequence of long-term demyelination. Lab Investig. 1989;60:714–25.
22. Griffiths I, Klugmann M, Anderson T, et al. Axonal swellings and degeneration in mice lacking the major proteolipid of myelin. Science. 1998;280(5369):1610–3.
23. MeyerFranke A, Kaplan MR, Pfrieger FW, Barres BA. Characterization of the signaling interactions that promote the survival and growth of developing retinal ganglion cells in culture. Neuron. 1995;15:805–19.
24. Wilkins A, Majed H, Layfield R, Compston A, Chandran S. Oligodendrocytes promote neuronal survival and axonal length by distinct intracellular mechanisms: a novel role for oligodendrocyte-derived glial cell line-derived neurotrophic factor. J Neurosci. 2003;23(12):4967–74.
25. Lappe-Siefke C, Goebbels S, Gravel M, et al. Disruption of Cnp1 uncouples oligodendroglial functions in axonal support and myelination. Nat Genet. 2003;33(3):366–74.
26. Edgar JM, McLaughlin M, Yool D, et al. Oligodendroglial modulation of fast axonal transport in a mouse model of hereditary spastic paraplegia. J Cell Biol. 2004;166(1):121–31.
27. Irvine KA, Blakemore WF. Remyelination protects axons from demyelination-associated axon degeneration. Brain. 2008;131(6):1464–77.
28. Gill SS, Patel NK, Hotton GR, et al. Direct brain infusion of glial cell line-derived neurotrophic factor in Parkinson disease. Nat Med. 2003;9(5):589–95.
29. Love S, Plaha P, Patel NK, Hotton GR, Brooks DJ, Gill SS. Glial cell line-derived neurotrophic factor induces neuronal sprouting in human brain. Nat Med. 2005;11(7):703–4.
30. Lang AE, Gill S, Patel NK, et al. Randomized controlled trial of intraputamenal glial cell line-derived neurotrophic factor infusion in Parkinson disease. Ann Neurol. 2006;59(3):459–66.
31. Hutchinson M, Gurney S, Newson R. GDNF in Parkinson disease: an object lesson in the tyranny of type II. J Neurosci Methods. 2007;163(2):190–2.
32. Patel NK, Gill SS. GDNF delivery for Parkinson's disease. Acta Neurochir Suppl. 2007; 97(Pt 2):135–54.

33. Du Y, Dreyfus CF. Oligodendrocytes as providers of growth factors. J Neurosci Res. 2002;68(6):647–54.
34. Wilkins A, Chandran S, Compston A. A role for oligodendrocyte-derived IGF-1 in trophic support of cortical neurons. Glia. 2001;36(1):48–57.
35. Wilkins A, Scolding N. Protecting axons in multiple sclerosis. Mult Scler. 2008;14(8):1013–25.
36. Frank JA, Richert N, Lewis B, et al. A pilot study of recombinant insulin-like growth factor-1 in seven multiple sderosis patients. Mult Scler. 2002;8(1):24–9.
37. Skaper SD. Peptide mimetics of neurotrophins and their receptors. Curr Pharm Des. 2011;17(25):2704–18.
38. Dawbarn D, Allen SJ. Neurotrophins and neurodegeneration. Neuropathol Appl Neurobiol. 2003;29(3):211–30.
39. Gilgun-Sherki Y, Panet H, Melamed E, Offen D. Riluzole suppresses experimental autoimmune encephalomyelitis: implications for the treatment of multiple sclerosis. Brain Res. 2003;989(2):196–204.
40. Waubant E, et al. A randomized controlled phase II trial of riluzole in early multiple sclerosis. Ann Clin Transl Neurol. 2014;1:340–7. doi:10.1002/acn3.60.
41. Gonsette RE. Oxidative stress and excitotoxicity: a therapeutic issue in multiple sclerosis? Mult Scler. 2008;14(1):22–34.
42. Loria F, Petrosino S, Hernangomez M, et al. An endocannabinoid tone limits excitotoxicity in vitro and in a model of multiple sclerosis. Neurobiol Dis. 2010;37(1):166–76.
43. Fitzpatrick JK, Downer EJ. Toll-like receptor signalling as a cannabinoid target in multiple sclerosis. Neuropharmacology. 2017;113:618–26. doi:10.1016/j.neuropharm.2016.04.009.
44. Jackson SJ, Baker D, Cuzner ML, Diemel LT. Cannabinoid-mediated neuroprotection following interferon-gamma treatment in a three-dimensional mouse brain aggregate cell culture. Eur J Neurosci. 2004;20(9):2267–75.
45. Jackson SJ, Diemel LT, Pryce G, Baker D. Cannabinoids and neuroprotection in CNS inflammatory disease. J Neurol Sci. 2005;233(1–2):21–5.
46. Pryce G, Ahmed Z, Hankey DJ, et al. Cannabinoids inhibit neurodegeneration in models of multiple sclerosis. Brain. 2003;126(Pt 10):2191–202.
47. Zajicek J, Fox P, Sanders H, et al. Cannabinoids for treatment of spasticity and other symptoms related to multiple sclerosis (CAMS study): multicentre randomised placebo-controlled trial. Lancet. 2003;362(9395):1517–26.
48. Zajicek J, et al. Effect of dronabinol on progression in progressive multiple sclerosis (CUPID): a randomised, placebo-controlled trial. Lancet Neurol. 2013;12:857–65. doi:10.1016/S1474-4422(13)70159-5.
49. Waxman SG. Mechanisms of disease: sodium channels and neuroprotection in multiple sclerosis-current status. Nat Clin Pract Neurol. 2008;4(3):159–69.
50. Bechtold DA, Kapoor R, Smith KJ. Axonal protection using flecainide in experimental autoimmune encephalomyelitis. Ann Neurol. 2004;55(5):607–16.
51. Black JA, Liu S, Hains BC, Saab CY, Waxman SG. Long-term protection of central axons with phenytoin in monophasic and chronic-relapsing EAE. Brain. 2006;129(12):3196–208.
52. Kapoor R, Davies M, Blaker PA, Hall SM, Smith KJ. Blockers of sodium and calcium entry protect axons from nitric oxide-mediated degeneration. Ann Neurol. 2003;53(2):174–80.
53. Shields SD, Butt RP, Dib-Hajj SD, Waxman SG. Oral administration of PF-01247324, a subtype-selective Nav1.8 blocker, reverses cerebellar deficits in a mouse model of multiple sclerosis. PLoS One. 2015;10:e0119067. doi:10.1371/journal.pone.0119067.
54. Kapoor R, Furby J, Hayton T, et al. Lamotrigine for neuroprotection in secondary progressive multiple sclerosis: a randomised, double-blind, placebo-controlled, parallel-group trial. Lancet Neurol. 2010;9(7):681–8.
55. Raftopoulos R, et al. Phenytoin for neuroprotection in patients with acute optic neuritis: a randomised, placebo-controlled, phase 2 trial. Lancet Neurol. 2016;15:259–69. doi:10.1016/s1474-4422(16)00004-1.
56. Saidha S, Calabresi PA. Phenytoin in acute optic neuritis: neuroprotective or not? Lancet Neurol. 2016;15:233–5. doi:10.1016/S1474-4422(16)00024-7.

57. Plane JM, Shen Y, Pleasure DE, Deng W. Prospects for minocycline neuroprotection. Arch Neurol. 2010;67(12):1442–8.
58. Yong W, Wells J, Giuliani F, Casha S, Power C, Metz LM. The promise of minocycline in neurology. Lancet Neurol. 2004;3(12):744–51.
59. Wilkins A, Nikodemova M, Compston A, Duncan I. Minocycline attenuates nitric oxide-mediated neuronal and axonal destruction in vitro. Neuron Glia Biol. 2004;1(3):297–305.
60. Metz LM, Zhang Y, Yeung M, et al. Minocycline reduces gadolinium-enhancing magnetic resonance imaging lesions in multiple sclerosis. Ann Neurol. 2004;55(5):756.
61. Metz LM, Li D, Traboulsee A, et al. Glatiramer acetate in combination with minocycline in patients with relapsing—remitting multiple sclerosis: results of a Canadian, multicenter, double-blind, placebo-controlled trial. Mult Scler. 2009;15(10):1183–94.
62. Sorensen PS, et al. Minocycline added to subcutaneous interferon beta-1a in multiple sclerosis: randomized RECYCLINE study. Eur J Neurol. 2016;23:861–70. doi:10.1111/ene.12953.
63. McPherson RJ, Juul SE. Recent trends in erythropoietin-mediated neuroprotection. Int J Dev Neurosci. 2008;26(1):103–11.
64. Sattler MB, Merkler D, Maier K, et al. Neuroprotective effects and intracellular signaling pathways of erythropoietin in a rat model of multiple sclerosis. Cell Death Differ. 2004;11(Suppl 2):S181–92.
65. Diem R, Sattler MB, Merkler D, et al. Combined therapy with methylprednisolone and erythropoietin in a model of multiple sclerosis. Brain. 2005;128(Pt 2):375–85.
66. Ehrenreich H, Fischer B, Norra C, et al. Exploring recombinant human erythropoietin in chronic progressive multiple sclerosis. Brain. 2007;130(Pt 10):2577–88.
67. Schreiber K, et al. High-dose erythropoietin in patients with progressive multiple sclerosis: a randomized, placebo-controlled, phase 2 trial. Mult Scler. 2017;23:675–85. doi:10.1177/1352458516661048.
68. Frank T, Schlachetzki JC, Goricke B, et al. Both systemic and local application of granulocyte-colony stimulating factor (G-CSF) is neuroprotective after retinal ganglion cell axotomy. BMC Neurosci. 2009;10:49.
69. Xiao BG, Lu CZ, Link H. Cell biology and clinical promise of G-CSF: immunomodulation and neuroprotection. J Cell Mol Med. 2007;11(6):1272–90.
70. Steffens S, Mach F. Anti-inflammatory properties of statins. Semin Vasc Med. 2004;4(4):417–22.
71. Stuve O, Prod'homme T, Slavin A, et al. Statins and their potential targets in multiple sclerosis therapy. Expert Opin Ther Targets. 2003;7(5):613–22.
72. Neuhaus O, Stuve O, Zamvil SS, Hartung HP. Are statins a treatment option for multiple sclerosis? Lancet Neurol. 2004;3(6):369–71.
73. Togha M, Karvigh SA, Nabavi M, et al. Simvastatin treatment in patients with relapsing-remitting multiple sclerosis receiving interferon beta 1a: a double-blind randomized controlled trial. Mult Scler. 2010;16(7):848–54.
74. Sorensen PS, Lycke J, Eralinna JP, et al. Simvastatin as add-on therapy to interferon beta-1a for relapsing-remitting multiple sclerosis (SIMCOMBIN study): a placebo-controlled randomised phase 4 trial. Lancet Neurol. 2011;10(8):691–701.
75. Lanzillo R, Orefice G, Quarantelli M, et al. Atorvastatin combined to interferon to verify the efficacy (ACTIVE) in relapsing-remitting active multiple sclerosis patients: a longitudinal controlled trial of combination therapy. Mult Scler. 2010;16(4):450–4.
76. Paul F, Waiczies S, Wuerfel J, et al. Oral high-dose atorvastatin treatment in relapsing-remitting multiple sclerosis. PLoS One. 2008;3(4):e1928.
77. Wang J, Xiao Y, Luo M, Zhang X, Luo H. Statins for multiple sclerosis. Cochrane Database Syst Rev. 2010;12:CD008386.
78. Lock C. Are "statins" beneficial or harmful in multiple sclerosis? Neurology. 2008;71(18):e54–5.
79. Goldman MD, Cohen JA. Statins to treat multiple sclerosis: friend or foe? Neurology. 2008;71(18):1386–7.
80. Birnbaum G, Cree B, Altafullah I, Zinser M, REDER AT. Combining beta interferon and atorvastatin may increase disease activity in multiple sclerosis. Neurology. 2008;71(18):1390–5.

81. Wang J, Xiao Y, Luo M, Luo H. Statins for multiple sclerosis. Cochrane Database Syst Rev. 2011;12:CD008386. doi:10.1002/14651858.CD008386.pub3.
82. Kamm CP, et al. Atorvastatin added to interferon beta for relapsing multiple sclerosis: a randomized controlled trial. J Neurol. 2012;259:2401–13. doi:10.1681/asn.2009111156.
83. Malkki H. Multiple sclerosis: could simvastatin slow down secondary progressive MS? Nat Rev Neurol. 2014;10:241. doi:10.1038/nrneurol.2014.61.
84. Chataway J, et al. Effect of high-dose simvastatin on brain atrophy and disability in secondary progressive multiple sclerosis (MS-STAT): a randomised, placebo-controlled, phase 2 trial. Lancet (London, England). 2014;**383**:2213–21. doi:10.1016/s0140-6736(13)62242-4.
85. Bunge MB, Bunge RP, Ris H. Ultrastructural study of remyelination in an experimental lesion in the adult cat spinal cord. J Biophys Biochem Cytol. 1961;10:67–94.
86. Perier O, Gregoire A. Electron microscopic features of multiple sclerosis lesions. Brain. 1965;88(5):937–52.
87. Blakemore WF. Remyelination of CNS axons by Schwann cells transplanted from the sciatic nerve. Nature. 1977;266(5597):68–9.
88. Scolding NJ. Strategies for repair and remyelination in demyelinating diseases. Curr Opin Neurol. 1997;10:193–200.
89. Bjartmar C, Trapp BD. Axonal and neuronal degeneration in multiple sclerosis: mechanisms and functional consequences. Curr Opin Neurol. 2001;14(3):271–8.
90. Smith KJ, McDonald WI. The pathophysiology of multiple sclerosis: the mechanisms underlying the production of symptoms and the natural history of the disease. Philos Trans R Soc Lond Ser B Biol Sci. 1999;354(1390):1649–73.
91. Hirst C, Ingram G, Pearson O, Pickersgill T, Scolding N, Robertson N. Contribution of relapses to disability in multiple sclerosis. J Neurol. 2008;255(2):280–7.
92. Lublin FD, Baier M, Cutter G. Effect of relapses on development of residual deficit in multiple sclerosis. Neurology. 2003;61(11):1528–32.
93. Garbern JY, Yool DA, Moore GJ, et al. Patients lacking the major CNS myelin protein, proteolipid protein 1, develop length-dependent axonal degeneration in the absence of demyelination and inflammation. Brain. 2002;125(Pt 3):551–61.
94. Itoyama Y, Webster HD, Richardson-EP J, Trapp BD. Schwann cell remyelination of demyelinated axons in spinal cord multiple sclerosis lesions. Ann Neurol. 1983;14(3):339–46.
95. Ludwin SK. Remyelination in the central nervous system and the peripheral nervous system. Adv Neurol. 1988;47:215–54.
96. Ogata J, Feigin I. Schwann cells and regenerated peripheral myelin in multiple sclerosis: an ultrastructural study. Neurology. 1975;25(8):713–6.
97. Zawadzka M, Rivers LE, Fancy SP, et al. CNS-resident glial progenitor/stem cells produce Schwann cells as well as oligodendrocytes during repair of CNS demyelination. Cell Stem Cell. 2010;6(6):578–90.
98. Morrissey TK, Kleitman N, Bunge RP. Human Schwann cells in vitro. II. Myelination of sensory axons following extensive purification and heregulin-induced expansion. J Neurobiol. 1995;28(2):190–201.
99. Rutkowski JL, Kirk CJ, Lerner MA, Tennekoon GI. Purification and expansion of human schwann cells in vitro. Nat Med. 1995;1:80–3.
100. Baron-Van Evercooren A, Blakemore W. Remyelination through engraftment. In: Lazzarini RA, editor. Myelin biology and disorders. New York: Elsevier; 2004. p. 143–72.
101. Lubetzki C, Williams A, Stankoff B. Promoting repair in multiple sclerosis: problems and prospects. Curr Opin Neurol. 2005;18(3):237–44.
102. Kocsis JD, Waxman SG. Schwann cells and their precursors for repair of central nervous system myelin. Brain. 2007;130(Pt 8):1978–80.
103. Woodhoo A, Sahni V, Gilson J, et al. Schwann cell precursors: a favourable cell for myelin repair in the Central Nervous System. Brain. 2007;130(8):2175–85.
104. Levi ADO, Bunge RP. Studies of myelin formation after transplantation of human Schwann cells into the severe combined immunodeficient mouse. Exp Neurol. 1994;130:41–52.

105. Brierley CM, Crang AJ, Iwashita Y, et al. Remyelination of demyelinated CNS axons by transplanted human schwann cells: the deleterious effect of contaminating fibroblasts. Cell Transplant. 2001;10(3):305–15.
106. Kohama I, Lankford KL, Preiningerova J, White FA, Vollmer TL, Kocsis JD. Transplantation of cryopreserved adult human Schwann cells enhances axonal conduction in demyelinated spinal cord. J Neurosci. 2001;21(3):944–50.
107. Bachelin C, Lachapelle F, Girard C, et al. Efficient myelin repair in the macaque spinal cord by autologous grafts of Schwann cells. Brain. 2005;128(Pt 3):540–9.
108. Langford LA, Porter S, Bunge RP. Immortalized rat Schwann cells produce tumours in vivo. J Neurocytol. 1988;17:521–9.
109. Franklin RJM, Blakemore WF. Requirements for Schwann cell migration within CNS environments: a viewpoint. Int J Dev Neurosci. 1993;11:641–9.
110. Harrison B. Schwann cell and oligodendrocyte remyelination in lysolecithin-induced lesions in irradiated rat spinal cord. J Neurol Sci. 1985;67(2):143–59.
111. Woodruff RH, Franklin RJ. Demyelination and remyelination of the caudal cerebellar peduncle of adult rats following stereotaxic injections of lysolecithin, ethidium bromide, and complement/anti-galactocerebroside: a comparative study. Glia. 1999;25(3):216–28.
112. Lavdas A, Franceschini I, Dubois-Dalcq M, Matsas R. Schwann cells genetically engineered to express PSA show enhanced migratory potential without impairment of their myelinating ability in vitro. Glia. 2006;53(8):868–78.
113. Jose AM. Multiple sclerosis: can Schwann cells wrap it up? Yale J Biol Med. 2002;75(2):113–6.
114. Franklin RJ, Barnett SC. Olfactory ensheathing cells. In: Lazzarini RA, editor. Myelin biology and disorders. New York: Elsevier; 2004. p. 371–84.
115. Raisman G, et al. Repair of central nervous system lesions by transplantation of olfactory ensheathing cells. Handb Clin Neurol. 2012;109:541–9. doi:10.1016/b978-0-444-52137-8.00033-4.
116. Lakatos A, Franklin RJ, Barnett SC. Olfactory ensheathing cells and Schwann cells differ in their in vitro interactions with astrocytes. Glia. 2000;32(3):214–25.
117. Lakatos A, Barnett SC, Franklin RJ. Olfactory ensheathing cells induce less host astrocyte response and chondroitin sulphate proteoglycan expression than Schwann cells following transplantation into adult CNS white matter. Exp Neurol. 2003;184(1):237–46.
118. Woodhall E, West AK, Chuah MI. Cultured olfactory ensheathing cells express nerve growth factor, brain-derived neurotrophic factor, glia cell line-derived neurotrophic factor and their receptors. Brain research. Mol Brain Res. 2001;88:203–13.
119. Boyd JG, Doucette R, Kawaja MD. Defining the role of olfactory ensheathing cells in facilitating axon remyelination following damage to the spinal cord. FASEB J. 2005;19(7):694–703.
120. Tabakow P, et al. Transplantation of autologous olfactory ensheathing cells in complete human spinal cord injury. Cell Transplant. 2013;22:1591–612. doi:10.3727/096368912X663532.
121. Rao Y, et al. Long-term outcome of olfactory Ensheathing cell transplantation in six patients with chronic complete spinal cord injury. Cell Transplant. 2013;22(Suppl 1):S21–5. doi:10.3727/096368913X672127.
122. Huang H, Xi H, Chen L, Zhang F, Liu Y. Long-term outcome of olfactory ensheathing cell therapy for patients with complete chronic spinal cord injury. Cell Transplant. 2012;21(Suppl 1):S23–31. doi:10.3727/096368912X633734.
123. Chen L, et al. A prospective randomized double-blind clinical trial using a combination of olfactory ensheathing cells and Schwann cells for the treatment of chronic complete spinal cord injuries. Cell Transplant. 2014;23(Suppl 1):S35–44. doi:10.3727/096368914X685014.
124. Sasaki M, Lankford KL, Radtke C, Honmou O, Kocsis JD. Remyelination after olfactory ensheathing cell transplantation into diverse demyelinating environments. Exp Neurol. 2011;229(1):88–98.
125. Kocsis JD, Lankford KL, Sasaki M, Radtke C. Unique in vivo properties of olfactory ensheathing cells that may contribute to neural repair and protection following spinal cord injury. Neurosci Lett. 2009;456(3):137–42.

126. Bonilla S, Alarcon P, Villaverde R, Aparicio P, Silva A, Martinez S. Haematopoietic progenitor cells from adult bone marrow differentiate into cells that express oligodendroglial antigens in the neonatal mouse brain. Eur J Neurosci. 2002;15(3):575–82.
127. Bonilla S, Silva A, Valdes L, Geijo E, Garcia-Verdugo JM, Martinez S. Functional neural stem cells derived from adult bone marrow. Neuroscience. 2005;133(1):85–95.
128. Koshizuka S, Okada S, Okawa A, et al. Transplanted hematopoietic stem cells from bone marrow differentiate into neural lineage cells and promote functional recovery after spinal cord injury in mice. J Neuropathol Exp Neurol. 2004;63(1):64–72.
129. Suzuki H, Taguchi T, Tanaka H, et al. Neurospheres induced from bone marrow stromal cells are multipotent for differentiation into neuron, astrocyte, and oligodendrocyte phenotypes. Biochem Biophys Res Commun. 2004;322(3):918–22.
130. Gordon D, Glover CP, Merrison AM, Uney JB, Scolding NJ. Enhanced green fluorescent protein-expressing human mesenchymal stem cells retain neural marker expression. J Neuroimmunol. 2008;193(1–2):59–67.
131. Terada N, Hamazaki T, Oka M, et al. Bone marrow cells adopt the phenotype of other cells by spontaneous cell fusion. Nature. 2002;416(6880):542–5.
132. Morikawa S, Mabuchi Y, Niibe K, et al. Development of mesenchymal stem cells partially originate from the neural crest. Biochem Biophys Res Commun. 2009;379(4):1114–9.
133. Nagoshi N, Shibata S, Kubota Y, et al. Ontogeny and multipotency of neural crest-derived stem cells in mouse bone marrow, dorsal root ganglia, and whisker pad. Cell Stem Cell. 2008;2(4):392–403.
134. Warrington AE, Barbarese E, Pfeiffer SE. Differential myelinogenic capacity of specific developmental stages of the oligodendrocyte lineage upon transplantation into hypomyelinating hosts. J Neurosci Res. 1993;34:1–13.
135. Groves AK, Barnett SC, Franklin RJM, et al. Repair of demyelinated lesions by transplantation of purified O-2A progenitor cells. Nature. 1993;362:453–5.
136. Windrem MS, Nunes MC, Rashbaum WK, et al. Fetal and adult human oligodendrocyte progenitor cell isolates myelinate the congenitally dysmyelinated brain. Nat Med. 2004;10(1):93–7.
137. Brustle O, Jones KN, Learish RD, et al. Embryonic stem cell-derived glial precursors: a source of myelinating transplants. Science. 1999;285(5428):754–6.
138. Glaser T, Perez-Bouza A, Klein K, Brustle O. Generation of purified oligodendrocyte progenitors from embryonic stem cells. FASEB J. 2005;19(1):112–4.
139. Chandran S, Compston A, Jauniaux E, Gilson J, Blakemore W, Svendsen C. Differential generation of oligodendrocytes from human and rodent embryonic spinal cord neural precursors. Glia. 2004;47(4):314–24.
140. Keirstead HS, Nistor G, Bernal G, et al. Human embryonic stem cell-derived oligodendrocyte progenitor cell transplants remyelinate and restore locomotion after spinal cord injury. J Neurosci. 2005;25(19):4694–705.
141. Nistor GI, Totoiu MO, Haque N, Carpenter MK, Keirstead HS. Human embryonic stem cells differentiate into oligodendrocytes in high purity and myelinate after spinal cord transplantation. Glia. 2005;49(3):385–96.
142. Vogel G. Cell biology. Ready or not? Human ES cells head toward the clinic. Science. 2005;308(5728):1534–8.
143. Nunes MC, Roy NS, Keyoung HM, et al. Identification and isolation of multipotential neural progenitor cells from the subcortical white matter of the adult human brain. Nat Med. 2003;9(4):439–47.
144. Pluchino S, Quattrini A, Brambilla E, et al. Injection of adult neurospheres induces recovery in a chronic model of multiple sclerosis. Nature. 2003;422(6933):688–94.
145. Pluchino S, Zanotti L, Rossi B, et al. Neurosphere-derived multipotent precursors promote neuroprotection by an immunomodulatory mechanism. Nature. 2005;436(7048):266–71.
146. Braude P, Minger SL, Warwick RM. Stem cell therapy: hope or hype? BMJ. 2005;330(7501):1159–60.

147. Scolding N. Stem-cell therapy: hope and hype. Lancet. 2005;365(9477):2073–5.
148. Hess PG. Risk of tumorigenesis in first-in-human trials of embryonic stem cell neural derivatives: ethics in the face of long-term uncertainty. Acc Res. 2009;16:175–98.
149. Rebuzzini P, Zuccotti M, Redi CA, Garagna S. Chromosomal abnormalities in embryonic and somatic stem cells. Cytogenet Genome Res. 2015;147:1–9. doi:10.1159/000441645.
150. Erdo F, Buhrle C, Blunk J, et al. Host-dependent tumorigenesis of embryonic stem cell transplantation in experimental stroke. J Cereb Blood Flow Metab. 2003;23(7):780–5.
151. Roy NS, Cleren C, Singh SK, Yang L, Beal MF, Goldman SA. Functional engraftment of human ES cell-derived dopaminergic neurons enriched by coculture with telomerase-immortalized midbrain astrocytes. Nat Med. 2006;12(11):1259–68.
152. Amariglio N, Hirshberg A, Scheithauer BW, et al. Donor-derived brain tumor following neural stem cell transplantation in an ataxia telangiectasia patient. PLoS Med. 2009;6(2):e29.
153. Jandial R, Snyder EY. A safer stem cell: on guard against cancer. Nat Med. 2009;15(9):999–1001.
154. Amariglio N, Rechavi G. On the origin of glioneural neoplasms after neural cell transplantation. Nat Med. 2010;16(2):157–8.
155. Keene CD, Chang RC, Leverenz JB, et al. A patient with Huntington's disease and long-surviving fetal neural transplants that developed mass lesions. Acta Neuropathol. 2009;117(3):329–38.
156. Bretzner F, Gilbert F, Baylis F, Brownstone RM. Target populations for first-in-human embryonic stem cell research in spinal cord injury. Cell Stem Cell. 2011;8(5):468–75.
157. Wirth E III, Lebkowski JS, Lebacqz K. Response to Frederic Bretzner et al. "Target populations for first-in-human embryonic stem cell research in spinal cord injury". Cell Stem Cell. 2011;8(5):476–8.
158. Solbakk JH, Zoloth L. The tragedy of translation: the case of "first use" in human embryonic stem cell research. Cell Stem Cell. 2011;8(5):479–81.
159. Paty DW, Arnold DL. The lesions of multiple sclerosis. N Engl J Med. 2002;346(3):199–200.
160. Scolding N. Adult stem cells and multiple sclerosis. Cell Prolif. 2011;44(Suppl 1):35–8.
161. Comi G. Is it clinically relevant to repair focal multiple sclerosis lesions? J Neurol Sci. 2008;265(1–2):17–20.
162. Scolding N, Franklin R, Stevens S, Heldin CH, Compston A, Newcombe J. Oligodendrocyte progenitors are present in the normal adult human CNS and in the lesions of multiple sclerosis. Brain. 1998;121(Pt 12):2221–8.
163. Wolswijk G. Chronic stage multiple sclerosis lesions contain a relatively quiescent population of oligodendrocyte precursor cells. J Neurosci. 1998;18(2):601–9.
164. Chang A, Nishiyama A, Peterson J, Prineas J, Trapp BD. NG2-positive oligodendrocyte progenitor cells in adult human brain and multiple sclerosis lesions. J Neurosci. 2000;20(17):6404–12.
165. Maeda Y, Solanky M, Menonna J, Chapin J, Li W, Dowling P. Platelet-derived growth factor-alpha receptor-positive oligodendroglia are frequent in multiple sclerosis lesions. Ann Neurol. 2001;49(6):776–85.
166. Chang A, Tourtellotte WW, Rudick R, Trapp BD. Premyelinating oligodendrocytes in chronic lesions of multiple sclerosis. N Engl J Med. 2002;346(3):165–73.
167. Wilson HC, Scolding NJ, Raine CS. Co-expression of PDGF alpha receptor and NG2 by oligodendrocyte precursors in human CNS and multiple sclerosis lesions. J Neuroimmunol. 2006;176(1–2):162–73.
168. Snethen H, Love S, Scolding N. Disease-responsive neural precursor cells are present in multiple sclerosis lesions. Regen Med. 2008;3(6):835–47.
169. Albert M, Antel J, Bruck W, Stadelmann C. Extensive cortical remyelination in patients with chronic multiple sclerosis. Brain Pathol. 2007;17(2):129–38.
170. Patani R, Balaratnam M, Vora A, Reynolds R. Remyelination can be extensive in multiple sclerosis despite a long disease course. Neuropathol Appl Neurobiol. 2007;33(3):277–87.

171. Evangelou N, DeLuca GC, Owens T, Esiri MM. Pathological study of spinal cord atrophy in multiple sclerosis suggests limited role of local lesions. Brain. 2005;128(Pt 1):29–34.
172. Chard D, Miller D. Is multiple sclerosis a generalized disease of the central nervous system? An MRI perspective. Curr Opin Neurol. 2009;22(3):214–8.
173. Filippi M, Rocca MA. MRI evidence for multiple sclerosis as a diffuse disease of the central nervous system. J Neurol. 2005;252(Suppl 5):v16–24.
174. Kutzelnigg A, Lucchinetti CF, Stadelmann C, et al. Cortical demyelination and diffuse white matter injury in multiple sclerosis. Brain. 2005;128(Pt 11):2705–12.
175. Korbling M, Estrov Z. Adult stem cells for tissue repair. N Engl J Med. 2003;349:570–82.
176. Phinney DG. Biochemical heterogeneity of mesenchymal stem cell populations: clues to their therapeutic efficacy. Cell Cycle. 2007;6(23):2884–9.
177. Rice CM, Scolding NJ. Adult stem cells—reprogramming neurological repair? Lancet. 2004;364(9429):193–9.
178. Zhang J, Li Y, Chen J, et al. Human bone marrow stromal cell treatment improves neurological functional recovery in EAE mice. Exp Neurol. 2005;195(1):16–26.
179. Gerdoni E, Gallo B, Casazza S, et al. Mesenchymal stem cells effectively modulate pathogenic immune response in experimental autoimmune encephalomyelitis. Ann Neurol. 2007;61(3):219–27.
180. Zappia E, Casazza S, Pedemonte E, et al. Mesenchymal stem cells ameliorate experimental autoimmune encephalomyelitis inducing T-cell anergy. Blood. 2005;106(5):1755–61.
181. Gordon D, Pavlovska G, Glover CP, Uney JB, Wraith D, Scolding NJ. Human mesenchymal stem cells abrogate experimental allergic encephalomyelitis after intraperitoneal injection and with sparse CNS infiltration. Neurosci Lett. 2008;448:71–3.
182. Akiyama Y, Radtke C, Honmou O, Kocsis JD. Remyelination of the spinal cord following intravenous delivery of bone marrow cells. Glia. 2002;39(3):229–36.
183. Akiyama Y, Radtke C, Kocsis JD. Remyelination of the rat spinal cord by transplantation of identified bone marrow stromal cells. J Neurosci. 2002;22(15):6623–30.
184. Hermann A, Gastl R, Liebau S, et al. Efficient generation of neural stem cell-like cells from adult human bone marrow stromal cells. J Cell Sci. 2004;117(19):4411–22.
185. Fu L, Zhu L, Huang Y, Lee TD, Forman SJ, Shih CC. Derivation of neural stem cells from mesenchymal stemcells: evidence for a bipotential stem cell population. Stem Cells Dev. 2008;17(6):1109–21.
186. Freedman MS, Bar-Or A, Atkins HL, et al. The therapeutic potential of mesenchymal stem cell transplantation as a treatment for multiple sclerosis: consensus report of the International MSCT Study Group. Mult Scler. 2010;16:503–10.
187. Martino G, Franklin RJ, Van Evercooren AB, Kerr DA. Stem cell transplantation in multiple sclerosis: current status and future prospects. Nat Rev Neurol. 2010;6:247–55.
188. Munoz JR, Stoutenger BR, Robinson AP, Spees JL, Prockop DJ. Human stem/progenitor cells from bone marrow promote neurogenesis of endogenous neural stem cells in the hippocampus of mice. Proc Natl Acad Sci U S A. 2005;102(50):18171–6.
189. Bao X, et al. Transplantation of Flk-1+ human bone marrow-derived mesenchymal stem cells promotes angiogenesis and neurogenesis after cerebral ischemia in rats. Eur J Neurosci. 2011;34:87–98. doi:10.1111/j.1460-9568.2011.07733.x.
190. Bai L, Caplan A, Lennon D, Miller RH. Human mesenchymal stem cells signals regulate neural stem cell fate. Neurochem Res. 2007;32(2):353–62.
191. Rivera FJ, Couillard-Despres S, Pedre X, et al. Mesenchymal stem cells instruct oligodendrogenic fate decision on adult neural stem cells. Stem Cells. 2006;24(10):2209–19.
192. Bai L, Lennon DP, Eaton V, et al. Human bone marrow-derived mesenchymal stem cells induce Th2-polarized immune response and promote endogenous repair in animal models of multiple sclerosis. Glia. 2009;57:1192–203.
193. Li Y, Chen J, Zhang CL, et al. Gliosis and brain remodeling after treatment of stroke in rats with marrow stromal cells. Glia. 2005;49(3):407–17.
194. Gao Q, Li Y, Shen L, et al. Bone marrow stromal cells reduce ischemia-induced astrocytic activation in vitro. Neuroscience. 2008;152(3):646–55.

195. Kim M, et al. Transplantation of human bone marrow-derived clonal mesenchymal stem cells reduces ffibrotic sscar fformation in a rat spinal cord injury model. J Tissue Eng Regen Med. 2017;34:87–98. doi:10.1002/term.2425.
196. Chen Q, Long Y, Yuan X, et al. Protective effects of bone marrow stromal cell transplantation in injured rodent brain: synthesis of neurotrophic factors. J Neurosci Res. 2005;80(5):611–9.
197. Garcia R, Aguiar J, Alberti E, de la Cuetara K, Pavon N. Bone marrow stromal cells produce nerve growth factor and glial cell line-derived neurotrophic factors. Biochem Biophys Res Commun. 2004;316(3):753–4.
198. Li Y, Chen J, Chen XG, et al. Human marrow stromal cell therapy for stroke in rat: neurotrophins and functional recovery. Neurology. 2002;59(4):514–23.
199. Ye M, Chen S, Wang X, et al. Glial cell line-derived neurotrophic factor in bone marrow stromal cells of rat. Neuroreport. 2005;16(6):581–4.
200. Wilkins A, Kemp K, Ginty M, Hares K, Mallam E, Scolding N. Human bone marrow-derived mesenchymal stem cells secrete brain-derived neurotrophic factor which promotes neuronal survival in vitro. Stem Cell Res. 2009;3:67–70.
201. Kemp K, Hares K, Mallam E, Heesom KJ, Scolding N, Wilkins A. Mesenchymal stem cell-secreted superoxide dismutase promotes cerebellar neuronal survival. J Neurochem. 2009;114:1569–80.
202. Kemp K, Gray E, Mallam E, Scolding N, Wilkins A. Inflammatory cytokine induced regulation of superoxide dismutase 3 expression by human mesenchymal stem cells. Stem Cell Rev. 2010;6:548–59.
203. Johansson CB, Youssef S, Koleckar K, et al. Extensive fusion of haematopoietic cells with Purkinje neurons in response to chronic inflammation. Nat Cell Biol. 2008;10(5):575–83.
204. Nygren JM, Liuba K, Breitbach M, et al. Myeloid and lymphoid contribution to non-haematopoietic lineages through irradiation-induced heterotypic cell fusion. Nat Cell Biol. 2008;10(5):584–92.
205. Kemp KC, et al. Purkinje cell injury, structural plasticity and fusion in patients with Friedreich's ataxia. Acta Neuropathol Commun. 2016;4:53. doi:10.1186/s40478-016-0326-3.
206. Kemp K, Wilkins A, Scolding N. Cell fusion in the brain: two cells forward, one cell back. Acta Neuropathol. 2014;128:629–38. doi:10.1111/bpa.12230.
207. Kemp K, Gray E, Wilkins A, Scolding N. Purkinje cell fusion and binucleate heterokaryon formation in multiple sclerosis cerebellum. Brain. 2012;135:2962–72.
208. Fox JM, Chamberlain G, Ashton BA, Middleton J. Recent advances into the understanding of mesenchymal stem cell trafficking. Br J Haematol. 2007;137(6):491–502.
209. Karp JM, Leng Teo GS. Mesenchymal stem cell homing: the devil is in the details. Cell Stem Cell. 2009;4(3):206–16.
210. Leibacher J, Henschler R. Biodistribution, migration and homing of systemically applied mesenchymal stem/stromal cells. Stem Cell Res Ther. 2016;7:7. doi:10.1111/bpa.12230.
211. Gordon D, Pavlovska G, Uney JB, Wraith DC, Scolding NJ. Human mesenchymal stem cells infiltrate the spinal cord, reduce demyelination, and localize to white matter lesions in experimental autoimmune encephalomyelitis. J Neuropathol Exp Neurol. 2010;69(11):1087–95.
212. Rice CM, Scolding N. Adult human mesenchymal cells proliferate and migrate in response to chemokines expressed in demyelination. Cell Adhes Migr. 2010;4:235–40.
213. da Silva ML, Chagastelles PC, Nardi NB. Mesenchymal stem cells reside in virtually all post-natal organs and tissues. J Cell Sci. 2006;119(Pt 11):2204–13.
214. Mosna F, Sensebe L, Krampera M. Human bone marrow and adipose tissue mesenchymal stem cells: a user's guide. Stem Cells Dev. 2010;19(10):1449–70.
215. Takakura N, Watanabe T, Suenobu S, et al. A role for hematopoietic stem cells in promoting angiogenesis. Cell. 2000;102(2):199–209.
216. Burt RK, Traynor AE, Oyama Y, Barr WG. Plasticity of hematopoietic stem cells: enough to induce tolerance and repair tissue? Arthritis Rheum. 2002;46(4):855–8.
217. Fu X, Sun X. Can hematopoietic stem cells be an alternative source for skin regeneration? Ageing Res Rev. 2009;8(3):244–9.

218. Zhou P, Wirthlin L, McGee J, Annett G, Nolta J. Contribution of human hematopoietic stem cells to liver repair. Semin Immunopathol. 2009;31(3):411–9.
219. Felfly H, et al. Hematopoietic stem cells: potential new applications for translational medicine. J Stem Cells. 2014;9:163–97.
220. Simmons PJ, Torok-Storb B. Identification of stromal cell precursors in human bone marrow by a novel monoclonal antibody, STRO-1. Blood. 1991;78(1):55–62.
221. Psaltis PJ, Paton S, See F, et al. Enrichment for STRO-1 expression enhances the cardiovascular paracrine activity of human bone marrow-derived mesenchymal cell populations. J Cell Physiol. 2010;223(2):530–40.
222. Stewart K, Monk P, Walsh S, Jefferiss CM, Letchford J, Beresford JN. STRO-1, HOP-26 (CD63), CD49a and SB-10 (CD166) as markers of primitive human marrow stromal cells and their more differentiated progeny: a comparative investigation in vitro. Cell Tissue Res. 2003;313(3):281–90.
223. Dennis JE, Carbillet JP, Caplan AI, Charbord P. The STRO-1+ marrow cell population is multipotential. Cells Tissues Organs. 2002;170(2–3):73–82.
224. Nasef A, Zhang YZ, Mazurier C, et al. Selected Stro-1-enriched bone marrow stromal cells display a major suppressive effect on lymphocyte proliferation. Int J Lab Hematol. 2009;31(1):9–19.
225. Hodgetts SI, et al. Human mesenchymal precursor cells (Stro-1(+)) from spinal cord injury patients improve functional recovery and tissue sparing in an acute spinal cord injury rat model. Cell Transplant. 2013;22:393–412. doi:10.3727/096368912x656081.
226. Bakondi B, Shimada IS, Perry A, et al. CD133 identifies a human bone marrow stem/progenitor cell sub-population with a repertoire of secreted factors that protect against stroke. Mol Ther. 2009;17(11):1938–47.
227. Harris JR, Fisher R, Jorgensen M, Kaushal S, Scott EW. CD133 progenitor cells from the bone marrow contribute to retinal pigment epithelium repair. Stem Cells. 2009;27(2):457–66.
228. Sasaki H, Ishikawa M, Tanaka N, et al. Administration of human peripheral blood-derived CD133+ cells accelerates functional recovery in a rat spinal cord injury model. Spine (Phila Pa 1976). 2009;34(3):249–54.
229. Kamei N, et al. Ex-vivo expanded human blood-derived CD133+ cells promote repair of injured spinal cord. J Neurol Sci. 2013;328:41–50. doi:10.1016/j.jns.2013.02.013.
230. Zuba-Surma EK, Kucia M, Ratajczak J, Ratajczak MZ. "Small stem cells" in adult tissues: very small embryonic-like stem cells stand up! Cytometry A. 2009;75(1):4–13.
231. Rice CM, Clavel C, Mazo M, Prosper F, Scolding N. Multipotent adult progenitor cell isolation and proliferation in cytokine and serum free medium conditioned by rat B104 cells. Br J Haematol. 2010;148:441–4.
232. Labedz-Maslowska A, Kamycka E, Bobis-Wozowicz S, Madeja Z, Zuba-Surma EK. Identification of new rat bone marrow-derived population of very small stem cell with Oct-4A and nanog expression by flow cytometric platforms. Stem Cells Int. 2016;2016:5069857. doi:10.1155/2016/5069857.
233. Jellema RK, et al. Multipotent adult progenitor cells for hypoxic-ischemic injury in the preterm brain. J Neuroinflammation. 2015;12:241. doi:10.1186/s12974-015-0459-5.
234. Walker PA, et al. Intravenous multipotent adult progenitor cell therapy after traumatic brain injury: modulation of the resident microglia population. J Neuroinflammation. 2012;9:228. doi:10.1186/s12974-015-0459-5.
235. Wagner W, Ho A. Mesenchymal stem cell preparations—comparing apples and oranges. Stem Cell Rev Rep. 2007;3(4):239–48.
236. Phinney DG, et al. Functional heterogeneity of mesenchymal stem cells: implications for cell therapy. J Cell Biochem. 2012;113:2806–12. doi:10.1002/jcb.24166.
237. Cogle CR, Yachnis AT, Laywell ED, et al. Bone marrow transdifferentiation in brain after transplantation: a retrospective study. Lancet. 2004;363(9419):1432–7.
238. Mezey E, Key S, Vogelsang G, Szalayova I, Lange GD, Crain B. Transplanted bone marrow generates new neurons in human brains. PNAS. 2003;100(3):1364–9.

239. Prockop DJ, Brenner M, Fibbe WE, et al. Defining the risks of mesenchymal stromal cell therapy. Cytotherapy. 2010;12(5):576–8.
240. Miura M, Miura Y, Padilla-Nash HM, et al. Accumulated chromosomal instability in murine bone marrow mesenchymal stem cells leads to malignant transformation. Stem Cells. 2006;24(4):1095–103.
241. Dahl JA, Duggal S, Coulston N, et al. Genetic and epigenetic instability of human bone marrow mesenchymal stem cells expanded in autologous serum or fetal bovine serum. Int J Dev Biol. 2008;52(8):1033–42.
242. Tonti GA, Mannello F. From bone marrow to therapeutic applications: different behaviour and genetic/epigenetic stability during mesenchymal stem cell expansion in autologous and foetal bovine sera? Int J Dev Biol. 2008;52(8):1023–32.
243. Pan Q, et al. Detection of spontaneous tumorigenic transformation during culture expansion of human mesenchymal stromal cells. Exp Biol Med (Maywood, NJ). 2014;239:105–15. doi:10.1177/1535370213506802.
244. Alves H, Munoz-Najar U, De Wit J, et al. A link between the accumulation of DNA damage and loss of multipotency of human mesenchymal stromal cells. J Cell Mol Med. 2000;14(12):2729–38.
245. Kretlow JD, Jin YQ, Liu W, et al. Donor age and cell passage affects differentiation potential of murine bone marrow-derived stem cells. BMC Cell Biol. 2008;9:60.
246. Crisostomo PR, Wang M, Wairiuko GM, et al. High passage number of stem cells adversely affects stem cell activation and myocardial protection. Shock. 2006;26(6):575–80.
247. Dominici M, Le BK, Mueller I, et al. Minimal criteria for defining multipotent mesenchymal stromal cells. The International Society for Cellular Therapy position statement. Cytotherapy. 2006;8(4):315–7.
248. Dominici M, Paolucci P, Conte P, Horwitz EM. Heterogeneity of multipotent mesenchymal stromal cells: from stromal cells to stem cells and vice versa. Transplantation. 2009;87(9 Suppl):S36–42.
249. Burt RK, Loh Y, Pearce W, et al. Clinical applications of blood-derived and marrow-derived stem cells for nonmalignant diseases. JAMA. 2008;299(8):925–36.
250. Grigoriadis N, Lourbopoulos A, Lagoudaki R, et al. Variable behavior and complications of autologous bone marrow mesenchymal stem cells transplanted in experimental autoimmune encephalomyelitis. Exp Neurol. 2011;230(1):78–89.
251. Snyder EY. The risk of putting something where it does not belong: mesenchymal stem cells produce masses in the brain. Exp Neurol. 2011;230(1):75–7.
252. Hunt DP, Irvine KA, Webber DJ, Compston DA, Blakemore WF, Chandran S. Effects of direct transplantation of multipotent mesenchymal stromal/stem cells into the demyelinated spinal cord. Cell Transplant. 2008;17(7):865–73.
253. Barbosa da Fonseca LM, Gutfilen B, Rosado de Castro PH, et al. Migration and homing of bone-marrow mononuclear cells in chronic ischemic stroke after intra-arterial injection. Exp Neurol. 2010;221(1):122–8.
254. Yoshihara T, Ohta M, Itokazu Y, et al. Neuroprotective effect of bone marrow-derived mononuclear cells promoting functional recovery from spinal cord injury. J Neurotrauma. 2007;24(6):1026–36.
255. Schachinger V, Erbs S, Elsasser A, et al. Improved clinical outcome after intracoronary administration of bone-marrow-derived progenitor cells in acute myocardial infarction: final 1-year results of the REPAIR-AMI trial. Eur Heart J. 2006;27(23):2775–83.
256. Wollert KC, Meyer GP, Lotz J, et al. Intracoronary autologous bone-marrow cell transfer after myocardial infarction: the BOOST randomised controlled clinical trial. Lancet. 2004;364(9429):141–8.
257. Lyra AC, Soares MB, da Silva LF, et al. Infusion of autologous bone marrow mononuclear cells through hepatic artery results in a short-term improvement of liver function in patients with chronic liver disease: a pilot randomized controlled study. Eur J Gastroenterol Hepatol. 2010;22(1):33–42.

258. Motukuru V, Suresh KR, Vivekanand V, Raj S, Girija KR. Therapeutic angiogenesis in Buerger's disease (thromboangiitis obliterans) patients with critical limb ischemia by autologous transplantation of bone marrow mononuclear cells. J Vasc Surg. 2008;48(6 Suppl):53S–60S.
259. Savitz SI, Misra V, Kasam M, et al. Intravenous autologous bone marrow mononuclear cells for ischemic stroke. Ann Neurol. 2011;70(1):59–69.
260. Hess DC, et al. Safety and efficacy of multipotent adult progenitor cells in acute ischaemic stroke (MASTERS): a randomised, double-blind, placebo-controlled, phase 2 trial. Lancet Neurol. 2017;16:360–8. doi:10.1016/S1474-4422(17)30046-7.
261. van der Bogt KE, Sheikh AY, Schrepfer S, et al. Comparison of different adult stem cell types for treatment of myocardial ischemia. Circulation. 2008;118(14 Suppl):S121–9.
262. Samdani AF, Paul C, Betz RR, Fischer I, Neuhuber B. Transplantation of human marrow stromal cells and mono-nuclear bone marrow cells into the injured spinal cord: a comparative study. Spine (Phila Pa 1976). 2009;34(24):2605–12.
263. Sasaki M, Honmou O, Akiyama Y, Uede T, Hashi K, Kocsis JD. Transplantation of an acutely isolated bone marrow fraction repairs demyelinated adult rat spinal cord axons. Glia. 2001;35(1):26–34.
264. Rice CM, Whone AL, Marks DI, Butler SB, Brooks DJ, Scolding NJ. A safety and feasibility study of intravenous autologous bone marrow stem cells in multiple sclerosis. J Neurol Neurosurg Psychiatry. 2007;78(9):1014–38.
265. Karussis D, Karageorgiou C, Vaknin-Dembinsky A, et al. Safety and immunological effects of mesenchymal stem cell transplantation in patients with multiple sclerosis and amyotrophic lateral sclerosis. Arch Neurol. 2010;67(10):1187–94.
266. Rice C, et al. Assessment of bone marrow-derived cellular therapy in progressive multiple sclerosis (ACTiMuS): study protocol for a randomised, placebo-controlled, stepped wedge study. Trials. 2015;16:463. doi:10.1186/s13063-015-0953-1.

Index

A. Wilkins (ed.), *Progressive Multiple Sclerosis*,
https://doi.org/10.1007/978-3-319-65921-3

O

P